RADIOGRAPHIC INTERPRETATION FOR THE DENTIST

RADIOGRAPHIC INTERPRETATION FOR THE DENTIST

S. N. BHASKAR, B.D.S., D.D.S., M.S., Ph.D.

Brigadier General, United States Army Dental Corps; Director of Personnel and Training, Office of the Surgeon General, United States Army; Associate Professor of Pathology, Georgetown University School of Dentistry, Washington, D. C.; Consultant in Oral Pathology to the Assistant Surgeon General and Chief of the Dental Corps, United States Army

SECOND EDITION

with 424 *illustrations*

THE C. V. MOSBY COMPANY

SAINT LOUIS 1975

SECOND EDITION

Printed in the United States of America

Distributed in Great Britain by Henry Kimpton, London

Library of Congress Cataloging in Publication Data

Bhaskar, S N
Radiographic interpretation for the dentist.

First ed. published in 1970 under title: Roentgenographic interpretation for the dentist.
Includes bibliographical references.
1. Teeth—Radiography. 2. Jaws—Radiography. I. Title. [DNLM: 1. Radiography, Dental. WN230 B575r]
RK309.B43 1975 617.6′07′572 74-14785
ISBN 0-8016-0684-5

CB/CB/B 9 8 7 6 5 4 3 2 1

To my wife
NORMA

and my sons
BILL, PHILIP, AND TOM

for many things

PREFACE

The first edition of this book was prepared to present a new, simple, and easy-to-consult approach to the interpretation of oral radiographs. This second edition is presented with the same purpose. Much of the material has been revised, and chapters on the radiographic interpretation of caries and periodontal diseases have been added. It is hoped that this edition, as did the first, will make it easier for the general practitioner to diagnose and treat lesions of the oral cavity.

Unlike his medical colleague, the dentist has the unusual opportunity, as well as the responsibility, of being his own radiologist. Not only must he take his own radiographs, but he must also interpret them.

With a few exceptions, radiographic interpretation of the oral cavity means the interpretation of lesions of the teeth and jaws. Since teeth are unique structures in the body and since the jawbones have numerous differences from other members of the skeleton, the interpretation of oral radiographs requires knowledge in dentistry and is a field unto itself.

Although as a rule the final diagnosis of any lesion can be made only after a tissue biopsy, a radiograph can reveal much to a clinician. When of good quality it can give so much information about a lesion that in many cases a tissue biopsy is necessary only to confirm the diagnosis, and in some cases its need may be altogether eliminated.

Because of rapidly accumulating knowledge, in dentistry no less than in other fields of human endeavor, the busy clinician is called on to be an expert in numerous areas of dental practice. Consequently, the demands on his time are many. For this reason, highly detailed, encyclopedic texts on any of the dental specialties are overwhelming and often of limited value to him. Since the general practitioner determines the level of dental practice and carries the greatest responsibility for the profession, it is the duty of every specialist to simplify and condense the most pertinent and practical part of his specialty and present it to him. The purpose of this text, therefore, is not to dwell on the minutiae related to oral radiography but to provide the clinician with a simple and reliable guide to radiographic interpretation. For techniques related to taking and processing oral radiographs the clinician must refer to one of a number of excellent texts on dental radiology.

Outside of my family life, my greatest satisfaction, pleasure, and purpose have been derived from the dental profession. In innumerable places in the United States, at countless times during and after lectures, I have not only received encouragement from my fellow dentists but have also learned many new things from them. In fact, the knowledge that I have gained from the general practitioners everywhere has far exceeded what I have been able to give in return. For the pride I feel in what I do, therefore, I owe a deep debt of gratitude to the dental profession; for the encouragement and inspiration I have received, I am grateful to my fellow dentists in all parts of the United States.

I was assisted in the preparation of the chapter on the radiographic interpretation of periodontal lesions by my associate Dr. Marvin P. Levin. I am grateful to this distinguished colleague for his assistance, consultation, and advice. Dr. Blahuta assisted me in the selection of radiographs used in the chapter on caries, and I am thankful to him for his willing cooperation.

This book was written during the hours I would normally have spent with my wife Norma and my sons Bill, Philip, and Tom. With gratitude and affection, therefore, I acknowledge their understanding and their unselfish cooperation.

S. N. BHASKAR

CONTENTS

PART ONE

NORMAL LANDMARKS

CHAPTER ONE

NORMAL RADIOGRAPHIC LANDMARKS

To interpret radiographs accurately, the dentist must bear in mind some of the normal features seen in intraoral, occlusal, and extraoral radiographs. Some of the most important of these landmarks are therefore described in this chapter.

- Structures associated with the teeth
  - Enamel
  - Dentin
  - Cementum
  - Bone
  - Pulp
  - Periodontal ligament
  - Lamina dura
  - Dental germ
- Landmarks in radiographs of the maxilla
  - Median suture
  - Incisive or anterior palatine foramen
  - Anterior nasal spine
  - Nasal septum
  - Nasal cavity (fossa)
  - Maxillary sinus
  - Lateral fossa
  - Zygomatic (malar) process of maxilla and zygomatic bone
  - Coronoid process of mandible
  - Hamulus and lateral plate of pterygoid process
- Landmarks in radiographs of the mandible
  - Mental fossa
  - Mental ridge
  - Lingual foramen
  - Genial tubercles
  - Mental foramen
  - Mandibular canal (inferior dental canal)
  - External oblique line
  - Internal oblique line
  - Mylohyoid ridge
  - Submaxillary gland fossa

Miscellaneous structures in oral radiographs
- Nutrient canals
- Hyoid bone
- Soft tissues
- Temporomandibular joint
- Styloid process
- Stylomandibular ligament
- Nasolacrimal canal
- Greater palatine foramen

STRUCTURES ASSOCIATED WITH THE TEETH

Enamel, dentin, cementum, and bone. Of the hard dental tissues the enamel is the most radiopaque structure (Fig. 1-1). This feature is often of important diagnostic value in distinguishing between lesions composed of bone tissue and lesions composed of enamel. Dentin is less radiopaque than enamel, and its radiopacity is the same as that of bone. Cementum, in most areas of the root surface, cannot be seen in the radiograph. Where cementum becomes excessive (hypercementosis), it can be identified, and its radiopacity appears to be of the same density as that of bone or dentin.

Although there are three basic types of bone tissue (p. 95), the bulk of the maxilla and mandible is composed of the mature lamellar bone. In the outer shell of the jaws, the mature lamellar bone is arranged in the form of a dense cortical plate, which, because of its density, is more radiopaque than the central area (Fig. 1-2). Within the shell of cortical bone, the lamellar bone tissue is arranged in the form of bone trabeculae. In the maxilla, the bone trabeculae are fine and arranged in a lacelike pattern, whereas in the mandible they are usually coarse and run in a horizontal pattern (Fig. 1-3). The arrangement of bone trabeculae in the jaws, however, varies greatly.

Pulp and periodontal ligament. The pulp and periodontal ligament appear radiolucent, and in radiographs the normal pulp chambers and canals, as well as the periodontal ligament, have smooth outlines (Fig. 1-4). Irregular outlines or boundaries in these structures may indicate pathology (Fig. 1-3, *A*).

Lamina dura. The lamina dura is the radiopaque border of bone surrounding the periodontal ligament (Fig. 1-4). It is composed of the so-called bundle bone (p. 95). This type of bone tissue gives attachment to ligaments and tendons in various areas of the skeleton and contains more calcium salts per unit area than any other type of bone (p. 95). The thickness of the lamina dura varies around different teeth of the same patient, in different areas of the same tooth, and at different times in life (Fig. 1-4). It may be entirely missing on one surface of the tooth or in some areas of the same side of the tooth (Fig. 1-4, *C*). Although localized or generalized absence of lamina dura is said to occur in hyperparathyroidism, osteomalacia, rickets, leukemia, multiple myeloma, Paget's disease, osteoporosis, osteopetrosis, ossifying fibroma, and fibrous dysplasia, its absence in isolated areas is often related to physiologic migration of teeth and is not necessarily associated with pathology.

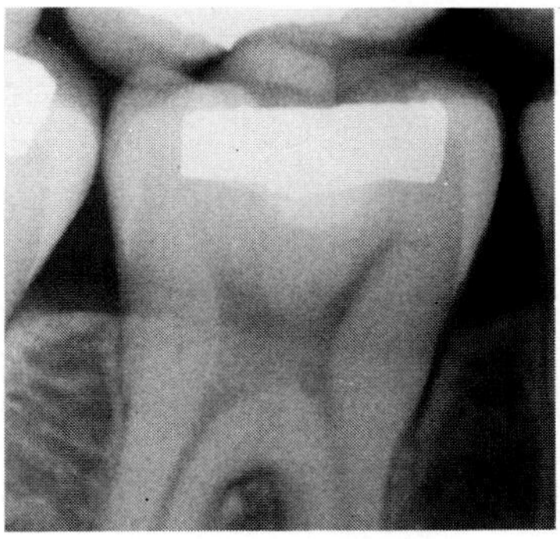

Fig. 1-1. Radiograph showing the relative radiopacity of bone, dentin, enamel, and restorative materials.

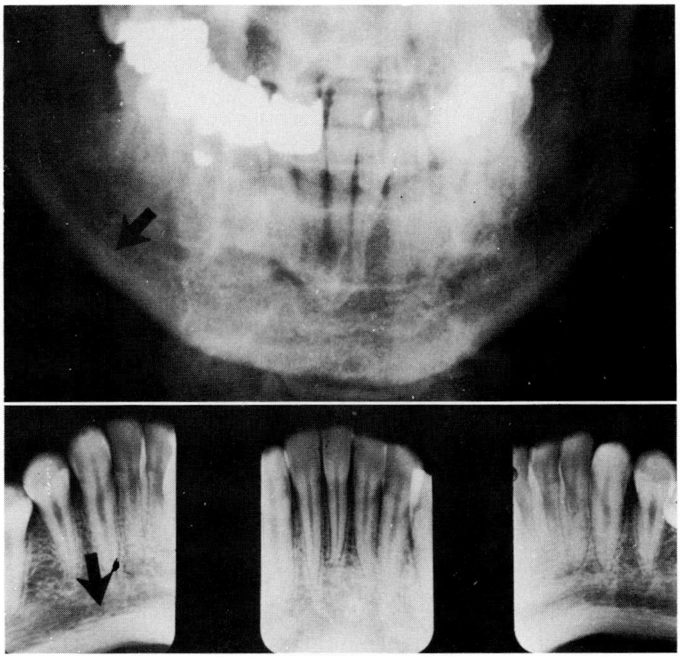

Fig. 1-2. Cortical plates of the jaws appear as a dense radiopacity (arrows).

A

B

C

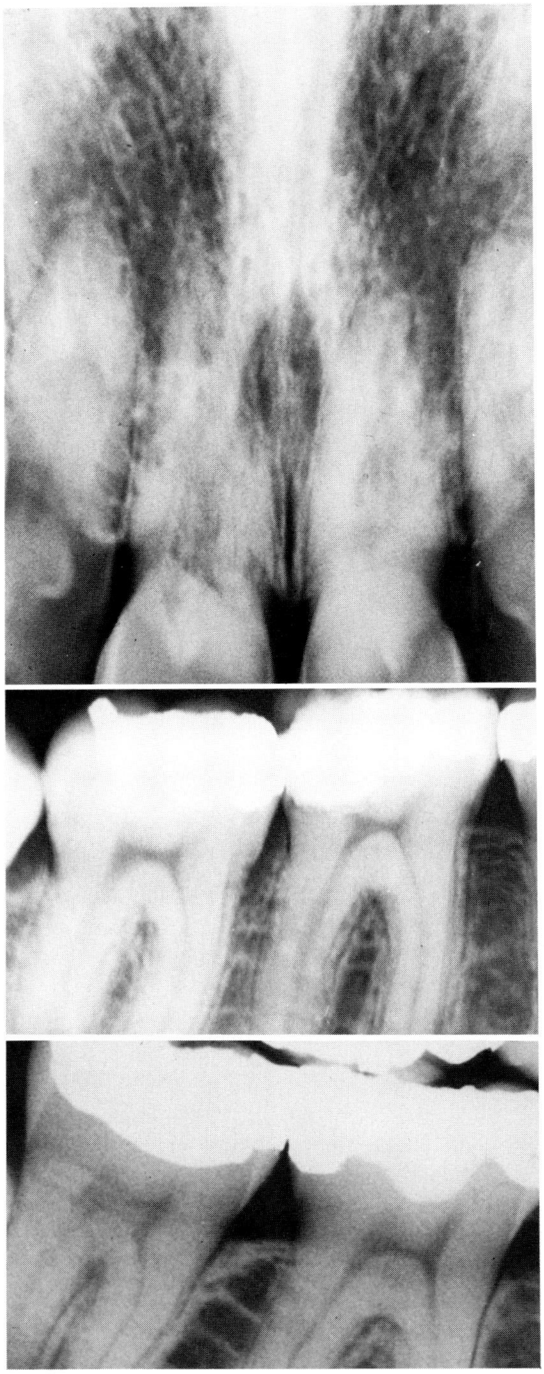

Fig. 1-3. Radiographs of the maxilla, **A,** and mandible, **B** and **C,** showing the arrangement of bone trabeculae. Note the lacelike pattern in **A** and the horizontal pattern in **B** and **C.** (Central incisors in **A** were ankylosed.)

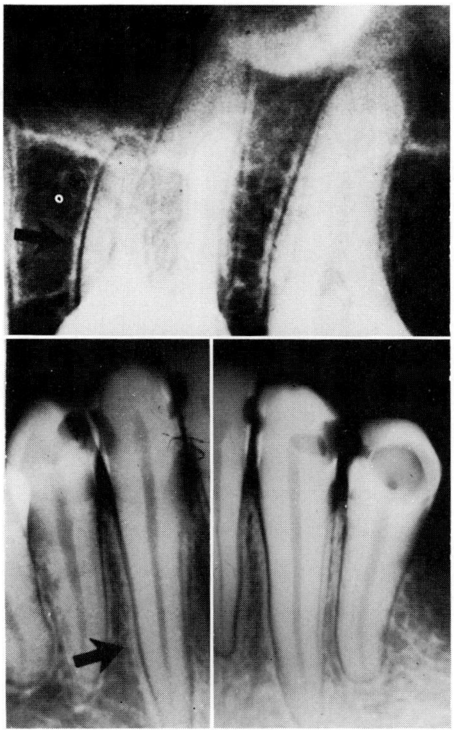

Fig. 1-4. **A** and **B,** Lamina dura is seen around teeth (arrows). **C,** Lamina dura cannot be identified around the bicuspid.

Dental germ. In the early stages the tooth germs appear as radiolucent areas (Fig. 1-5). With the beginning calcification of enamel and dentin, small radiopaque areas appear in the radiolucency. Since calcification begins at cusp tips (growth centers), dental germs with varying amounts of crown formation appear as circumscribed radiolucencies with inverted V- or U-shaped radiopaque foci (Fig. 1-6). After the beginning of root formation, radiolucent zones can be seen at the root tips (Fig. 1-7). These areas represent the growing dental papillae. The lateral and the occlusal areas of developing teeth are also surrounded by radiolucencies that represent the dental follicle (Fig. 1-7). When the tooth approaches eruption, this radiolucency surrounding the crown may become very prominent. Unless this area is very large, it does not represent pathology (p. 119).

Since the development of the third molar teeth occurs much later than the development of the other teeth, the dental germs of these molars have been mistaken for a "cyst" or a "tumor" and excised by error. Since the development of these teeth can sometimes be delayed (Fig. 1-5), the presence of a radiolucency in the third molar area in patients who are in the second or early third decade of life should not always be assumed to represent pathology.

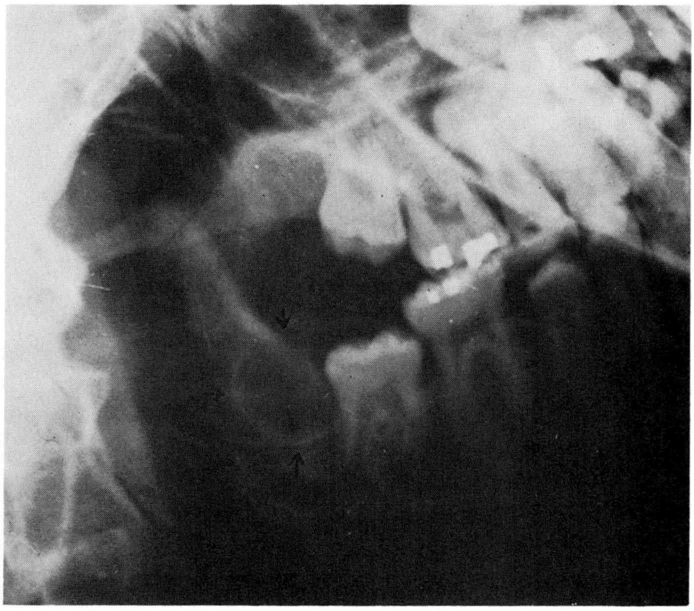

Fig. 1-5. Tooth germ of the third molar appears as a radiolucent area. It was misdiagnosed as a cyst and removed.

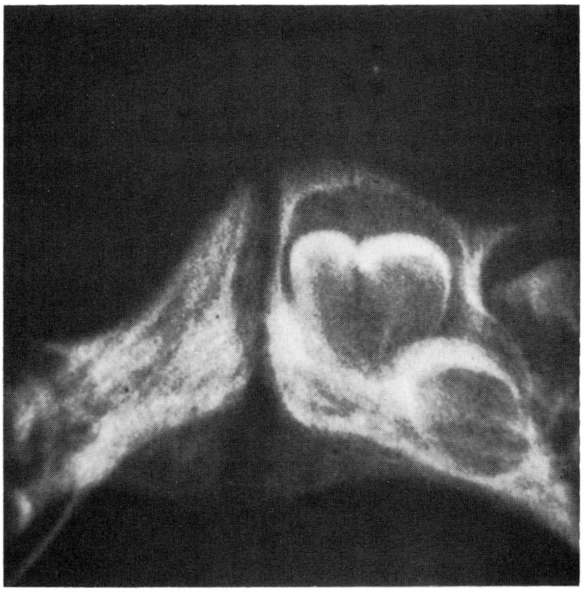

Fig. 1-6. Symphyseal region of the mandible in a fetus, showing the unfused median suture. Incisor tooth germs show beginning "caps" of calcification of growth centers.

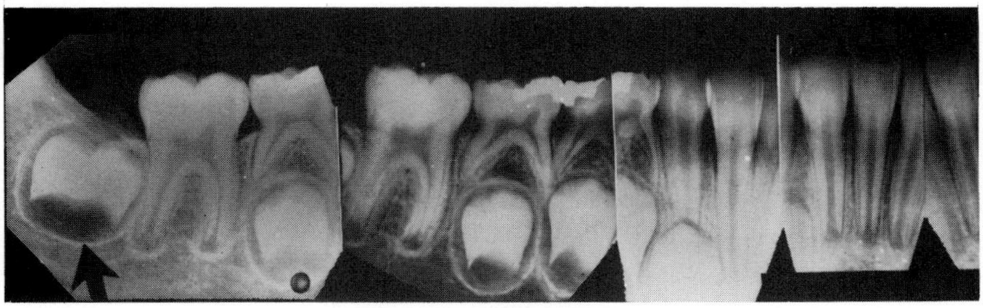

Fig. 1-7. Radiolucency in the apical area of developing tooth (arrow) represents the growing dental papilla. Similar areas are seen in other tooth germs. The radiolucency around the occlusal and lateral aspects of the crown is the dental follicle.

A

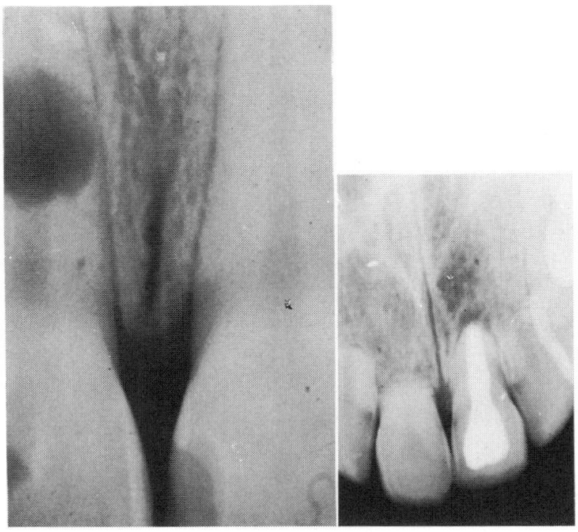

B

Fig. 1-8. Median suture of the maxilla appears as a linear radiolucent area in **A** and **B**. **A,** Tooth shows internal resorption. **B,** Root resorption is seen.

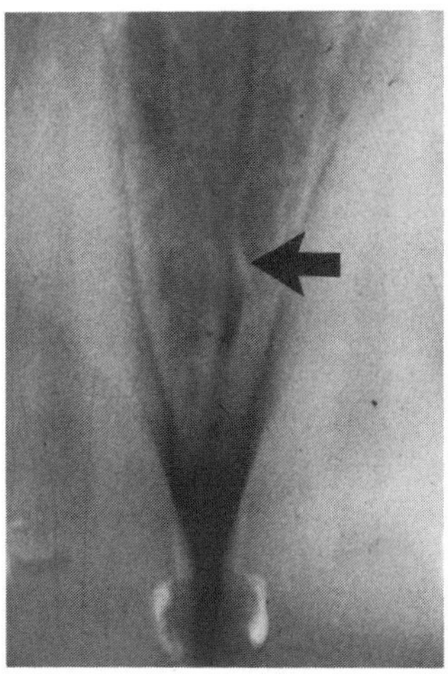

Fig. 1-9. Median suture of the maxilla (arrow).

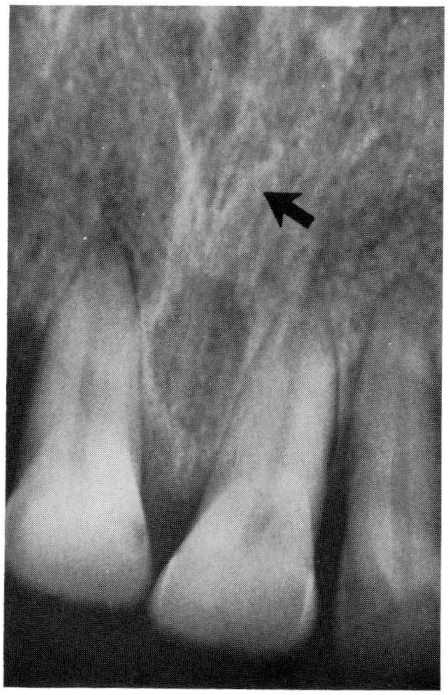

Fig. 1-10. Large incisive foramen and V-shaped nasal spine (arrow).

LANDMARKS IN RADIOGRAPHS OF THE MAXILLA

Median suture. In radiographs of young patients, the median suture of the maxilla may appear as a radiolucent line between the central incisors (Figs. 1-8 and 1-9).

Incisive or anterior palatine foramen. The incisive palatine foramen is usually an oval radiolucency, the location of which depends on the angulation at which the radiograph is taken (Fig 1-10). Although there is usually a single radiolucency, there may be more than one shadow, and the foramen may be round, heart-shaped, or diamond-shaped. Additional radiolucencies may represent the foramina of Scarpa (for the nasopalatine nerves) or the foramina of Stensen (for the nasopalatine artery). The radiolucency of the incisive foramen is generally located between or above the maxillary central incisors. The incisive canal is sometimes seen connected to the incisive foramen. The size of the foramen varies greatly, and making the distinction between a large incisive foramen and a small incisive canal cyst is often difficult. It has been suggested that radiolucencies up to 6 mm. wide may be considered normal. When there is doubt, however, aspiration of the area assists in a differential diagnosis. If aspiration yields a fluid of any kind, the lesion may be assumed to be a cyst.

Anterior nasal spine. The anterior nasal spine appears as a V-shaped radiopacity that is seen in the inferior aspect of the nasal fossae. It is located above the incisive foramen and may be superimposed on it (Fig. 1-10).

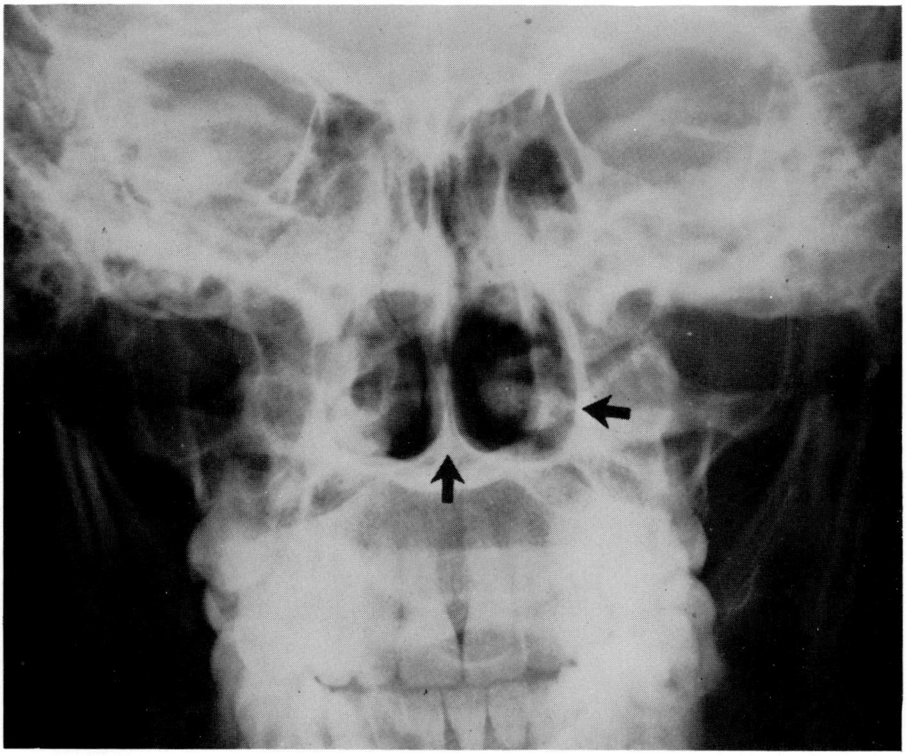

Fig. 1-11. Anteroposterior view of the midportion of the skull, showing the nasal fossae, the median nasal septum (lower arrow), and the inferior concha (right arrow).

Nasal septum. The nasal septum separates the two nasal fossae, is located in the midline, and appears as a gray or white shadow above the central incisors (Fig. 1-11).

Nasal cavity (fossa). The nasal fossae, or nasal cavities, appear as bilateral radiolucencies in radiographs of the incisor area (Fig. 1-11). In radiographs of the cuspid area, the floor of the nasal cavity usually overlaps the radiolucency of the maxillary sinus, whereas in radiographs of the bicuspid and molar area, it is not normally observed (Figs. 1-12 and 1-13). In some cases, however, it may be seen high above the floor of the sinus (Fig. 1-14). In anteroposterior extraoral radiographs, the nasal fossae appear as pear-shaped radiolucencies. From the lateral wall of each of them, the inferior concha projects medially and appears as a radiopaque structure (Fig. 1-11).

Maxillary sinus. The maxillary sinus begins its development at birth and starts to enlarge so that at puberty its floor is at about the same level as the floor of the nasal cavity. The expansion of the sinus continues, and its floor reaches below that of the nose. Radiographically, the sinus is not seen until after 5 years of age, but after this time it is a dominant radiolucency in radiographs of the maxillary

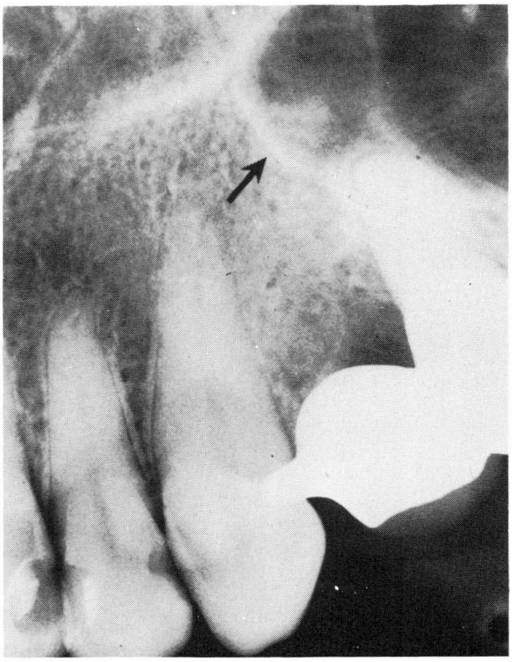

Fig. 1-12. Anterior boundary of the maxillary sinus almost reaches the cuspid root area (arrow) and meets the nasal floor in an inverted Y-shaped pattern. This is an important landmark in intraoral radiographs of this area.

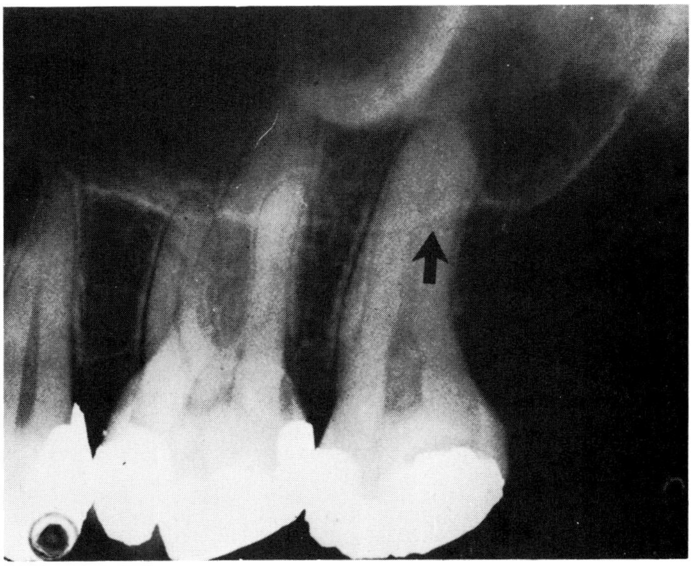

Fig. 1-13. Floor of the maxillary sinus (arrow) extends to the tuberosity. The crescent-shaped radiopacity above the molar roots is the zygomatic process of the maxilla. The nasal floor cannot be seen.

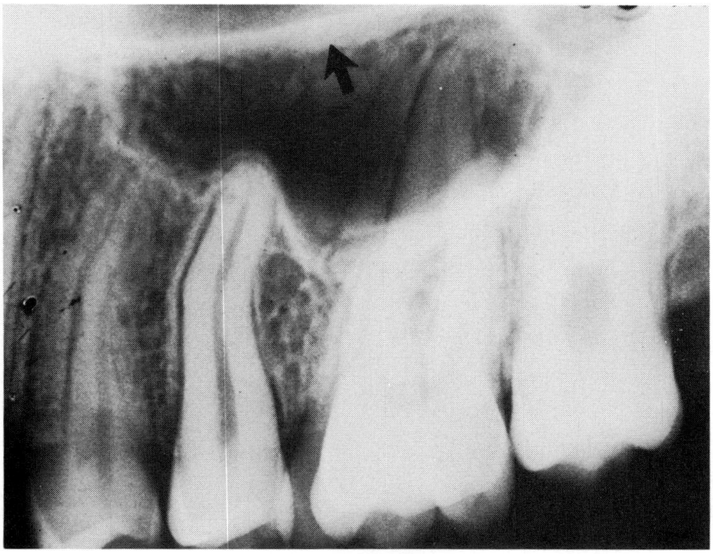

Fig. 1-14. Intraoral radiograph showing the floor of the maxillary sinus. The floor of the nasal cavity can also be identified (arrow).

bicuspid and molar areas. As a rule it extends from the bicuspid area to the tuberosity (Figs. 1-12 to 1-15). In most cases its anterior boundary may extend to the cuspid root and very rarely to the lateral incisor (Figs. 1-14 and 1-16). Its floor lies above the apices of teeth or may dip between their roots for various depths (Figs. 1-13 to 1-15). The overall morphology of this structure, however, varies widely. The radiolucency is often divided into compartments by radiopaque lines representing bony septa (Fig. 1-17). Although usually there is a single septum, multiple septa that completely or incompletely compartmentalize the antrum may be seen. Occasionally, spurs or ridges of bone project from the sinus wall and may appear as radiopacities that can be mistaken for roots or foreign bodies. The right and left antrum may be of equal size, or they may be grossly dissimilar (Fig. 1-18). In radiographs of the cuspid area, the boundaries of the maxillary sinus and the nasal cavity cross each other in an inverted Y-shaped pattern, and this feature is often a very prominent landmark of this area (Figs. 1-12 and 1-16).

After the loss of teeth and the alveolar process of the maxilla, the floor of the maxillary sinus begins to recede and may once again reach the level of the nasal floor.

Lateral fossa. In some individuals the bony depression in the labial cortical bone of the maxillary lateral incisor area, called the *lateral fossa,* is quite prominent. In such cases a radiograph of the area shows a zone of diminished density that should not be mistaken for pathology (Fig. 1-16).

Zygomatic (malar) process of maxilla and zygomatic bone. In intraoral radio-

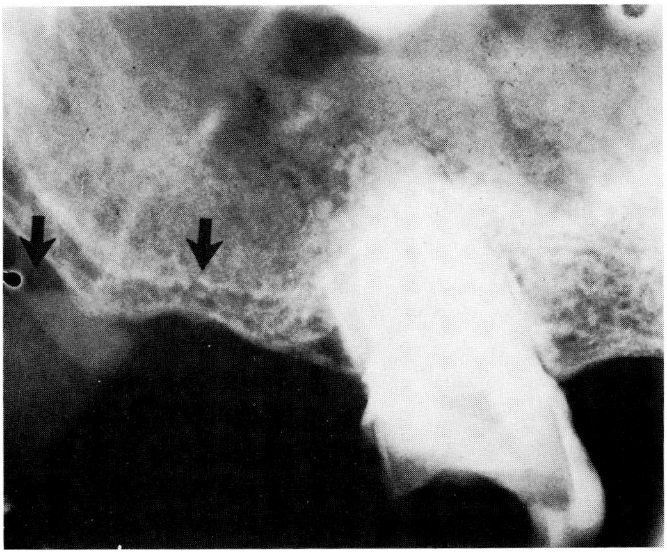

Fig. 1-15. Coronoid process of the mandible appears in radiographs of the maxillary molar area (left arrow). The maxillary sinus (right arrow) reaches into the maxillary tuberosity.

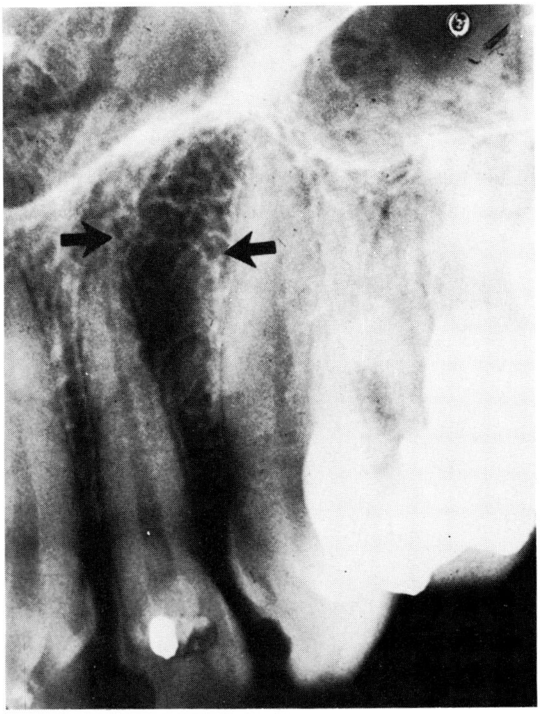

Fig. 1-16. Lateral fossa (arrows) appears as a radiolucent area in the region of the maxillary lateral incisor. The maxillary sinus (radiolucency on right) and the floor of the nasal cavity (left) join in an inverted Y-shaped pattern.

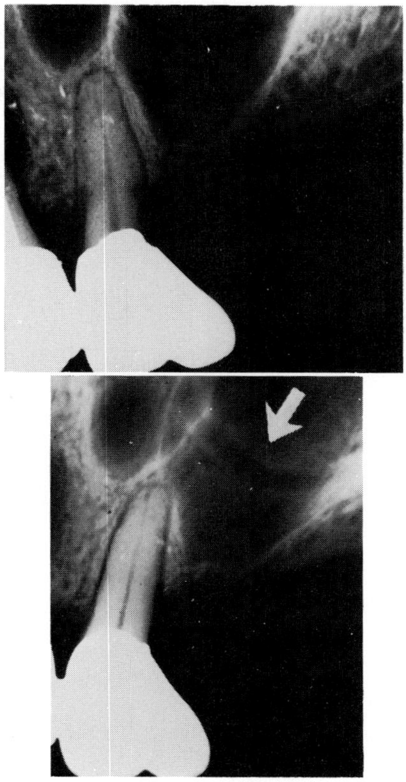

Fig. 1-17. Two views of the same maxillary sinus, showing the presence of two compartments. The bottom illustration shows the shadow of a groove made by a nutrient canal in the sinus wall (arrow).

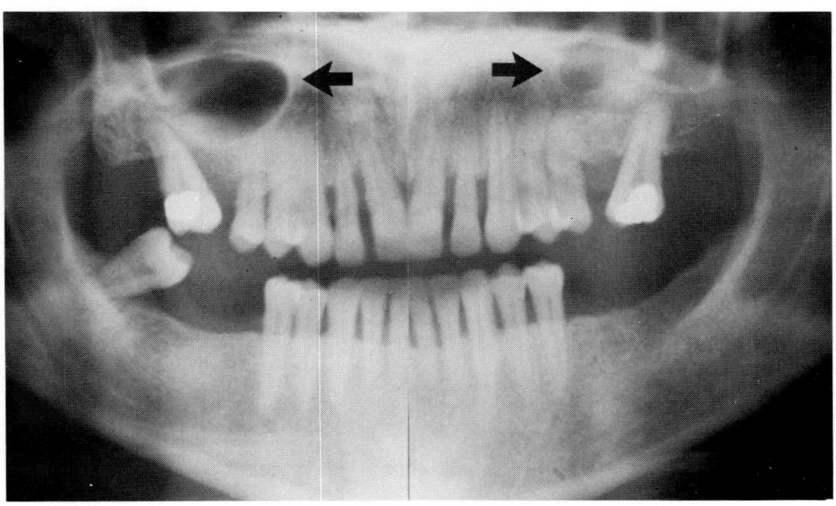

Fig. 1-18. Panoramic radiograph of the jaws, showing marked dissimilarity between the right and left maxillary sinuses (arrows). The patient had no clinical symptoms.

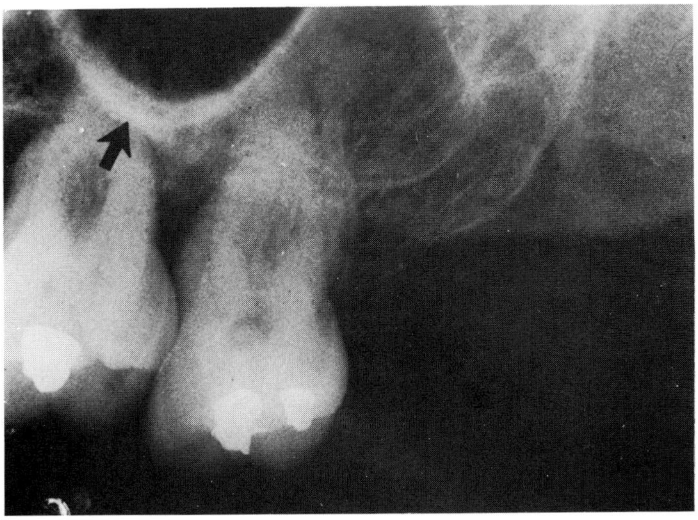

Fig. 1-19. U-shaped radiopacity (arrow) represents the zygomatic process of the maxilla.

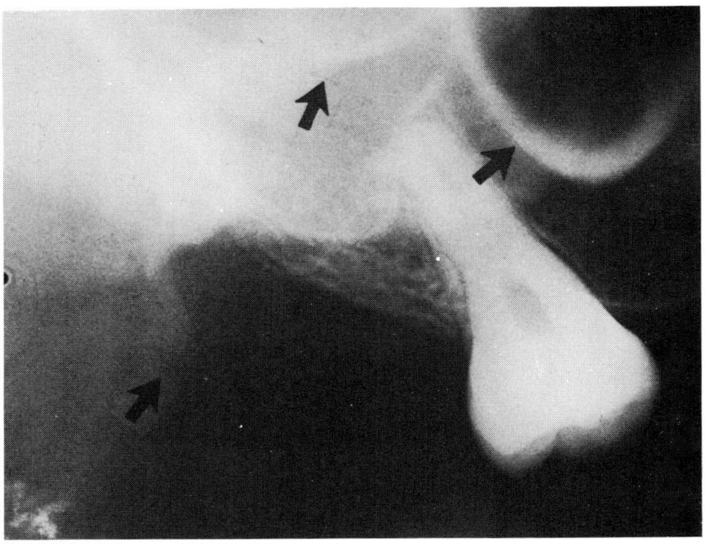

Fig. 1-20. U-shaped radiopacity is the zygomatic process of the maxilla (right arrow), and the radiopacity extending posteriorly from it represents the zygomatic bone (middle arrow). The lateral pterygoid plate appears below and behind the tuberosity (lower arrow).

graphs the zygomatic process of the maxilla appears as a U-shaped radiopacity overlying the larger radiolucency of the antrum (Figs. 1-19 and 1-20). The U-shaped radiopacity represents the attachment of the zygomatic bone to the maxilla. In the apical films of the molar area, the *zygomatic arch* appears as a radiopaque band extending posteriorly from the U-shaped radiopacity of the zygomaticomaxillary junction (Fig. 1-20).

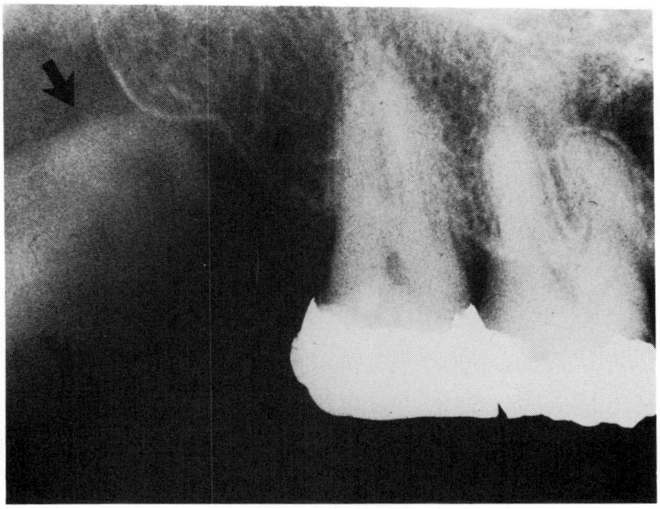

Fig. 1-21. Coronoid process of the mandible appears in radiograph of the maxillary third molar area (arrow).

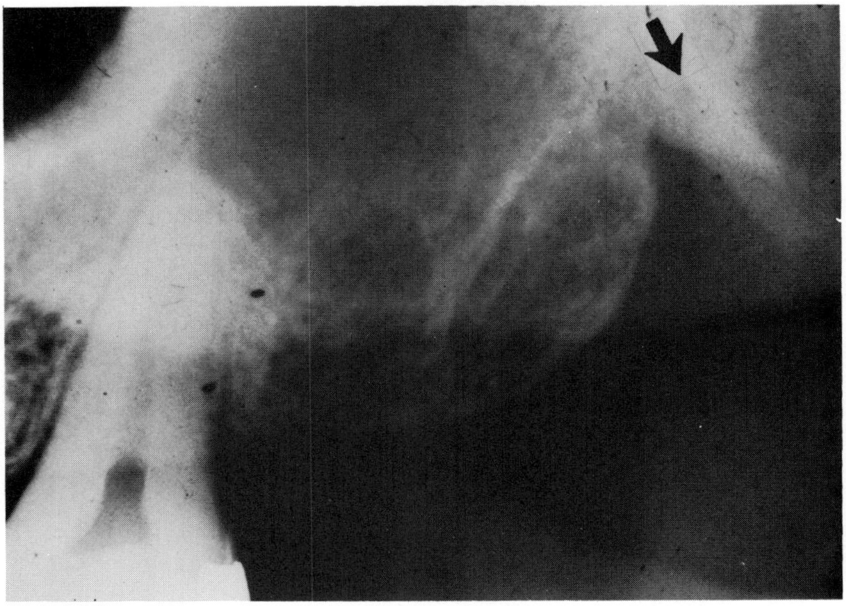

Fig. 1-22. Hamulus appears behind the maxillary tuberosity (arrow). The lateral pterygoid plate is located anterior and superior to it but cannot be identified.

Coronoid process of mandible. The coronoid process of the mandible appears as a triangular structure in radiographs of the posterior maxillary teeth and is easily identified (Figs. 1-15 and 1-21).

Hamulus and lateral plate of pterygoid process. The pterygoid process of the sphenoid bone has two plates—a broad, short lateral plate, and a long medial plate. The inferior end of the lateral plate is wide and round, and can sometimes be seen as a radiopacity behind the maxillary tuberosity (Fig. 1-20). The inferior end of the medial plate ends in a thin, curved process called the hamulus, or the pterygoid hamulus. This structure is sometimes seen behind and below the radiopacity of the lateral pterygoid plate (Fig. 1-22). Whereas the hamulus is often seen in radiographs of the maxillary tuberosity area, the lateral pterygoid plate is not easy to identify (Fig. 1-22).

LANDMARKS IN RADIOGRAPHS OF THE MANDIBLE

Mental fossa. The mental fossa are slight depressions in bone on the labial aspect of the mandibular lateral incisors, and in radiographs of the lower anterior teeth, they may sometimes appear as areas of diminished radiopacity (Fig. 1-23). They may be seen on one or both sides of the midline and do not represent pathology.

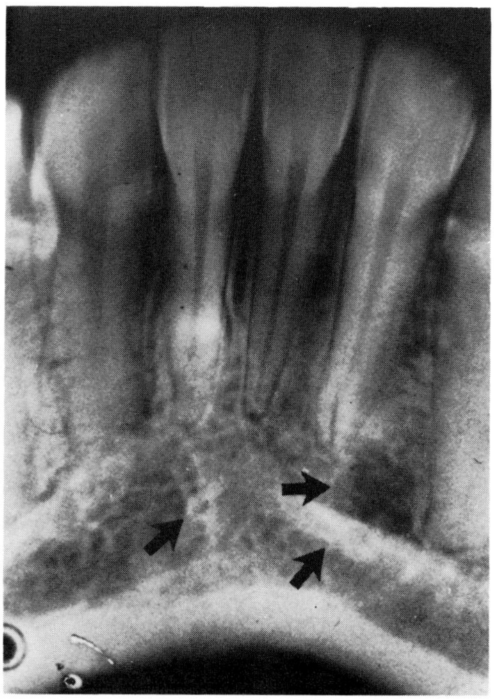

Fig. 1-23. Intraoral film of lower anterior area, showing the mental fossa (upper arrow) and the mental ridge (lower right arrow). The lingual foramen is barely visible in the midline (left arrow).

Mental ridge. The mental ridge is a bony prominence extending from the midline of the mandible to the area of the premolars. Located on the labial side, it arches downward and backward from the midline, and its density and prominence vary widely. It is best seen in intraoral radiographs of the lower incisor area (Figs. 1-23 and 1-24).

Lingual foramen. In radiographs of the lower incisor area, the lingual foramen is seen as a single radiolucent area located in the midline of the mandible. Its size and prominence, however, vary widely (Figs. 1-23 to 1-25).

Genial tubercles. In radiographs of the lower incisor area, genial tubercles are sometimes seen as radiopaque zones located on either side of the incisive foramen (Fig. 1-25). They can be better visualized in occlusal radiographs.

Mental foramen. Radiographs of the bicuspid and cuspid area of the mandible show a radiolucency that represents the mental foramen. Its position, as well as the position of the other anatomic landmarks, can be changed by altering the angulation of the x rays. It may be oval, round, or irregular in shape, and varies from a few millimeters to a centimeter in size. Usually it is

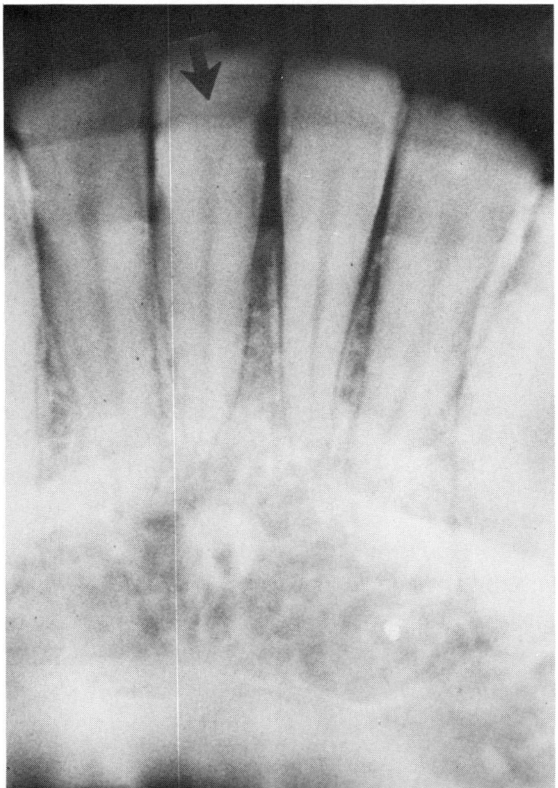

Fig. 1-24. Radiolucent lingual foramen and radiopaque mental ridges (linear structures). Also note the lip line (arrow).

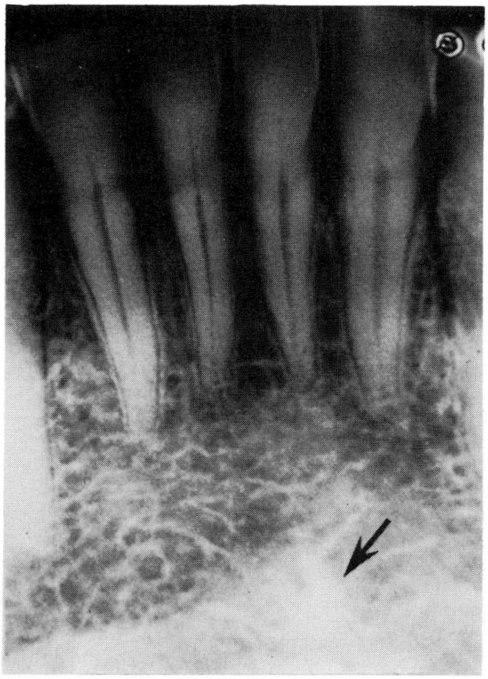

Fig. 1-25. Genial tubercles appear as radiopaque areas around the barely visible lingual foramen (arrow).

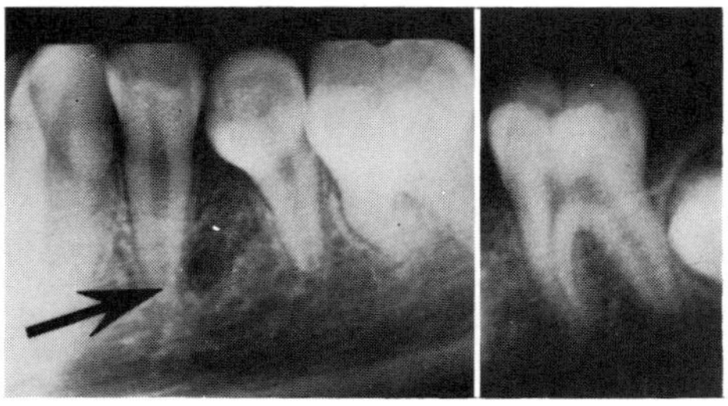

Fig. 1-26. Mental foramen (arrow).

located below and distal to the apex of the first bicuspid, and sometimes its connection with the inferior dental canal can be visualized (Figs. 1-26 and 1-27).

Mandibular canal (inferior dental canal). The mandibular canal, or inferior dental canal, runs as a radiolucent structure from the mandibular foramen in the ramus to the mental foramen where the canal turns upward and ends at the opening (Fig. 1-27). On rare occasions, however, it can be seen to continue beyond the area of the mental foramen and is located apical to the lower incisors (Fig. 1-28). The mandibular foramen is a funnel-shaped area of radiolucency that varies greatly in size and location (Fig. 1-29). The inferior dental canal is bordered by slightly radiopaque margins, and it is located at varying sites between

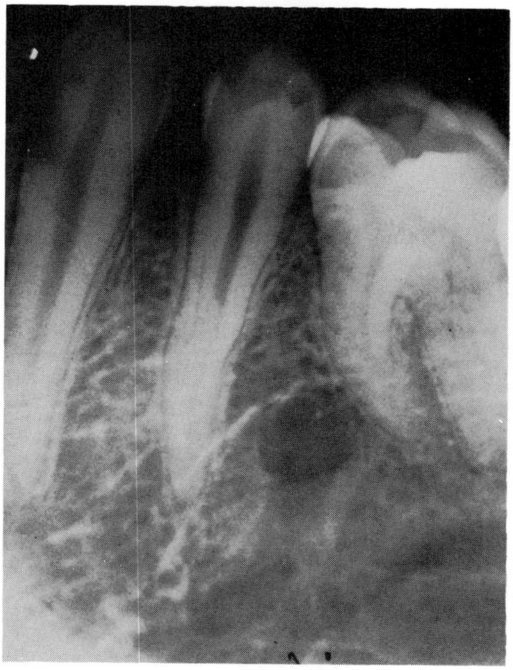

Fig. 1-27. Mental foramen and its connection with the inferior dental canal.

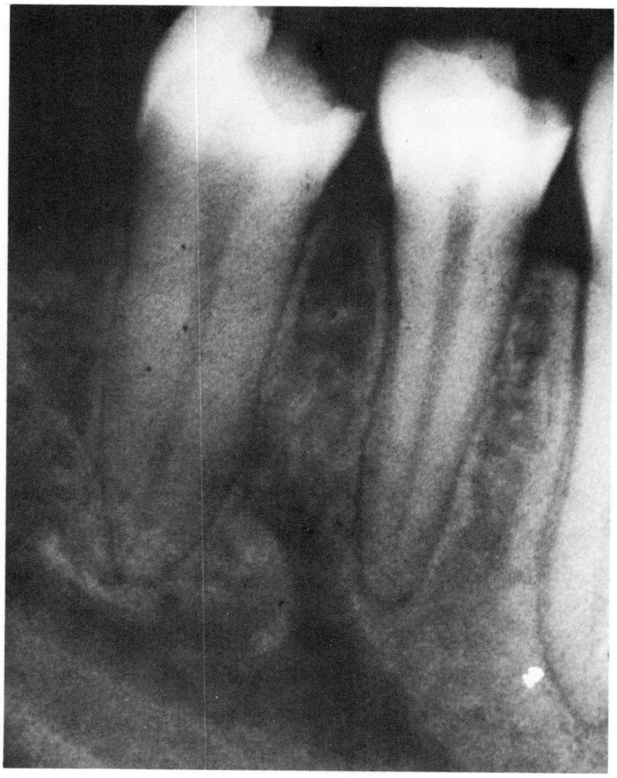

Fig. 1-28. The inferior dental canal in the bicuspid area extends between the roots of the teeth toward the mental foramen (not seen) and also continues forward toward the apices of incisors (right).

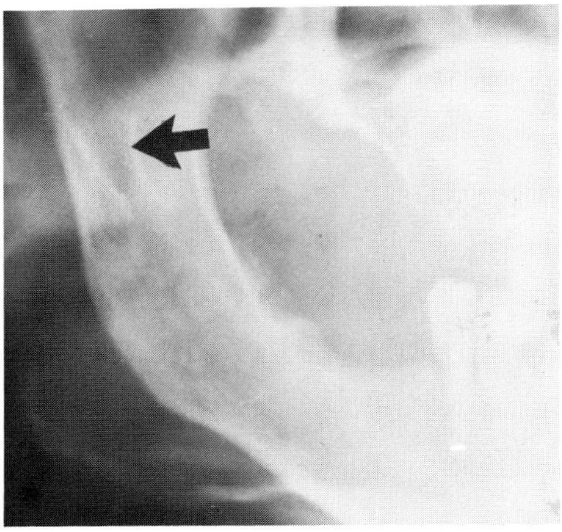

Fig. 1-29. The funnel-shaped mental foramen can be seen in the ramus of the mandible (arrow).

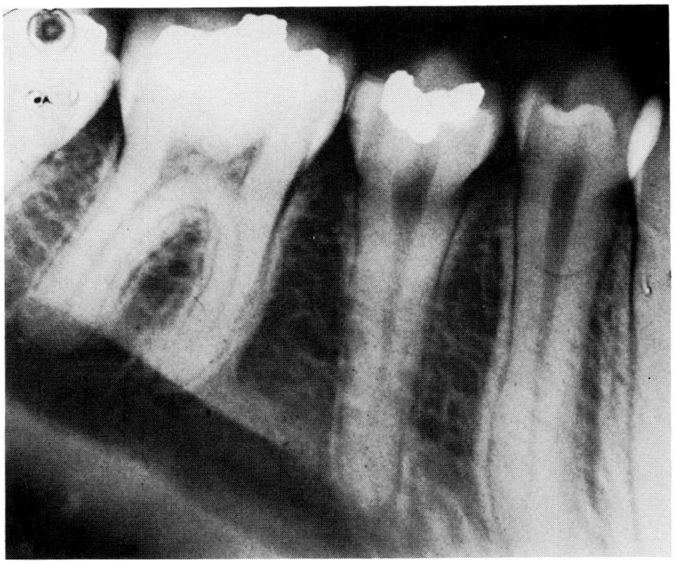

Fig. 1-30. Inferior dental canal. Note the prominent periodontal shadow in the apical area of first molar roots. The radiopaque upper border of the canal is caused by the mylohyoid ridge.

the inferior border of the mandible and the apices of the bicuspids and molars (Figs. 1-30 to 1-32). In some cases the radiographs may show root apices extending into the canal. They are, however, surrounded by the lamina dura. When the roots of the third or second molar are superimposed on the inferior dental canal, the width of the periodontal membrane at the root apex may be widened (Fig. 1-33). The widening of the apical periodontal shadow, seen when the apex of the central incisor is superimposed over the incisive foramen or when

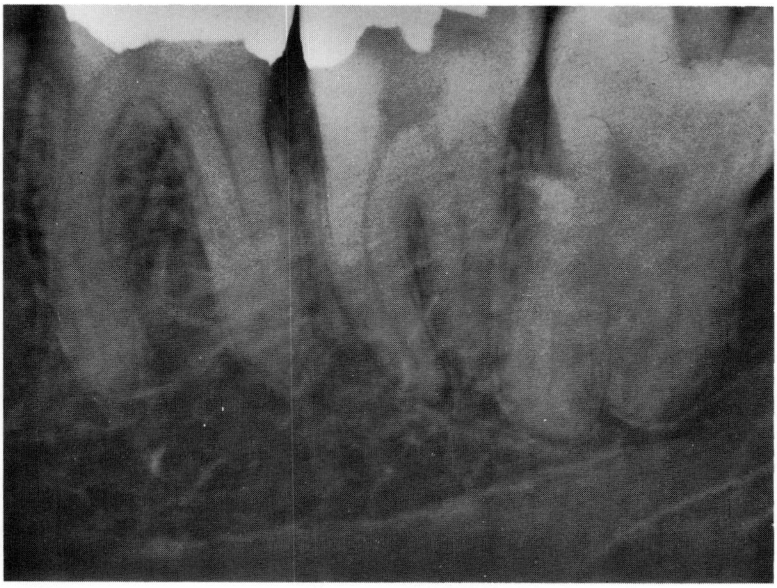

Fig. 1-31. Inferior dental canal. The radiolucency at the apical area of the distal root of the third molar does not represent a pathologic condition.

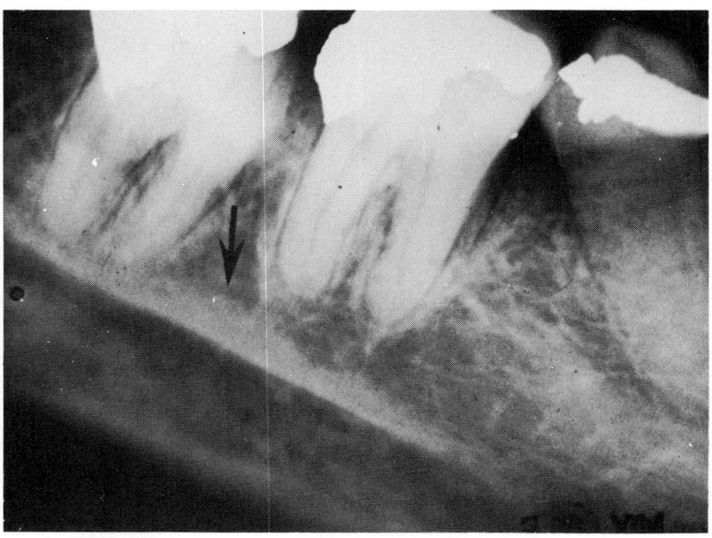

Fig. 1-32. Inferior dental canal. Its lower border is not clearly delineated. The radiopacity at the upper border represents the mylohyoid ridge (arrow).

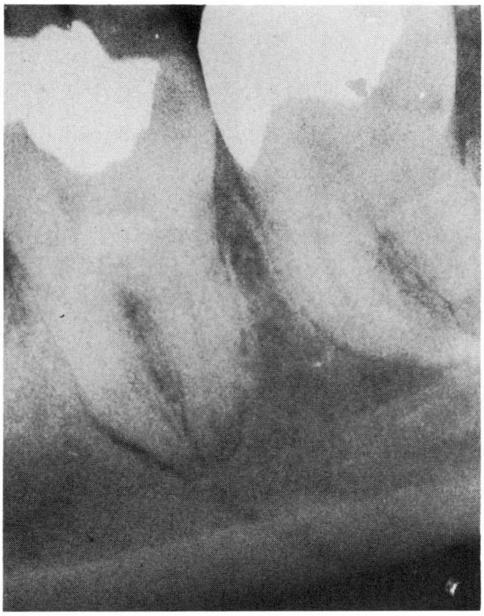

Fig. 1-33. Apical area of the first molar is superimposed on the inferior dental canal and shows a widening of the periodontal membrane shadow.

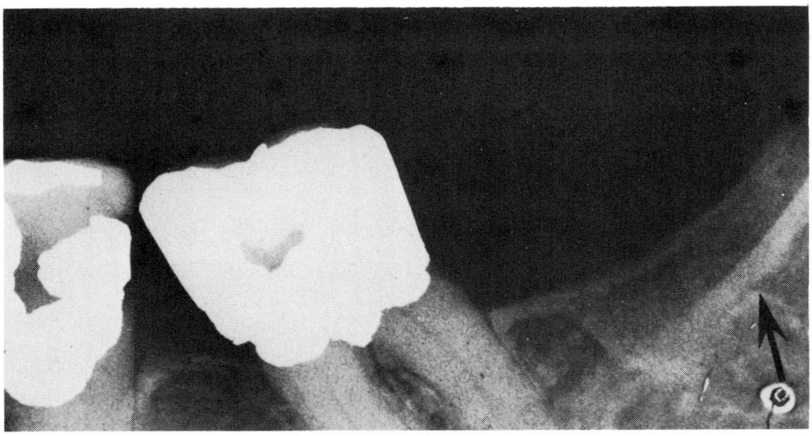

Fig. 1-34. External oblique line appears as a radiopaque structure in the radiographs of the mandibular molar area.

the apex of a tooth is superimposed on the antrum, is similar. The cause of this phenomenon is not known. It is, however, always limited to the superimposed part of the periodontal membrane space and does not indicate pathology.

External oblique line. Radiographs of the posterior mandibular teeth often show a radiopaque structure that corresponds to the anterior border of the ramus and descends to the area of the third molar. This is the external oblique line (Figs. 1-34 and 1-35).

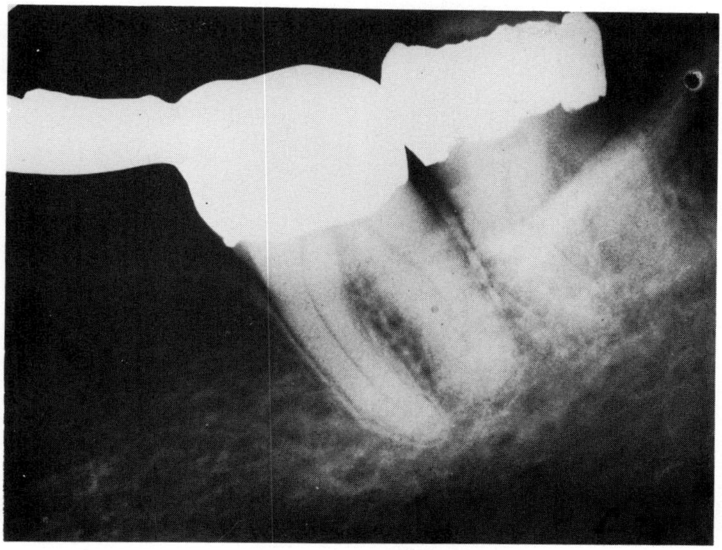

Fig. 1-35. Radiopaque external oblique line overlaps the third molar and becomes continuous with a larger radiopacity, the mylohyoid ridge.

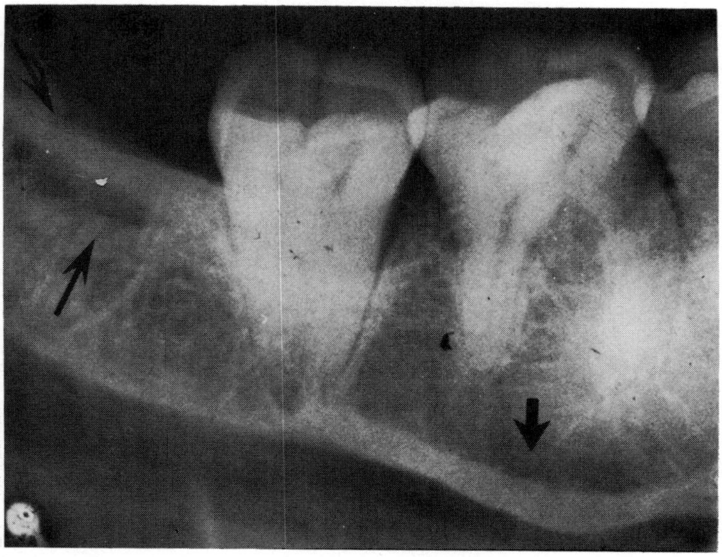

Fig. 1-36. Radiopaque external (upper left arrow) and internal (lower left arrow) oblique lines enclose the radiolucent *retromolar triangle*. The arrow on right marks the mylohyoid ridge.

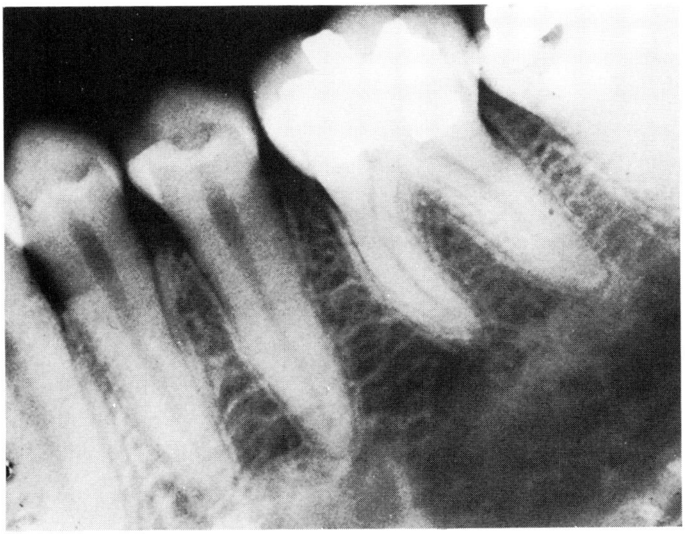

Fig. 1-37. Radiolucent area below the first lower molar roots represents the submandibular fossa.

Internal oblique line. The internal oblique line is a radiopaque structure that descends downward and forward from the coronoid process. It is located below the external oblique line, but it is not as prominent and is placed in a more horizontal position (Fig. 1-36). It may stop in the third molar area or become continuous with the mylohyoid line. The internal and external oblique lines, when pronounced, enclose an area of radiolucency, the *retromolar triangle* (Fig. 1-36).

Mylohyoid ridge. Also called the *mylohyoid line,* the mylohyoid ridge is seen as a radiopaque structure below the external oblique line (Fig. 1-36). It passes downward and forward from the ramus and gradually fades in the alveolar process or the body of the mandible of the bicuspid area. Since it varies widely in prominence, its radiopacity and length is not consistent (Figs. 1-32, 1-35, and 1-36).

Submaxillary gland fossa. The submaxillary gland fossa, or *submandibular fossa,* is an anatomic landmark. This area of reduced thickness of the bone below the lower posterior teeth is caused by a depression on the lingual side of the mandible and represents the position of the submaxillary gland. In the radiographs of the lower posterior teeth, it appears as a zone of relative radiolucency below the molars (Figs. 1-37 and 1-38). When excessively prounounced, it may be mistaken for a radiolucent "lesion."

MISCELLANEOUS STRUCTURES IN ORAL RADIOGRAPHS

Nutrient canals. Nutrient canals contain blood vessels and are seen most frequently in the incisor area of the mandible, followed by the bicuspid area, and finally the maxillary bicuspid region (Figs. 1-39 and 1-40). They appear as radiolucent, linear shadows between the roots of the teeth and have no resemblance to

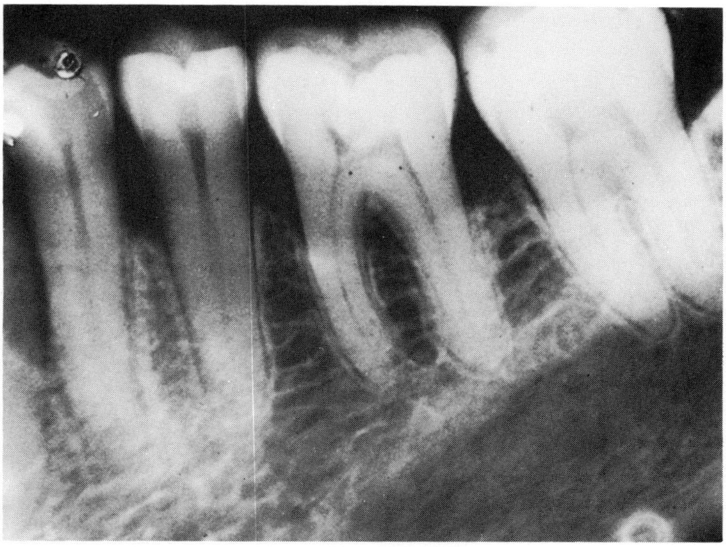

Fig. 1-38. Submandibular fossa is represented by the radiolucent area below the second lower molar roots and extends almost to the second bicuspid area.

A

B

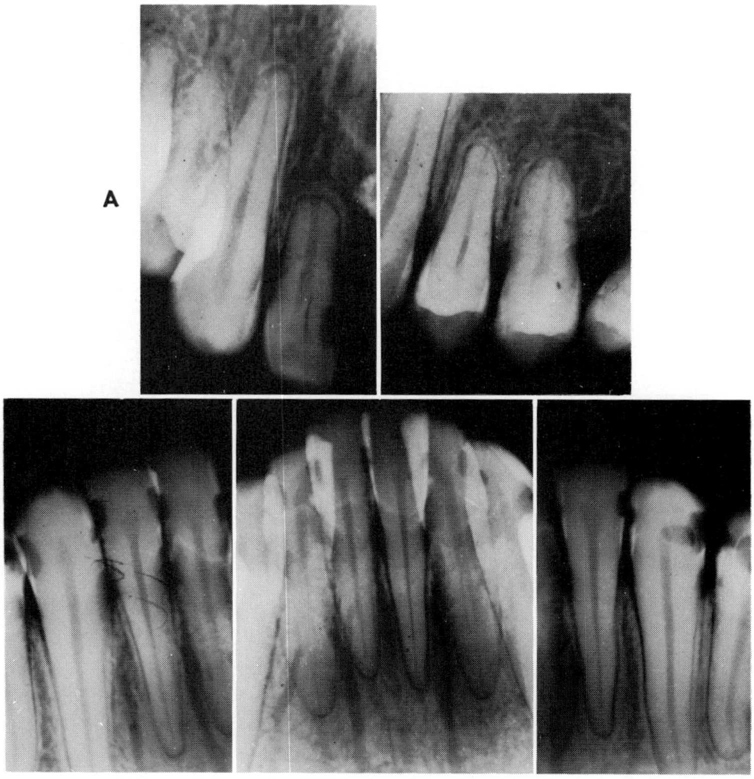

Fig. 1-39. Nutrient canals (radiolucent linear shadows between roots of teeth) in the maxillary, **A,** and mandibular, **B,** radiographs. Usually these canals cannot be seen to the very tip of the alveolar crest.

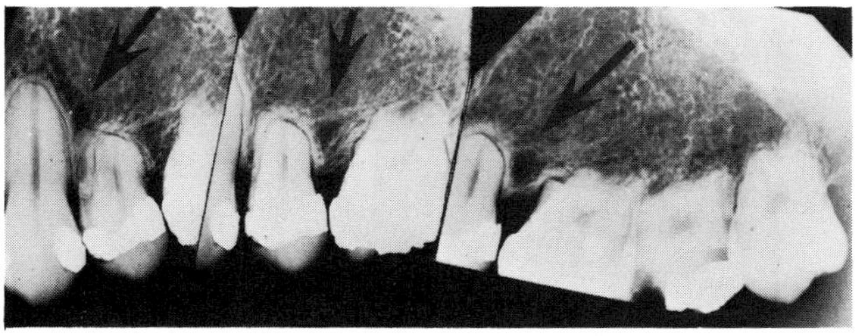

Fig. 1-40. Circular radiolucent shadows in maxillary radiographs, each illustrating a nutrient canal (arrows).

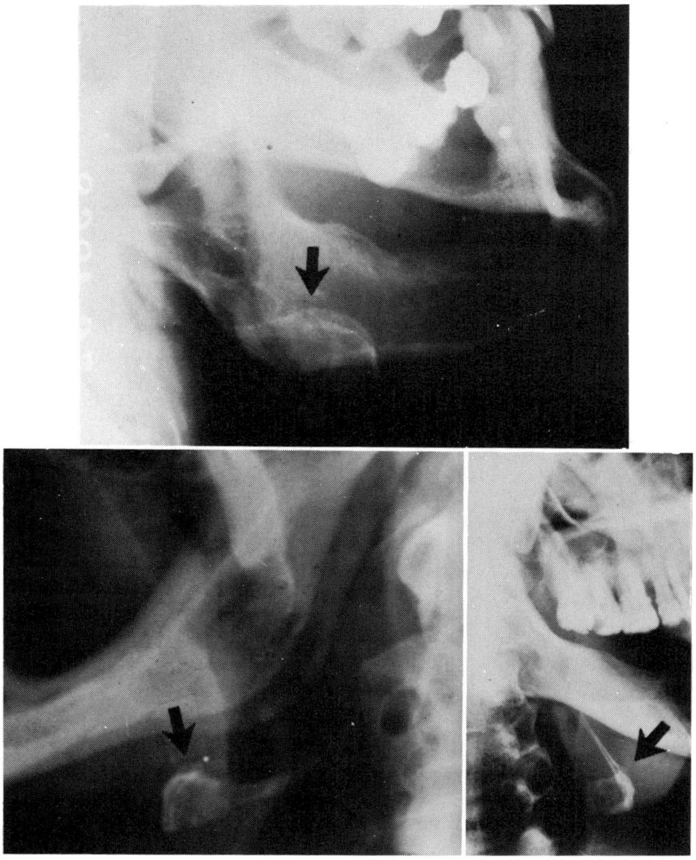

Fig. 1-41. In extraoral radiographs, radiopacity of the hyoid bone (arrows) appears below the mandible. Its location with regard to the jaw depends on the angulation of the film.

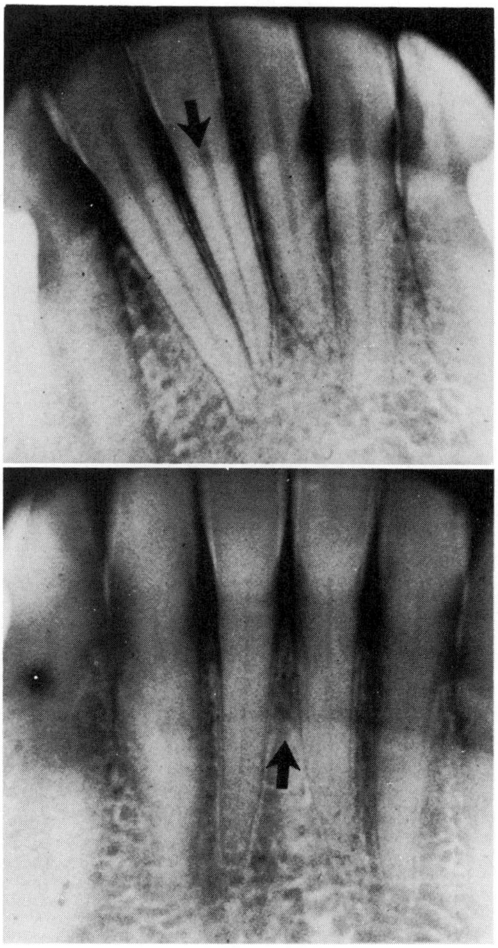

Fig. 1-42. "Lip line" appears at different levels across the lower anterior radiographs (arrows).

any pathologic radiolucency. Usually they do not extend to the crest of the bony septa (Fig. 1-39). On occasion these structures may be seen in the wall of the maxillary sinus (Fig. 1-17).

Hyoid bone. In lateral extraoral radiographs the hyoid bone appears as a radiopaque structure. Its location depends on the angulation, and it may be found below the lower border of the mandible or may be superimposed on the posterior part of the mandibular body (Fig. 1-41).

Soft tissues. Soft tissues of the face affect the radiographic appearance of the dento-osseous structures. Thick tissues (cheeks, for example) affect the radiographic quality adversely. The lip appears in radiographs of the anterior teeth, and its edge represents the so-called lip line. It sometimes affects the radiographs in such a way that the portion of teeth not covered by it appears darker than the

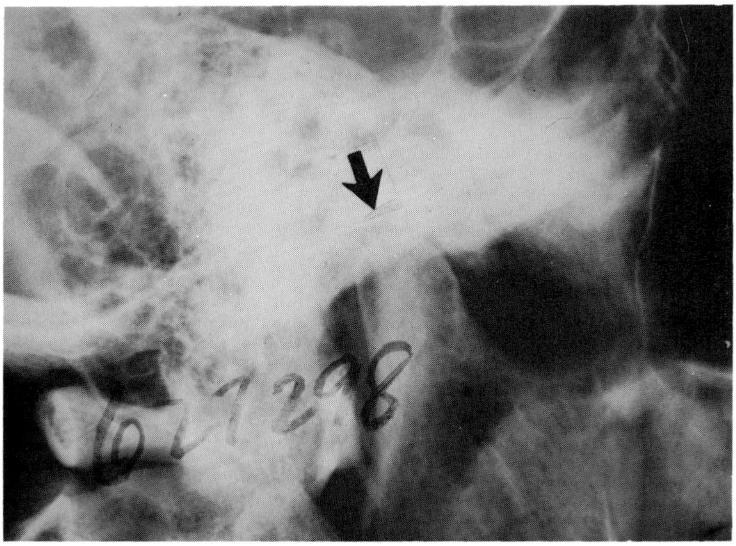

Fig. 1-43. Temporomandibular joint in a lateral extraoral radiograph.

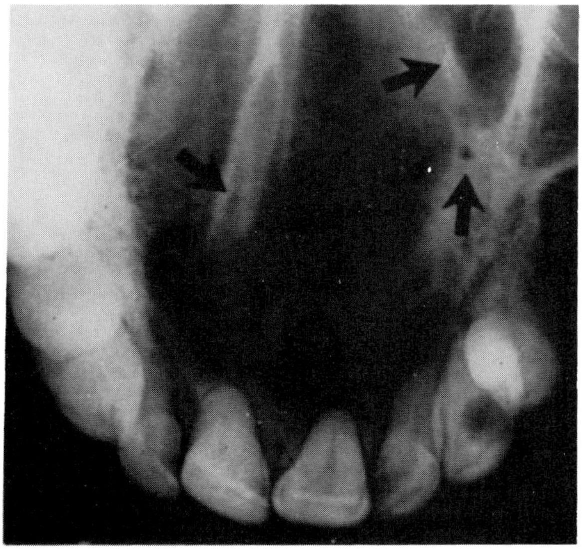

Fig. 1-44. Occlusal radiograph of the maxilla, showing the radiolucencies of a large fissural cyst (left arrow), the nasolacrimal canal (top arrow), and the greater palatine foramen (lower arrow). A nutrient canal is seen between the central incisors.

covered area (Fig. 1-42). The lip line may be seen above the incisal edges, and unless recognized, it can complicate accurate interpretation of radiographs.

Temporomandibular joint. The temporomandibular joint appears in lateral extraoral radiographs and is easily recognized (Fig. 1-43).

Styloid process and stylomandibular ligament. The styloid process of the temporal bone can sometimes be seen in lateral head radiographs behind the posterior margin of the mandible. On rare occasions this process, as well as the calcified stylomandibular ligament, may be seen as a single radiopaque unit.

Nasolacrimal canal. The nasolacrimal canal is not usually visible in apical radiographs of the maxillary teeth. In occlusal views of the maxilla, however, it appears as a round or oval radiolucency that may be 4 to 8 mm. in diameter and is located in the posterior part of the hard palate area (Fig. 1-44).

Greater palatine foramen. Occlusal radiographs of the maxilla often show these structures as small radiolucencies (Fig. 1-44).

REFERENCES

Bender, I. B.: Roentgenographic significance of the lamina dura in systemic disease, J. Albert Einstein Med. Center **9:**82, 1961.

Benkow, H. H.: Interpretive pitfalls in radiodontics, Dent. Radiogr. Photogr. **34:**86, 1961.

Brynolf, I.: Improved viewing facilities for better roentgenodiagnosis, Oral Surg. **32:** 808, 1971.

Ennis, L. M., Berry, H. M., and Phillips, J. E.: Dental roentgenology, ed. 6, Philadelphia, 1967, Lea & Febiger.

Etter, L. E.: Atlas of roentgen anatomy of the skull, Springfield, Ill., 1955, Charles C Thomas, Publisher.

Lovett, D. W.: Nutrient canals—a roentgenographic study, J. Am. Dent. Assoc. **37:** 671, 1948.

Meschan, I.: An atlas of normal radiographic anatomy, ed. 2, Philadelphia, 1959, W. B. Saunders Co.

Parfitt, G. J.: An investigation of the normal variations in alveolar bone trabeculations, Oral Surg. **15:**1453, 1962.

Phillips, J. D., and Shawkat, A. H.: A study of the radiographic appearance of osseous defects on panoramic and conventional films, Oral Surg. **36:**745, 1973.

Sicher, H., and DuBrul, E. L.: Oral anatomy, ed. 6, St. Louis, 1975, The C. V. Mosby Co.

Stafne, E. C.: Oral roentgenographic diagnosis, ed. 3, Philadelphia, 1973, W. B. Saunders Co.

Updegrave, W. J.: Normal radiodontic anatomy, Dent. Radiogr. Photogr. **31:** 57, 1958.

Updegrave, W. J.: Visualizing the mandibular ramus in panoramic radiograph, Oral Surg. **31:**422, 1971.

Waggener, D. T.: Relationships of third molar roots to the mandibular canal, Oral Surg. **12:**853, 1959.

Wuehrmann, A. H., and Manson-Hing, L. R.: Dental radiology, ed. 3, St. Louis, 1973, The C. V. Mosby Co.

PART TWO

TEETH

The radiographic interpretation of teeth and the immediate area around the teeth will be discussed under three separate headings. Chapter 2 will deal with *changes in the shape and number of teeth,* Chapter 3 with *caries,* and Chapter 4 with the radiographic interpretation of *periodontal diseases.* For the sake of organization only those lesions that are related to gingival and periodontal diseases will be considered in Chapter 4. Although anatomically and in a strict sense the periapical lesions also involve the periodontal tissues, they will be included in the section on the radiographic interpretation of the jaws.

CHAPTER TWO

CHANGES IN NUMBER AND SHAPE OF TEETH

Abnormalities of the coronal portions of erupted teeth can be diagnosed by a clinical examination. For a diagnosis of the changes in the root portion or in the unerupted teeth, the radiograph is the only diagnostic aid.

The radiograph may show an alteration in the number of teeth, in their shape, or in their internal architecture. The radiologic interpretation of teeth can therefore be classified as follows:

- Changes in number of teeth
  - Natal and neonatal teeth
  - Accessory and supernumerary teeth
  - Postpermanent dentition, or third dentition
  - Anodontia
- Changes in shape of teeth
  - Microdontia
  - Macrodontia
  - Gemination
  - Fusion
  - Concrescence
  - Dens in dente
  - Dilaceration
  - Fracture
  - Enamel agenesis
  - Hereditary enamel hypoplasia
  - Hereditary enamel hypocalcification
  - Systemic and local enamel hypoplasia
  - Systemic and local enamel hypocalcification
  - Turner tooth
  - Dentinogenesis imperfecta and shell teeth
  - Odontodysplasia
  - Taurodontia
  - Cementum aplasia
  - Hypercementosis
  - Abrasion

- Attrition
- External resorption
- Ankylosis
- Caries

Changes in root canal
- Narrow root canals
- Pulp stones
- Lateral canals
- Internal resorption

Miscellaneous lesions
- Calculus
- Malocclusion

CHANGES IN NUMBER OF TEETH

Natal and neonatal teeth. Natal and neonatal teeth either are present at birth or erupt soon after. The radiograph shows deciduous teeth that erupted prematurely, or predecidious toothlike structures. In some instances, however, natal or neonatal teeth may be clinically present, although the radiograph shows no evidence of tooth structure. Such "teeth" are keratinized masses and do not contain enamel or dentin. Natal and neonatal teeth are most often seen in the mandibular incisor area.

Accessory and supernumerary teeth. Teeth that are in excess of the normal complement are called *accessory* or *supernumerary*. They may be visible clinically or may be seen only in the radiographs. When they resemble a normal tooth they are called *supernumerary,* whereas if they do not have the normal outline, the term *accessory* is used. Accessory and supernumerary teeth are most often seen in the incisor, bicuspid, and molar area of the maxilla but can occur anywhere. On rare occasions these teeth can be discovered early in their development and are repre-

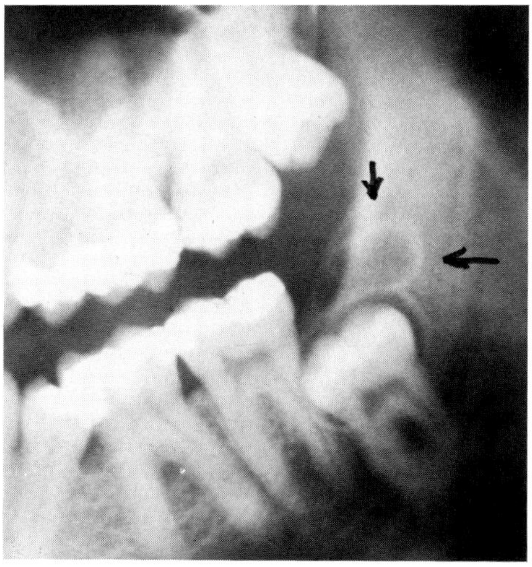

Fig. 2-1. Radiograph showing the tooth germ of a fourth mandibular molar.

sented only as radiolucencies in the radiographs (Fig. 2-1). At this stage, however, their differential diagnosis from other radiolucent conditions is not easy.

Numerous supernumerary or accessory teeth are found in such developmental disturbances as *cleidocranial dysostosis, craniofacial dysostosis,* and *mandibulofacial dysostosis.* Radiographs in these conditions show underdevelopment of the upper face and multiple unerupted teeth or toothlike structures (Fig. 2-2, *B*). These diseases are similar except that in cleidocranial dysostosis, the clavicle is missing (Fig. 2-2, *A*).

Postpermanent dentition, or third dentition. On rare occasions a permanent tooth may be followed by yet another tooth of normal morphology. Such teeth represent postpermanent dentition (Fig. 2-3).

Anodontia. Reduction in the normal complement of teeth is called *anodontia.* It may be *true* anodontia, in which teeth fail to develop, or *false* anodontia, in which they develop but fail to erupt. The distinction between true and false anodontia can therefore be made only after the examination of radiographs.

When only one or a few teeth are missing, the condition is called *partial* anodontia (Fig. 2-4); when all teeth are missing, it is called *total* anodontia (Fig. 2-5). When a single tooth is missing, it is usually a maxillary lateral or mandibular bicuspid, or a third molar tooth (Fig. 2-4). Total or partial anodontia is seen in a hereditary disturbance called *ectodermal dysplasia* (Figs. 2-5 and 2-6). False

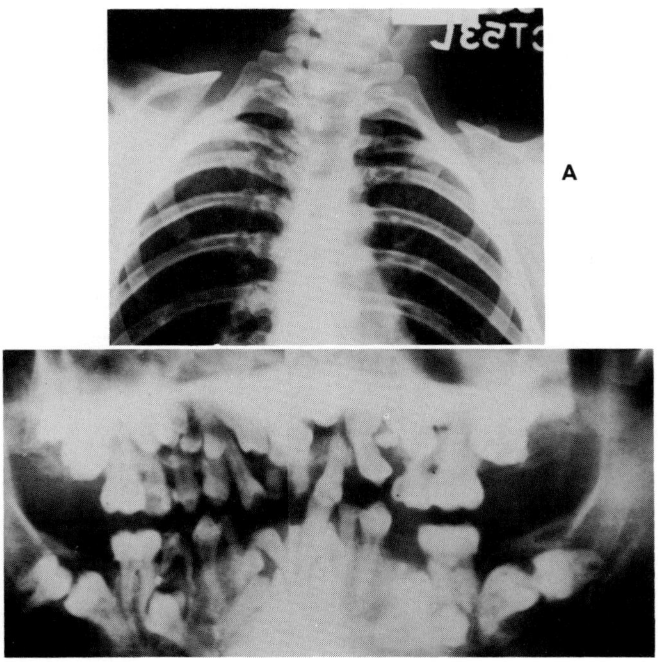

A

B

Fig. 2-2. Cleidocranial dysostosis. **A,** Absence of the clavicle. **B,** Multiple unerupted teeth can be seen.

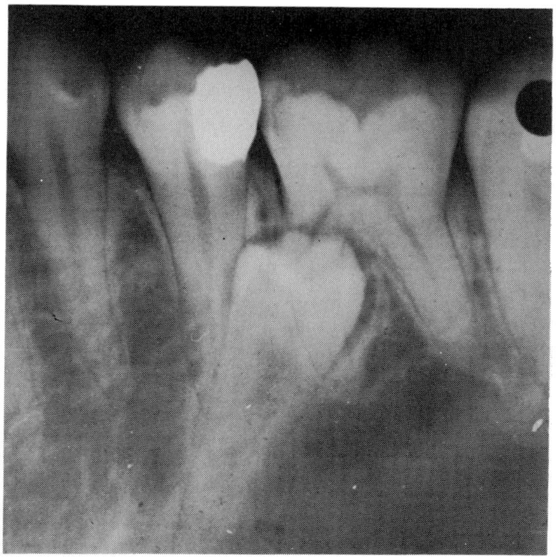

Fig. 2-3. Postpermanent, or "third," dentition is represented by a normal-appearing unerupted second bicuspid tooth.

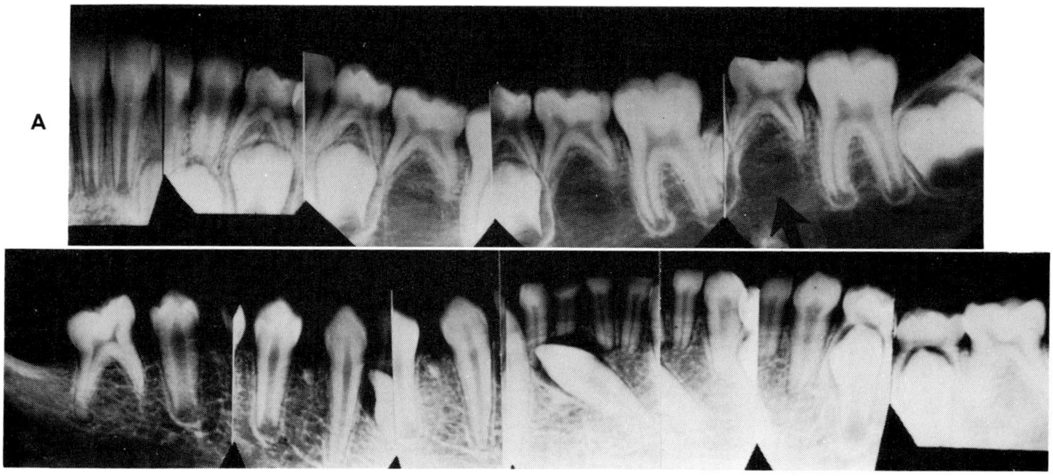

Fig. 2-4. Two cases of partial anodontia. **A,** Radiographs showing a missing lower second bicuspid (arrow). **B,** Absence of many permanent teeth.

anodontia is seen in impactions, but some of the best examples of this condition occur in *cleidocranial, craniofacial,* and *mandibulofacial dysostoses,* in which multiple teeth are present but fail to erupt (Fig. 2-2, *B*).

CHANGES IN SHAPE OF TEETH

Microdontia. In microdontia the radiograph shows a small tooth. This condition usually involves the maxillary lateral incisor or the maxillary third molar teeth.

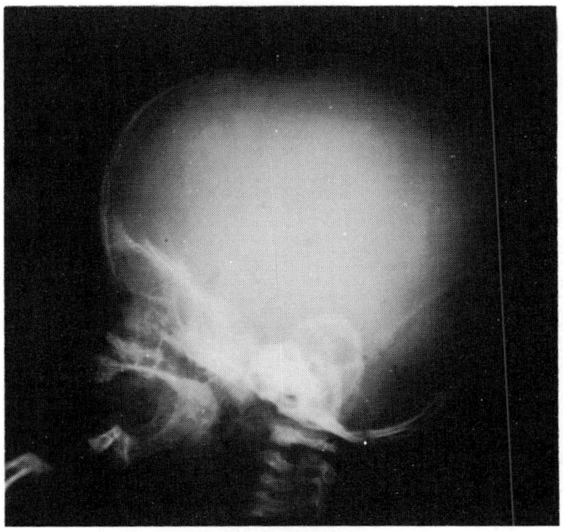

Fig. 2-5. Total anodontia in a case of ectodermal dysplasia. The radiopacity in the lower left corner of the figure is the radiopacity of the finger of an attendant who was holding the patient's jaws.

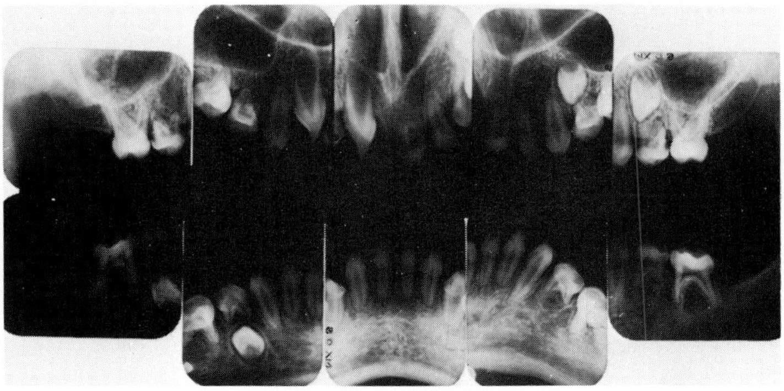

Fig. 2-6. Anodontia in ectodermal dysplasia. Many permanent teeth are missing.

Macrodontia. In macrodontia a larger-than-normal tooth is seen in the radiograph. The maxillary central incisor, cuspid, and mandibular second bicuspid are usually affected.

Gemination. In gemination the radiograph shows a tooth with a single root canal and either a large crown or two crowns (Figs. 2-7 and 2-8). These structures arise from a single dental germ.

Fusion. In fusion a tooth has two root canals and either a large crown or two crowns. A distinction between fusion and gemination can be made only with a radiograph and is based on the number of root canals (Fig. 2-9). Many times, however, this distinction is academic.

Concrescence. Unerupted, independently formed teeth may become fused by cementum. This fusion can be seen in the radiographs and is called concrescence (Fig. 2-10).

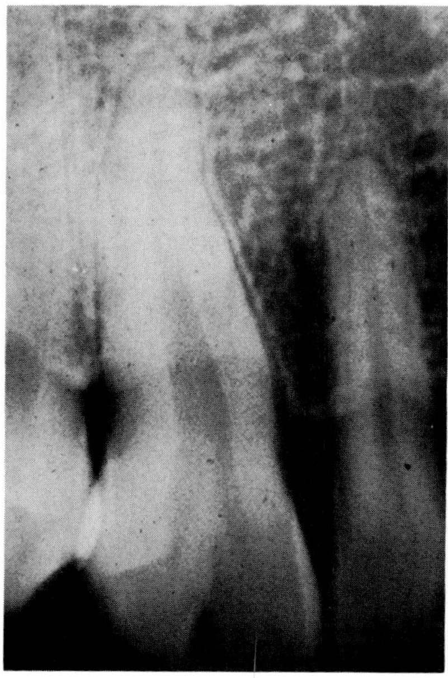

Fig. 2-7

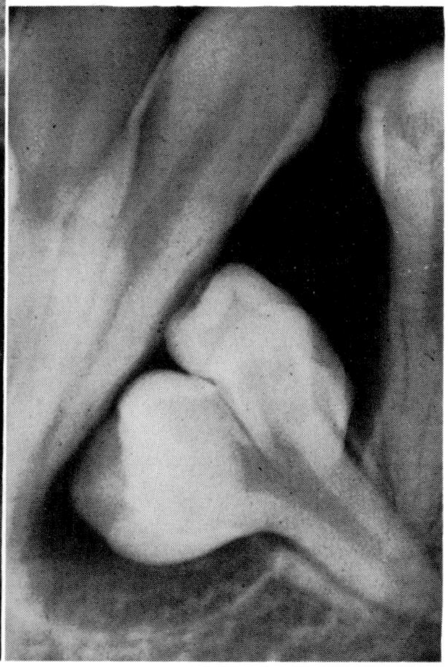

Fig. 2-8

Fig. 2-7. Gemination.
Fig. 2-8. Gemination. The tooth shows two crowns and a single root.

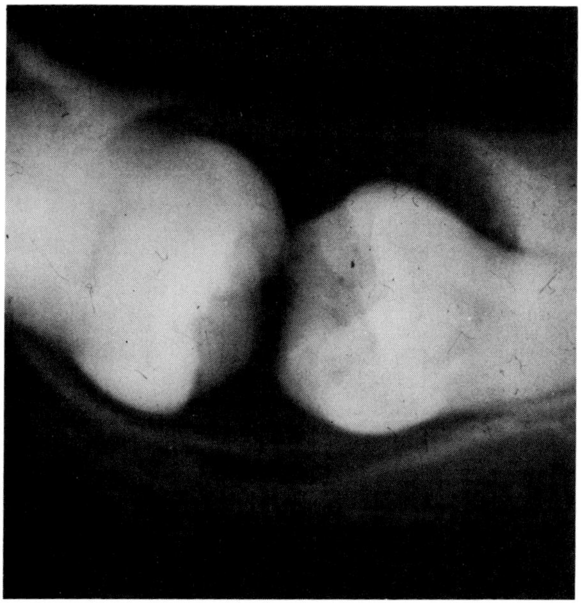

Fig. 2-9. Fusion. Two tooth germs have partially fused to form a structure that has two crowns and roots.

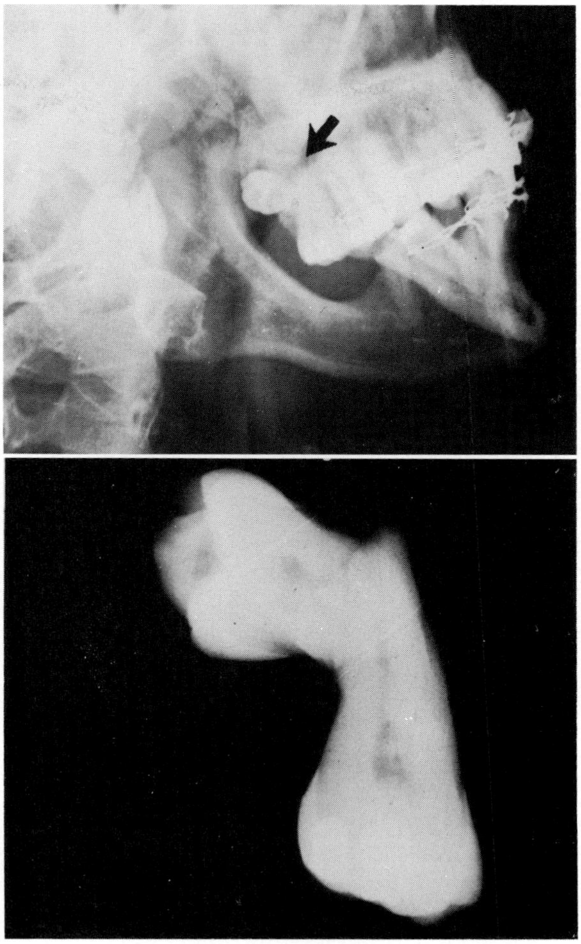

Fig. 2-10. Concrescence. Maxillary second molar and unerupted third molar have become united (arrow).

Dens in dente. When the radiograph shows a tooth the crown of which contains another small "toothlike" structure, the condition is called dens in dente (Figs. 2-11 and 2-12). Such teeth occur most often in the maxillary lateral incisor area. Since clinically they may appear normal, their true nature can be discovered only in radiographs. The pulps of these teeth usually become necrotic, and their periapical region often shows a radiolucent lesion that represents a dental granuloma or cyst. In dens in dente, therefore, endodontic therapy is usually necessary.

Dilaceration. In dilaceration there is a distortion of the usual relationship between the root and the crown. The radiograph is the only means of diagnosis, and it reveals an abnormality in the angulation of the root (Fig. 2-13).

Fracture. Fracture can be seen in the radiographs as a breakage in the continuity of the tooth (Fig. 2-14). However, fractures are not always apparent in

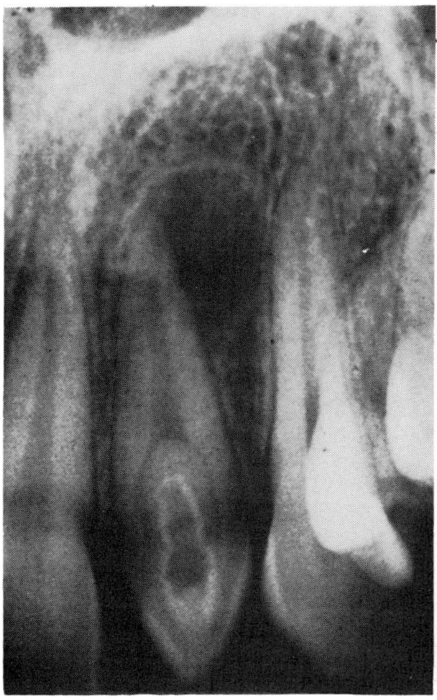

Fig. 2-11

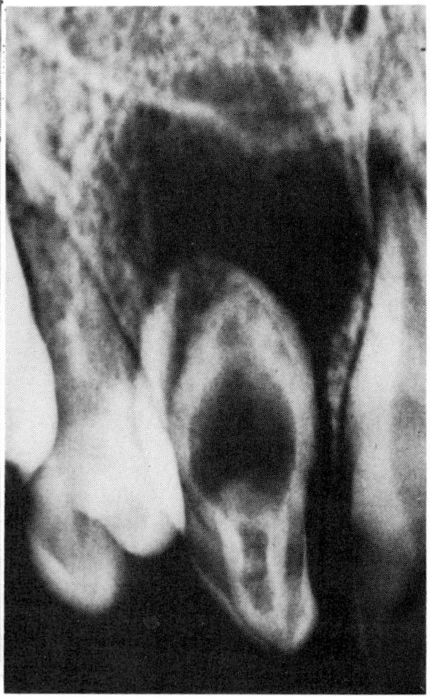

Fig. 2-12

Fig. 2-11. Dens in dente. Radiograph of a lateral incisor, showing a radiopaque toothlike structure within its crown.

Fig. 2-12. Deformed, dilated dens in dente. These structures take various forms in radiographs. The most important criterion is the presence of densely radiopaque enamel within the pulp chamber. Note the radiolucency at the apex of the tooth.

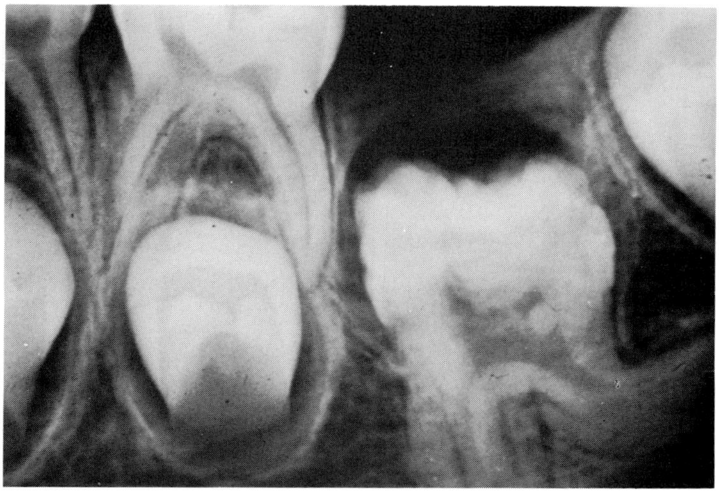

Fig. 2-13. Dilaceration. Radiograph shows the bent distal root of the first permanent molar.

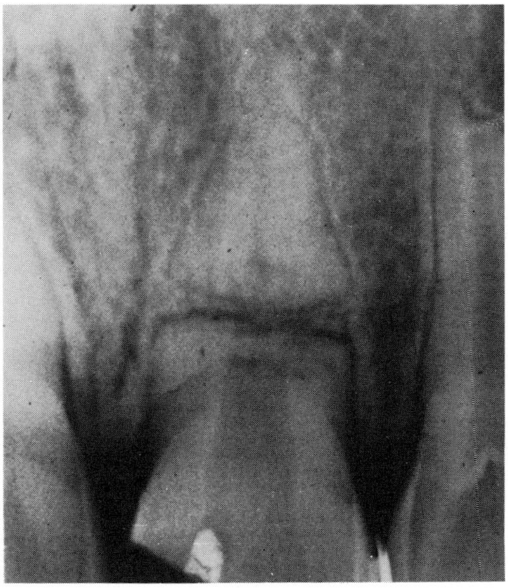

Fig. 2-14. Fracture usually appears as a radiolucent linear abnormality. Some fractures, however, may not be visible in radiographs.

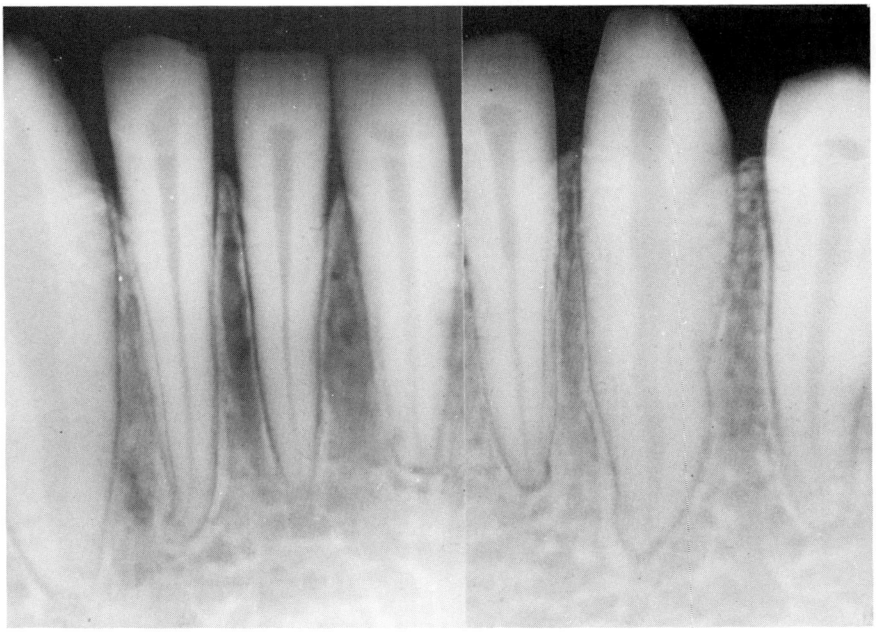

Fig. 2-15. Radiographs of teeth in a patient with apparent enamel agenesis. The crowns do not show the characteristic radiopaque enamel covering.

radiographs, and clinical symptoms of pain, history of trauma, and presence of mobility should all be considered in a differential diagnosis.

Enamel agenesis. In extremely rare cases of enamel agenesis, radiographs show an absence of enamel (Fig. 2-15). Although clinically and in the radiographs enamel cannot be identified, microscopically these cases usually do reveal a thin layer of enamel.

Hereditary enamel hypoplasia. When the radiographs show a reduction in the width of the entire coronal enamel, the condition usually represents hereditary enamel hypoplasia. Whereas the enamel appears pitted and moth-eaten, the rest of the tooth structure is normal. This condition is sometimes referred to as *amelogenesis imperfecta,* and it affects both the deciduous and permanent teeth (Fig. 2-16).

Hereditary enamel hypocalcification. In hereditary enamel hypocalcification the enamel covering of the teeth shows markedly reduced radiopacity. This condition affects both the deciduous and permanent dentitions and is sometimes referred to as *hereditary brown teeth.*

Systemic and local enamel hypoplasia. Radiographs of enamel hypoplasia are characterized by a reduction of the thickness of enamel at one or more isolated areas of the crown. Local enamel hypoplasia affects single teeth and is related to a *local* disturbance. When the defect is related to a transitory systemic disease, it affects those areas of the crowns of teeth which are undergoing development at that time. This condition is called *systemic* enamel hypoplasia. Only the severe cases of systemic and local enamel hypoplasia can be seen in radiographs.

Systemic and local enamel hypocalcification. In radiographs systemic and local enamel hypocalcification are not distinguishable from systemic and local hypoplasia.

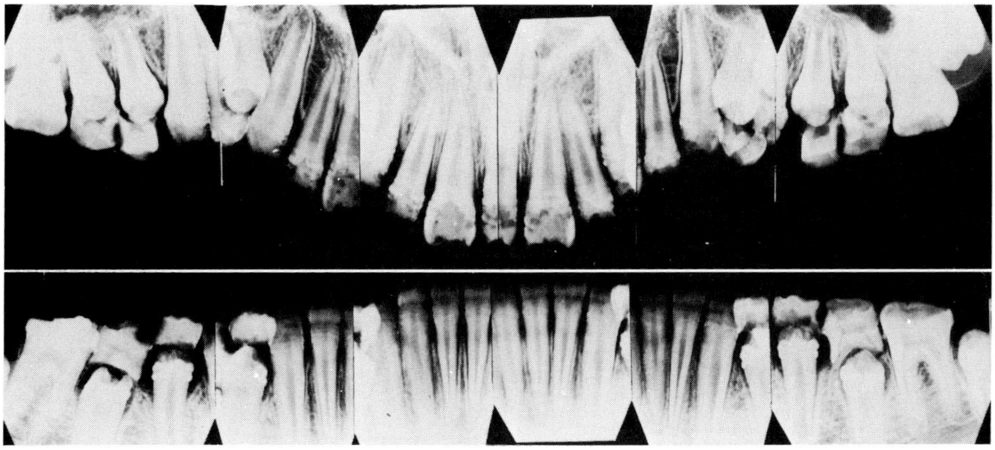

Fig. 2-16. Enamel hypoplasia of deciduous and permanent dentition appears as reduction in the thickness and radiopacity of the enamel, as well as changes in the normal contour of the tooth surface.

Turner tooth. Permanent teeth developing under a nonvital deciduous tooth with an apical lesion may develop severe local hypoplasia of enamel. In a radiograph of such a tooth, irregularities of the normal contours of the crown can be seen. The tooth is referred to as a *Turner tooth* (Fig. 2-17).

Dentinogenesis imperfecta and shell teeth. Dentinogenesis imperfecta affects the deciduous and permanent dentition or only the permanent dentition. The teeth have narrow roots and bulbous crowns (Figs. 2-18 and 2-19). In the early stage the pulp chambers are wide (Fig. 2-20, *A* and *B*), but in later stages they are severely narrowed or completely obliterated (Fig. 2-18). In a variation of dentinogenesis imperfecta, the pulp chambers remain large and the roots are incompletely formed or absent. This condition is called *shell teeth* (Fig. 2-20, *C*). In some cases of dentinogenesis imperfecta the apices of teeth show radiolucent areas *resembling* dental granulomas or radicular cysts (Fig. 2-21). These teeth, however, are vital, and the radiolucencies represent only normal connective tissue without evidence of pathology. The mechanism of development of these connective tissue foci is not known.

Odontodysplasia. In odontodysplasia the radiographs of the erupted and unerupted deciduous and/or permanent teeth, of one or more quadrants, have a moth-eaten appearance (Fig. 2-22). The pulp chambers are wider than normal. The enamel has severe hypoplasia, and the dentin is poorly calcified. Since all parts of the tooth are affected in this condition, it has been called *odontodysplasia.* These teeth should not be extracted.

Taurodontia. Radiographs of taurodontia (also called taurodontism) show a tooth with a long crown and short roots, giving it a characteristic appearance (Figs.

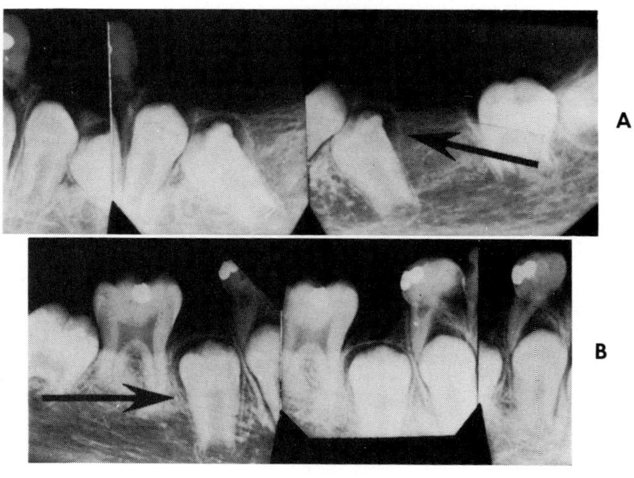

Fig. 2-17. Turner tooth. As compared to the normal side, **B,** the shape of the second bicuspid on the right side, **A,** is deformed (arrows). This deformation is the result of a periapical lesion that was associated with the second right deciduous molar.

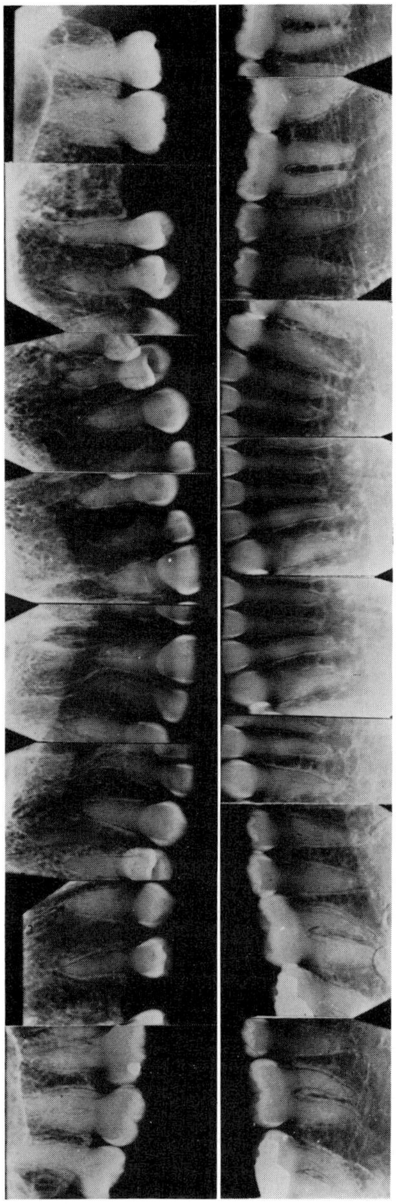

Fig. 2-18. Dentinogenesis imperfecta. Radiographs of a case in late stage. Pulp canals have become completely obliterated. Note wide crowns.

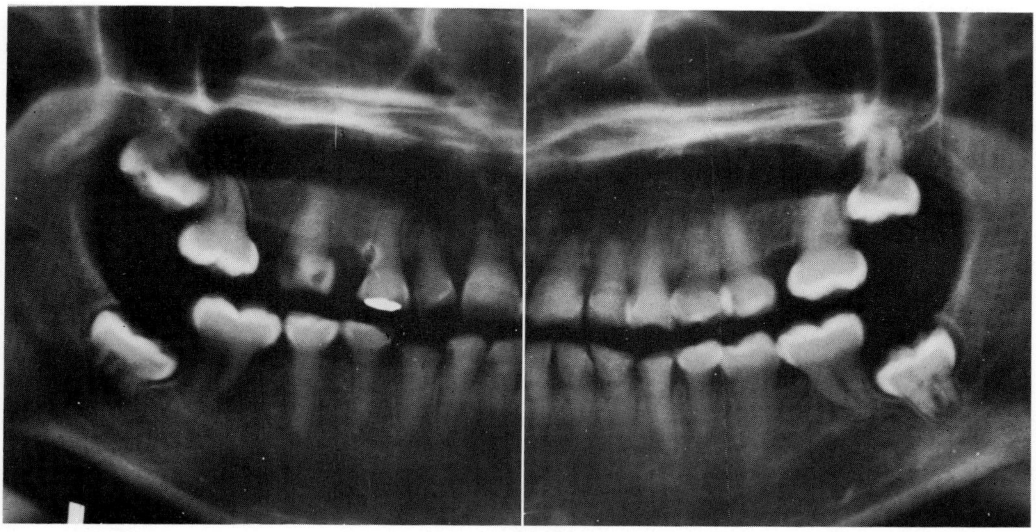

Fig. 2-19. Dentinogenesis imperfecta. Radiographs reveal short, pointed roots and absence or narrowing of root canals.

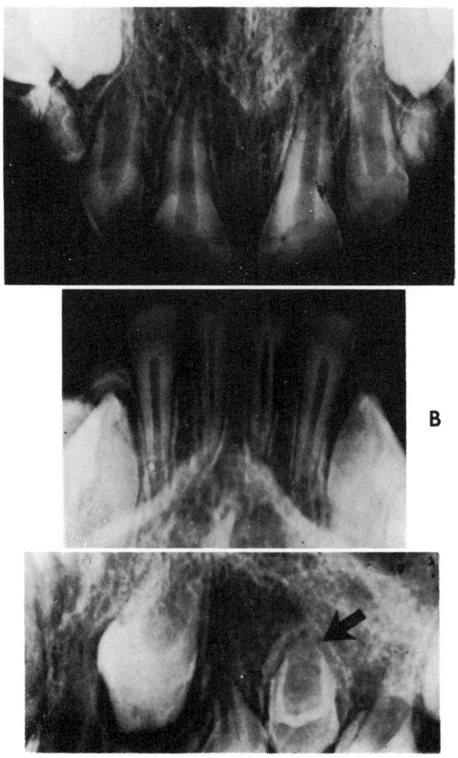

A

B

C

Fig. 2-20. A and **B,** Early stages of dentinogenesis imperfecta show wide pulp chambers. **C,** The so-called shell teeth can be seen.

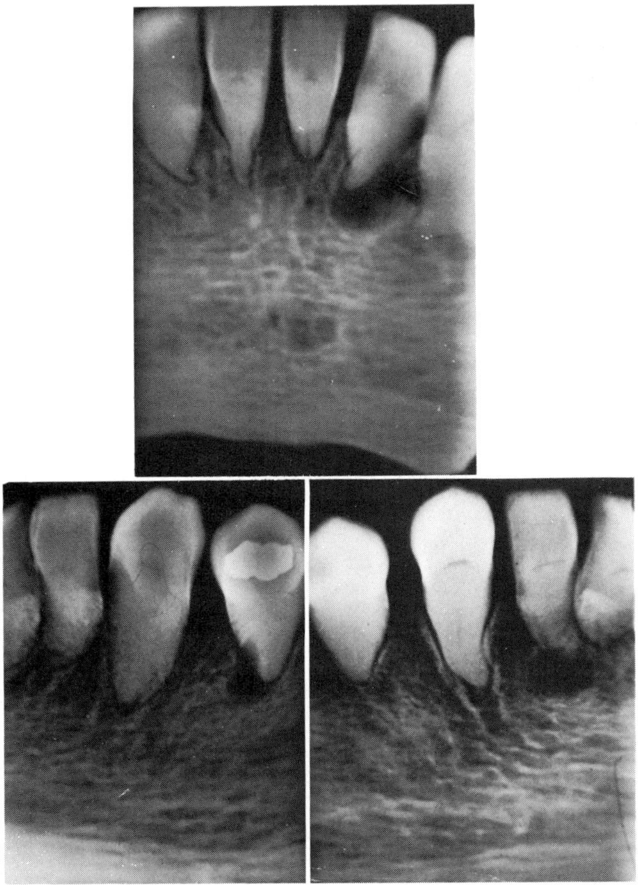

Fig. 2-21. In some cases the apical radiographs of teeth with dentinogenesis imperfecta show circumscribed radiolucent areas, which do not represent dental granulomas or cysts.

2-23 and 2-24). In later stages the pulp chamber and canals of these teeth may become completely obliterated (Fig. 2-24). Taurodontia is a hereditary disturbance.

Cementum aplasia. Radiographs showing cementum aplasia usually do not reveal any striking abnormality, but the teeth exfoliate spontaneously. When microscopically examnied, they show either an absence or a very thin layer of cementum.

Hypercementosis. Bulbous radiopaque enlargement of the root tips is diagnostic of hypercementosis (Fig. 2-25). Although any tooth may be affected, it usually involves the upper bicuspids and the lower first molars. This condition, primarily seen in permanent teeth, is said to occur in periapical granulomas, Paget's disease (p. 178), acromegaly, giantism, and occlusal trauma. In many cases, however, no cause can be demonstrated. In spite of the enlargement of the root, the periodontal ligament is maintained and can be identified in the radiographs (Fig. 2-25).

Abrasion. Wearing down of root structures by prosthetic appliances, tooth-

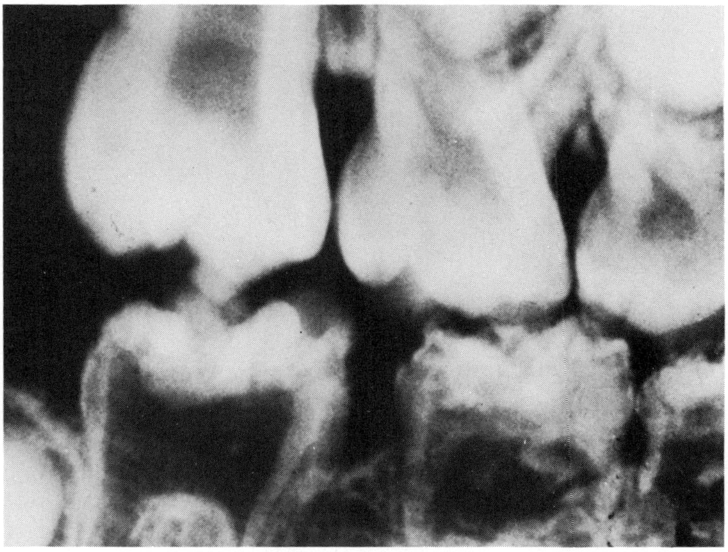

Fig. 2-22. Radiograph of odontodysplasia of lower posterior teeth shows "moth-eaten" appearance. Maxillary teeth are normal.

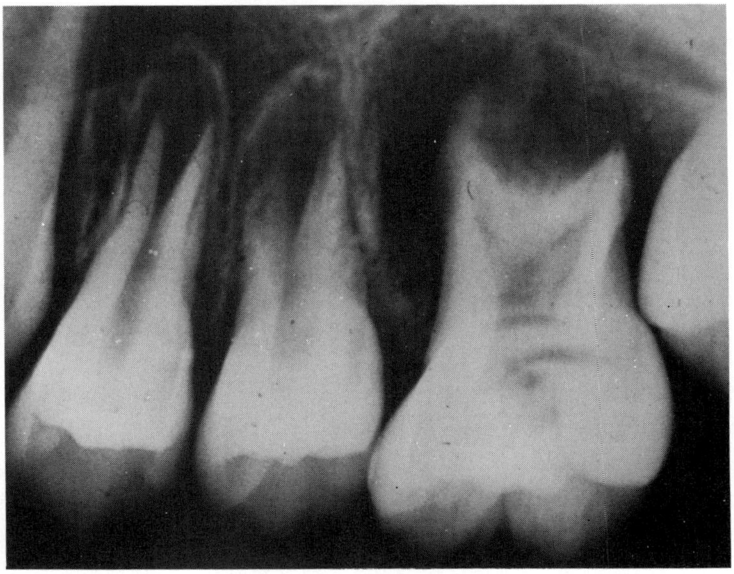

Fig. 2-23. Taurodontia (taurodontism) can be diagnosed only from radiographs. Long crowns and short roots are characteristic.

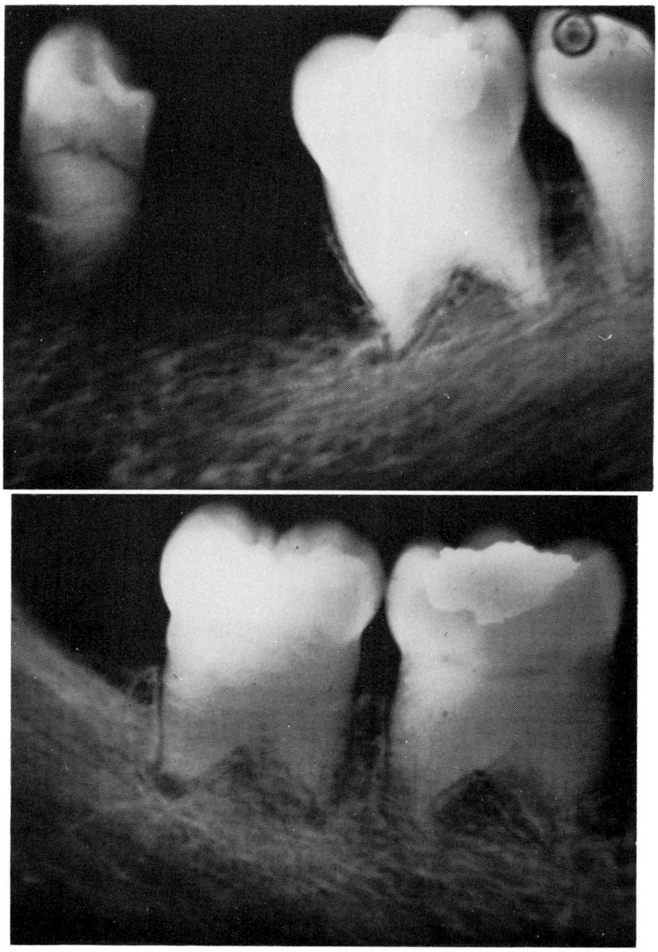

Fig. 2-24. Late stages of taurodontia (taurodontism). Note absence of root canals and short roots.

brushes, dental floss, toothpicks, or other mechanical means can alter the shape of the teeth. This deformity, called abrasion, is apparent in the radiographs (Fig. 2-26).

Attrition. Occlusal wear can easily be identified in radiographs (Fig. 2-19).

External resorption. External resorption of teeth appears as an irregularity in the normal contour of the root (Figs. 2-27 and 2-28, *A*). Comparison with earlier radiographs assists in diagnosis. Resorption may be uniform and may produce gradual blunting of the root apex, or it may begin on the sides of the root and give a moth-eaten appearance to the radicular radiograph (Figs. 2-27 to 2-32). It is seen in transplanted and reimplanted teeth, orthodontically moved teeth (Fig. 2-29), and teeth that have been irradiated. On occasion it is without any known

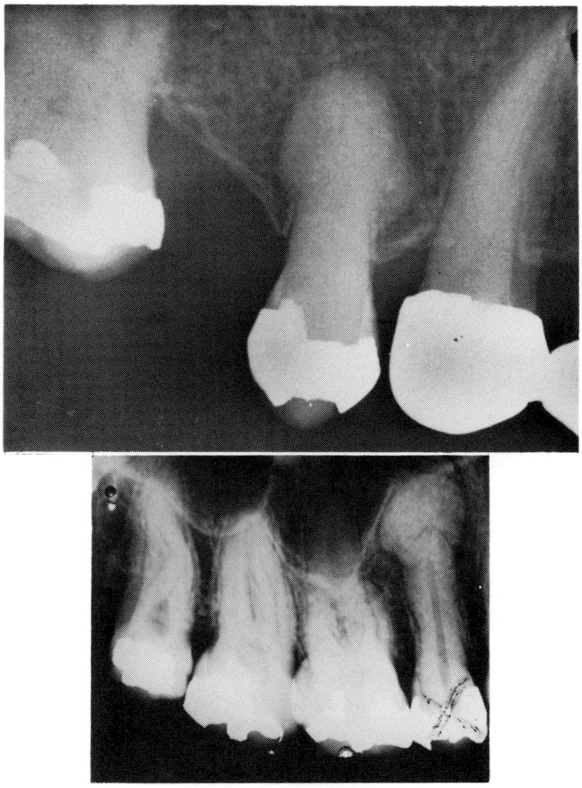

Fig. 2-25. Radiopacity of hypercementosis is continuous with the root tip.

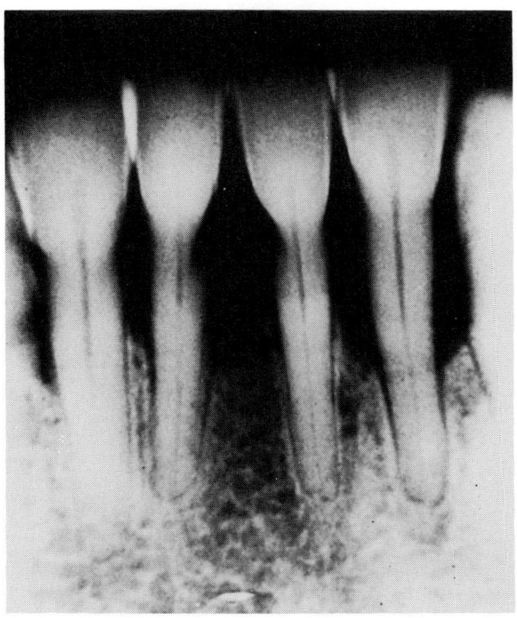

Fig. 2-26. Abrasion in the roots of the lower incisor appears as notches and was produced by toothpicks. Note the narrowed root canals.

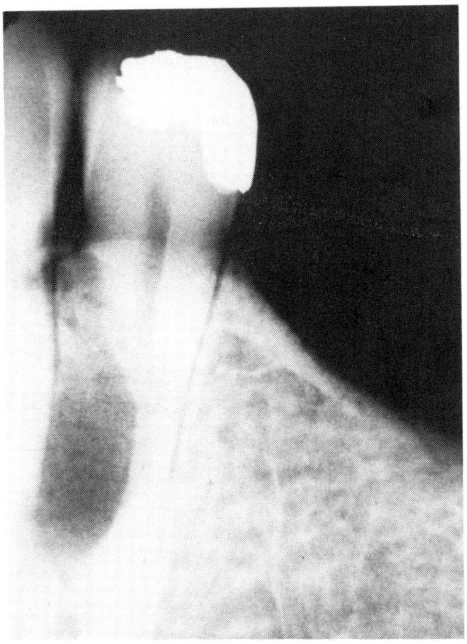

Fig. 2-27. External resorption in a bicuspid.

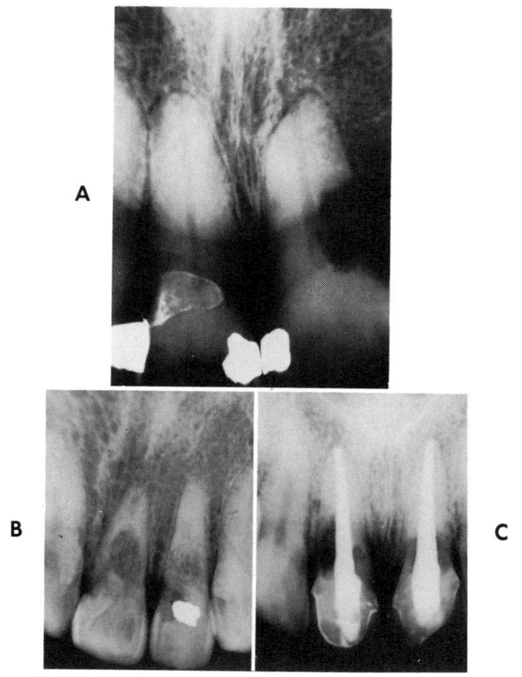

Fig. 2-28. A, External resorption. **B,** Internal resorption in the central incisors extended to the surface of the roots, and from these radiographs could not be unequivocally distinguished from external resorption. **C,** The endodontically treated teeth shown in **B.**

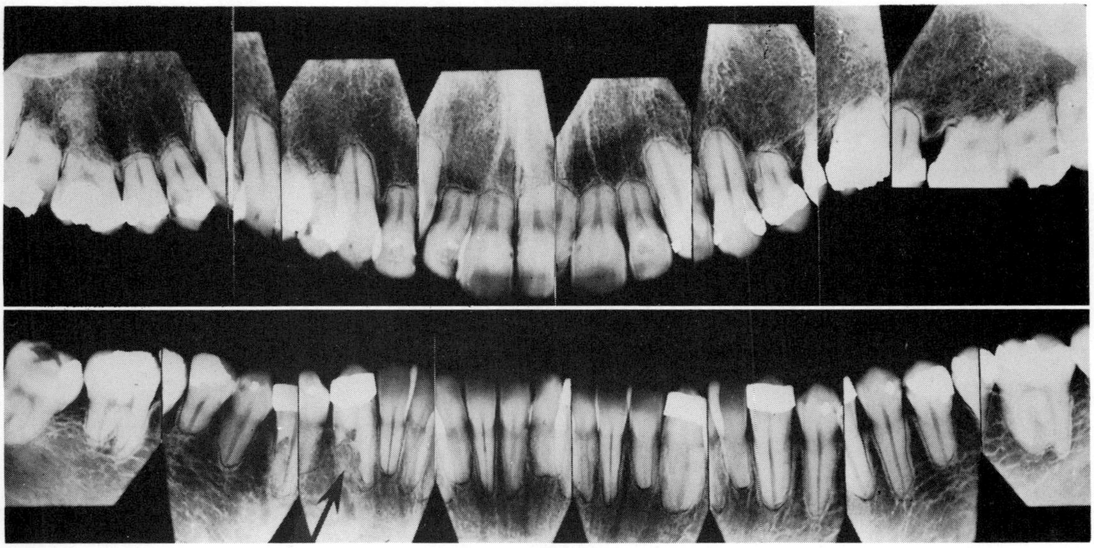

Fig. 2-29. Intraoral radiographs of an orthodontically treated patient, showing generalized root resorption and an area of ankylosis (arrow).

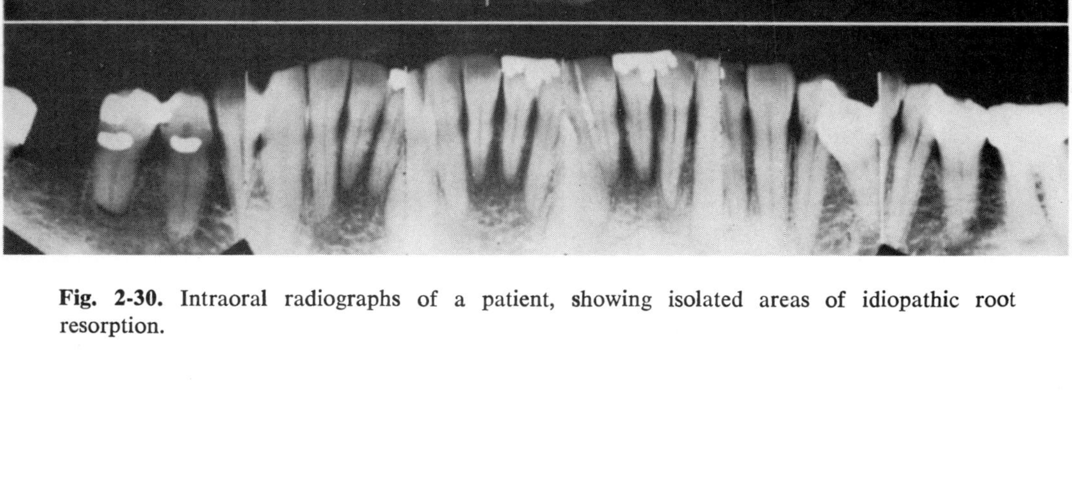

Fig. 2-30. Intraoral radiographs of a patient, showing isolated areas of idiopathic root resorption.

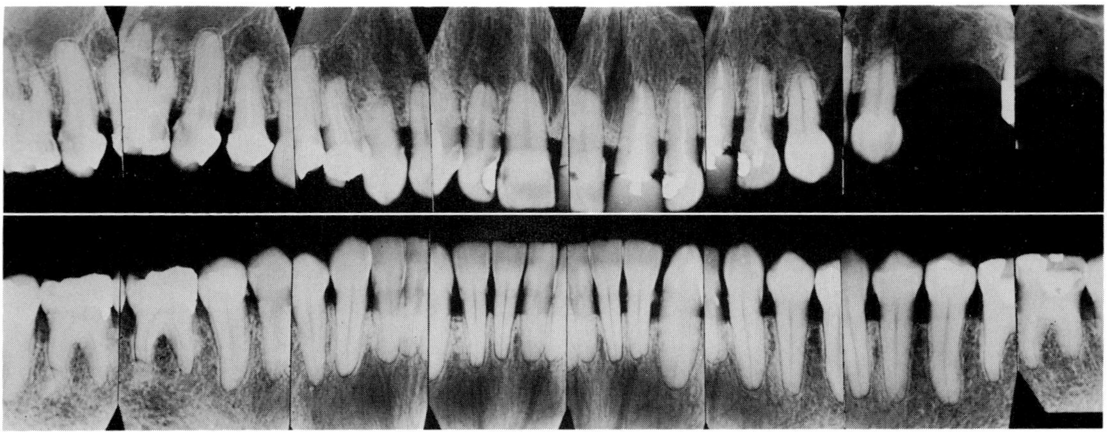

Fig. 2-31. Generalized root resorption in a patient with acromegaly (hyperpituitarism).

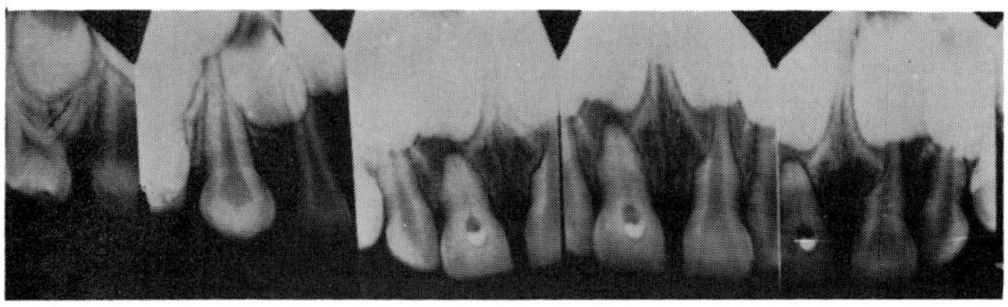

Fig. 2-32. Radiographs showing physiologic root resorption of deciduous teeth.

cause (idiopathic), or it may accompany endocrine disorders (Figs. 2-30 and 2-31). In the latter case, root resorption occurs on multiple teeth.

Although the radiograph is the only means of diagnosis, it is not always a conclusive means of distinguishing external from internal resorption of teeth.

Physiologic root resorption of deciduous teeth precedes the eruption of the permanent successors and is easily recognized in radiographs (Fig. 2-32).

Ankylosis. Fusion of a tooth to the surrounding bone is called ankylosis. Teeth with minimal areas of ankylosis show no abnormality in radiographs. When ankylosis is extensive, however, the periodontal membrane cannot be identified, the root has a moth-eaten appearance, and bone appears fused with dentin (Fig. 2-33).

Caries. The carious lesion, whether in the enamel, dentin, or cementum, is characterized by a relative reduction in the radiopacity of the respective tissue and will be discussed in Chapter 3.

CHANGES IN ROOT CANAL

Narrow root canals. Obliteration or narrowing of root canals is usually seen in old age and is the result of the formation of secondary dentin. In addition, teeth

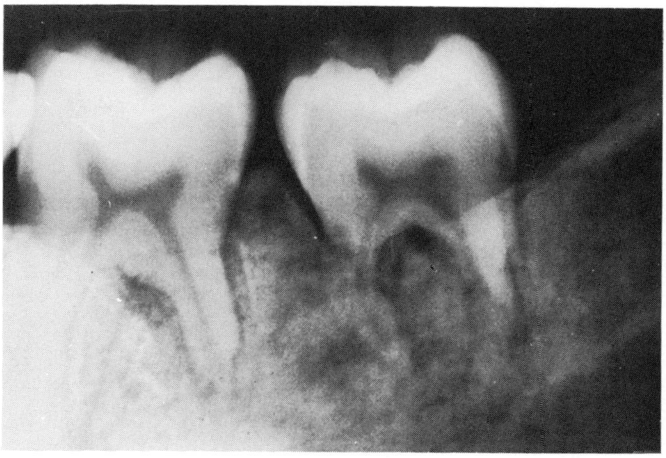

Fig. 2-33. In ankylosis the radiograph shows an absence of periodontal membrane radiolucency. In some cases root resorption is also present. This lesion was associated with an ossifying fibroma (note diffuse radiopacity in the molar area).

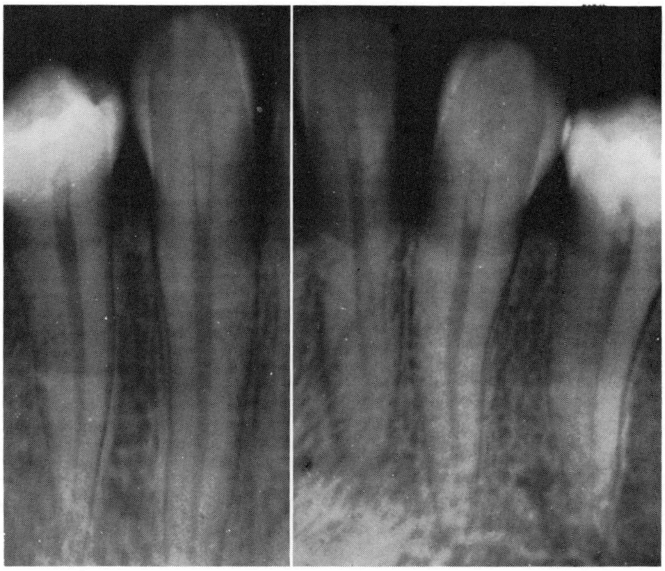

Fig. 2-34. Radiopaque masses in the pulp chambers and the root canals of these teeth represent calcifications.

with deep caries, attrition, abrasion, pulp-capping procedures, healed fractures, or dentinogenesis imperfecta may show absence or narrowing of root canals (Figs. 2-18, 2-19, and 2-26). Although they may show radiographic evidence of complete obliteration of the root canals, and although the usual vitality tests may elicit little or no response, these teeth still maintain their vitality and should not be treated.

Pulp stones. Radiographs show only a small minority of pulp calcifications.

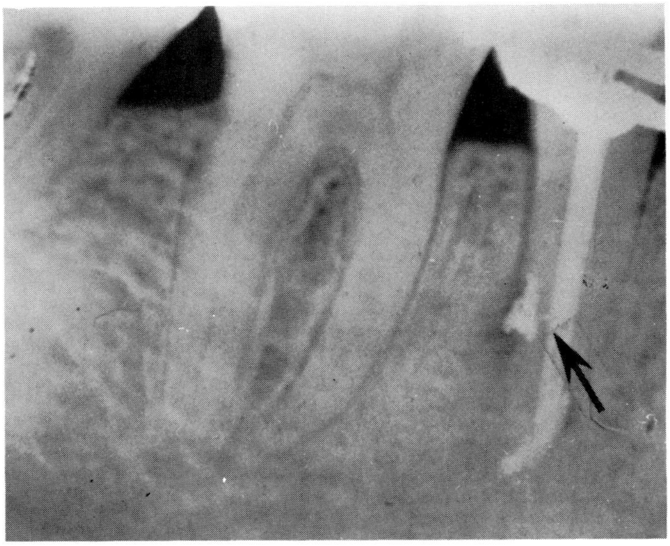

Fig. 2-35. In this radiograph of an endodontically treated second bicuspid the lateral canal is outlined by the gutta-percha filling, and the excess can be seen in the distal periodontium (arrow).

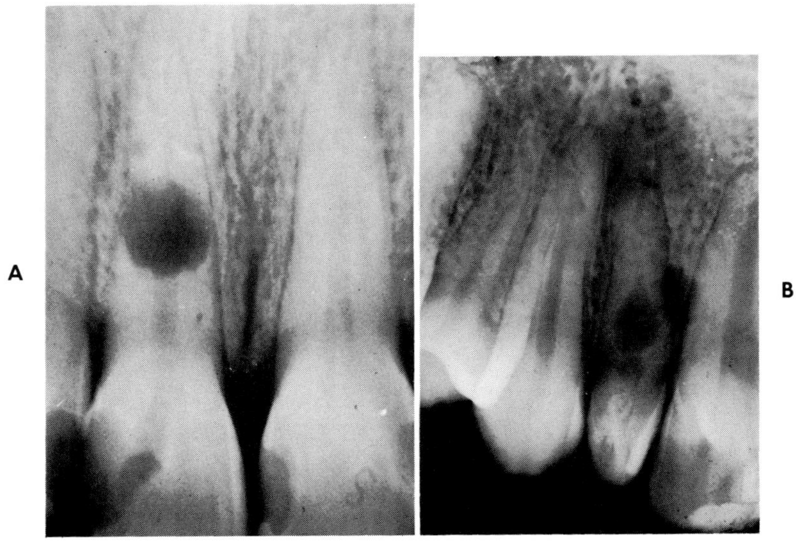

Fig. 2-36. Internal resorption in a central incisor, **A,** and in dens in dente, **B.**

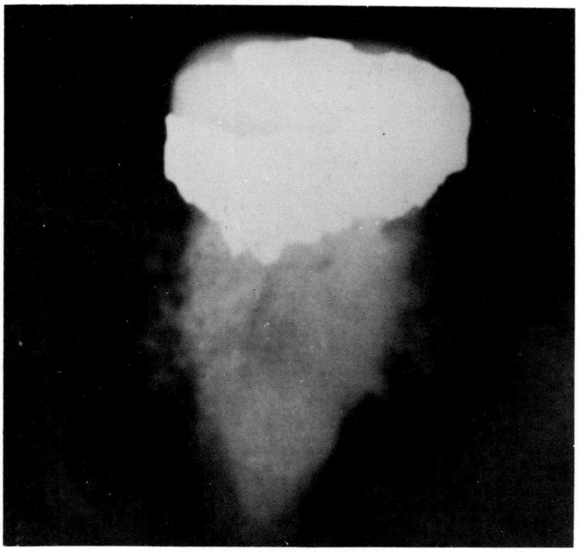

Fig. 2-37. Calculus appears as radiopaque excrescences on the root of the tooth. The bone around the tooth has almost completely disappeared.

They appear as circumscribed or linear radiopaque areas in the pulp chamber or the pulp (root) canal (Fig. 2-34). In some cases the radiopacity is diffuse and the pulp may appear completely obliterated (Figs. 2-19 and 2-21).

Lateral canals. Lateral canals may appear in the radiograph as dark lines, but usually they elude radiographic detection. In teeth that have received endodontic therapy, however, they may become delineated by the filling material (Fig. 2-35).

Internal resorption. An irregularity in the usual smooth radiographic outline of the root canal or the pulp chamber implies internal resorption (Fig. 2-36). A comparison with an earlier, preresorption radiograph confirms the diagnosis. Sometimes internal resorption produces complete destruction of the dentin wall and extends to the periodontal ligament. In such cases it is not possible to distinguish between internal and external resorption. Furthermore, areas of external resorption may become superimposed on the pulp and present as areas of internal resorption (Fig. 2-28, *B*). Since internal resorption should be treated promptly by root canal filling, and since external resorption requires no treatment, the distinction between these two conditions is important. Radiographs taken at two or three angulations are often of diagnostic value.

MISCELLANEOUS LESIONS

Calculus. Dental calculus appears as radiopaque excrescences around the cervical areas of teeth, and it offers no diagnostic problem (Fig. 2-37).

Malocclusion. Malpositioning of teeth is best diagnosed in radiographs. The type and degree of malocclusion, however, vary widely.

REFERENCES

Alexander, W. N., Lilly, G. E., and Irby, W. B.: Odontodysplasia, Oral Surg. **22:** 814, 1966.

Amos, E. R.: Incidence of the small dens-in-dente, J. Am. Dent. Assoc. **51:**31, 1955.

Archer, W. H., and Henderson, S. G.: Cleidocranial dysostosis: report of two cases, Oral Surg. **4:**1201, 1951.

Bhaskar, S. N.: Synopsis of oral pathology, ed. 4, St. Louis, 1972, The C. V. Mosby Co.

Chaudhry, A. P., Wittich, H. C., Stickel, F. R., and Holland, M. R.: Odontogenesis imperfecta: report of a case, Oral Surg. **14:**1099, 1961.

Elzay, R. P., and Robinson, C. T.: Dentinal dysplasia, Oral Surg. **23:**338, 1967.

Goldstein, E.: Taurodontism: familial tendencies demonstrated in eleven of fourteen case reports, Oral Surg. **36:**131, 1973.

Gyenes, V., de Grosz, I., and Toth, I.: Some observations concerning mandibulofacial dysostosis (Franceschetti's syndrome), Oral Surg. **16:**68, 1963.

Kalliala, E., and Taskinen, P. J.: Cleidocranial dysostosis, Oral Surg. **15:**808, 1962.

Kelln, E. E., Chaudhry, A. P., and Gorlin, R. F.: Oral manifestations of Crouzon's disease, Oral Surg. **13:**1245, 1960.

Mena, C. A.: Taurodontism, Oral Surg. **32:** 812, 1971.

Metro, P. S.: Mandibulofacial dysostosis (Treacher-Collins syndrome), Oral Surg. **20:**583, 1965.

Metro, P. S.: Taurodontism: a dental rarity in modern man, Oral Surg. **20:**263, 1965.

Peterson, A.: A case of dentinal dysplasia and/or calcification of the dental papilla, Oral Surg. **33:**1014, 1972.

Rushton, M. A.: A new form of dentinal dysplasia: shell teeth, Oral Surg. **7:**453, 1954.

Rushton, M. A.: Anomalies of human dentin, Br. Dent. J. **98:**431, 1955.

Stenvik, A., Zachrisson, B. U., and Svatun, B.: Taurodontism and concomitant hypodontia in siblings, Oral Surg. **33:**841, 1972.

Ulmansky, M., and Hermal, J.: Double dens-in-dente in a single tooth, Oral Surg. **17:**92, 1964.

Vandes Linden, L. W. J., and Van Aken, J.: The origin of localized increased radiopacity in dentin, Oral Surg. **35:**862, 1973.

Wege, W. R.: Idiopathic internal resorption, Oral Surg. **36:**443, 1973.

Zegarelli, E. V., Kutscher, A. H., Applebaum, E., and Archard, H. O.: Odontodysplasia, Oral Surg. **16:**187, 1963.

CHAPTER THREE

RADIOGRAPHIC FEATURES OF DENTAL CARIES

Occlusal caries
Interproximal caries
Labial, buccal, lingual, and palatal caries
Cementum caries
Recurrent caries
Indirect pulp-capping shadow
Radiation caries

Of all the diagnostic purposes for which a dentist uses radiographs, the detection of carious lesions is the most common. Advanced carious lesions of the occlusal, cervical, and other exposed portions of a tooth are not difficult to diagnose. The purpose of a radiograph, therefore, is to diagnose early carious lesions or those which lie hidden under restorations, in soft tissues, or in the interproximal areas. It is estimated that the use of bite-wing radiographs increases caries detection by about 80% over detection by clinical examination. For detection of caries, bite-wing x-ray films are most desirable. The frequency with which they should be made depends on the relative caries susceptibility of the patient. Usually, bite-wing radiographs for caries detection are begun at about 4 to 5 years of age and are continued for the life of the dentition.

Occlusal caries. Beginning occlusal caries in unfilled teeth is diagnosed earlier with explorer than in a radiograph. In the latter it becomes apparent when the lesion has transgressed the fissure and has reached the dentinoenamel junction. In some cases, however, it may appear as a darkening of the occlusal fissure (Fig. 3-1). When occlusal caries reaches the dentinoenamel junction, it appears as a dark line; as it progresses into the dentin, it expands as a diffuse radiolucent lesion (Fig. 3-2). As contrasted with the cervical decay, the margins of the occlusal carious radiolucencies are ill defined (Fig. 3-2). In the enamel the carious lesion of the fissure has a triangular appearance in such a way that the base of the triangle is at the dentinoenamel junction.

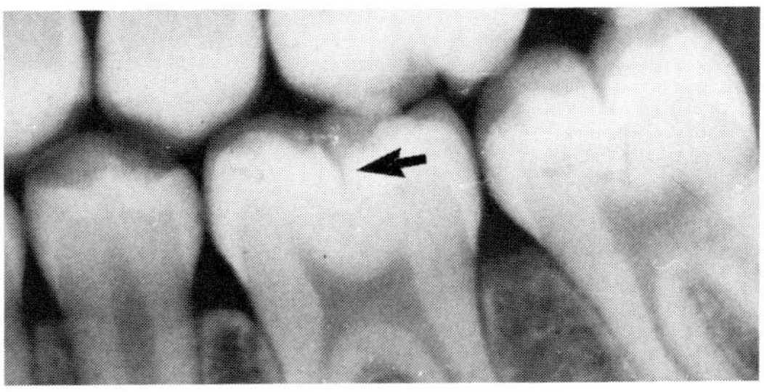

Fig. 3-1. Early caries of the occlusal fissure (first molar) can be seen as a dark line that does not yet extend to the dentin (arrow).

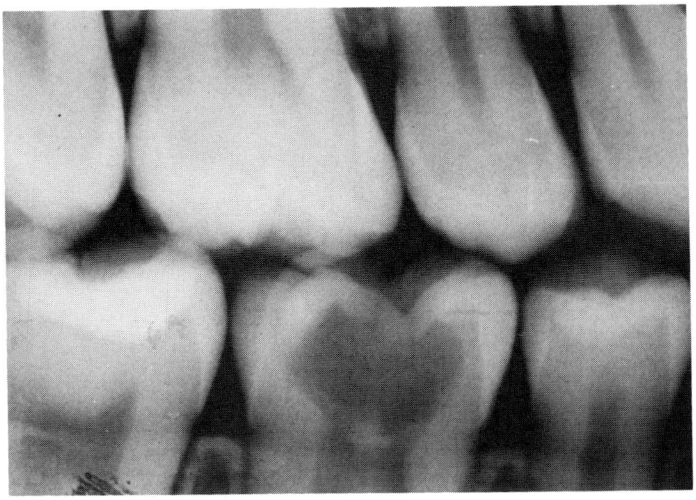

Fig. 3-2. Advanced carious lesion of dentin.

Interproximal caries. Early interproximal carious lesions are seen as small notches in the enamel (Fig. 3-3). The most common site is just apical to the contact area. As the lesion progresses it assumes a triangular shape, with the base of the triangle on the surface and the apex toward the dentinoenamel junction (Figs. 3-4 and 3-5). At the dentinoenamel junction the lesion spreads laterally and progresses toward the pulp (Figs. 3-6 to 3-8). The proximal decay of the dentin therefore has a wide base at the dentinoenamel junction, and the apex is toward the pulp (Fig. 3-6).

Labial, buccal, lingual, and palatal caries. Carious lesions of these surfaces occur along the cervical area and in the radiographs have distinct borders. This appearance is due to the fact that caries progresses along the direction of enamel rods, which in the cervical region run approximately parallel to each other. Since in bite-wing radiographs the occlusal and cervical lesions may appear in the same area of the crown, the clear, punched-out appearance of cervical decay, as com-

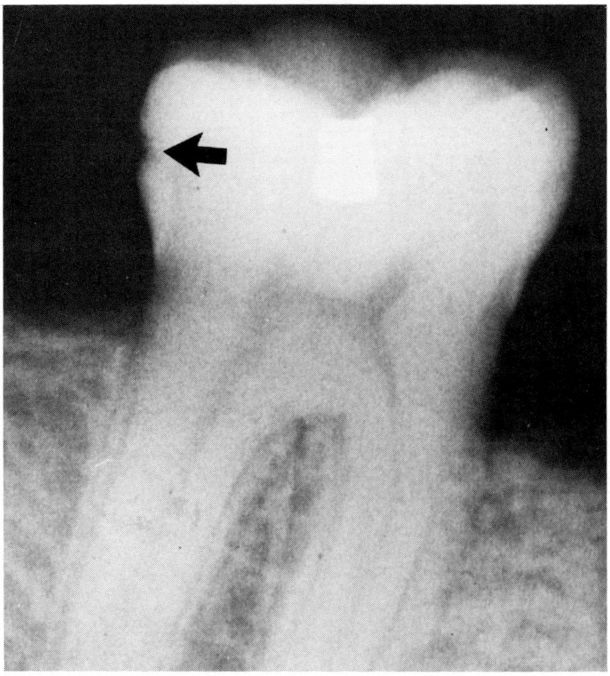

Fig. 3-3. Early interproximal caries appears as a notching of the enamel (arrow).

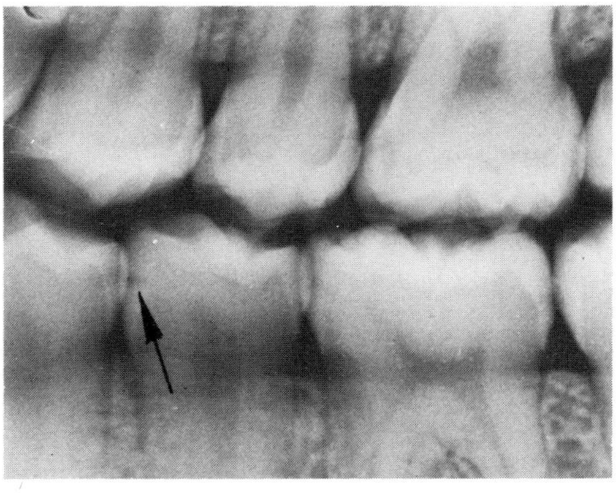

Fig. 3-4. Interproximal carious lesion of enamel is seen as a triangular radiolucency (arrow). The base of the triangle is on the enamel surface and the apex is toward the dentin.

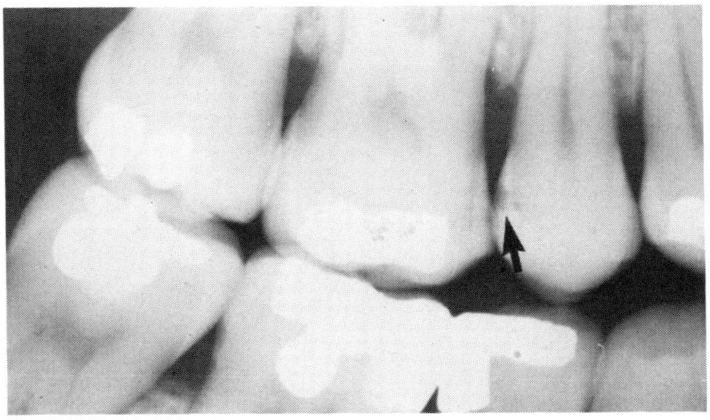

Fig. 3-5. Carious lesion of enamel that has extended to the dentinoenamel junction (arrow).

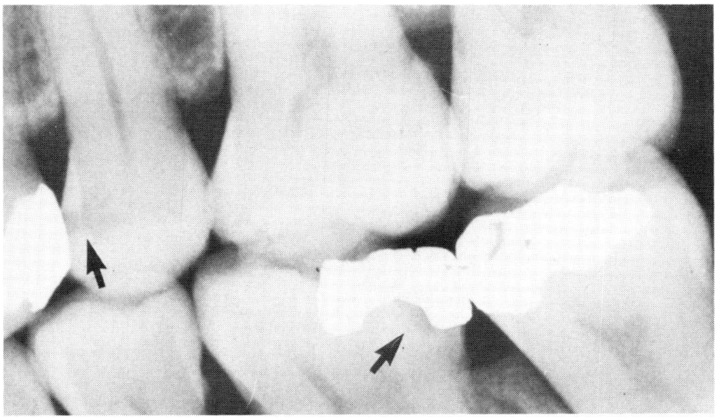

Fig. 3-6. Carious lesion of enamel and dentin in the upper second bicuspid. Also note recurrent caries under the lower molar restoration.

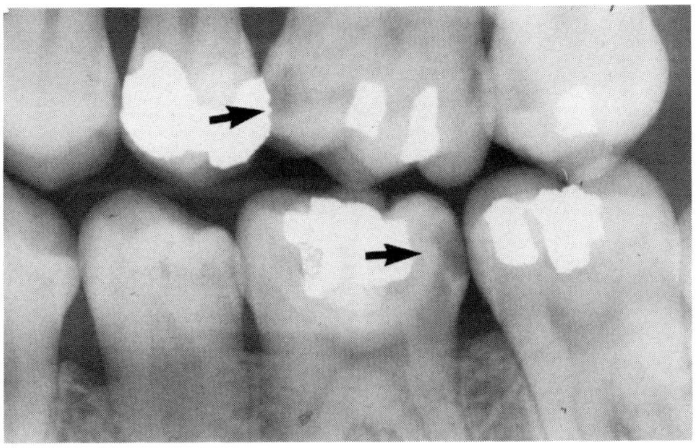

Fig. 3-7. Carious lesions of the dentin can be seen in the upper and lower first molars.

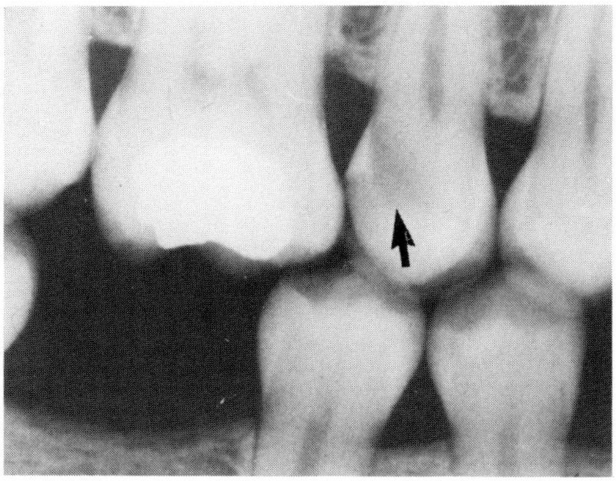

Fig. 3-8. Advanced diffuse undermining lesion of dentin in the upper second bicuspid.

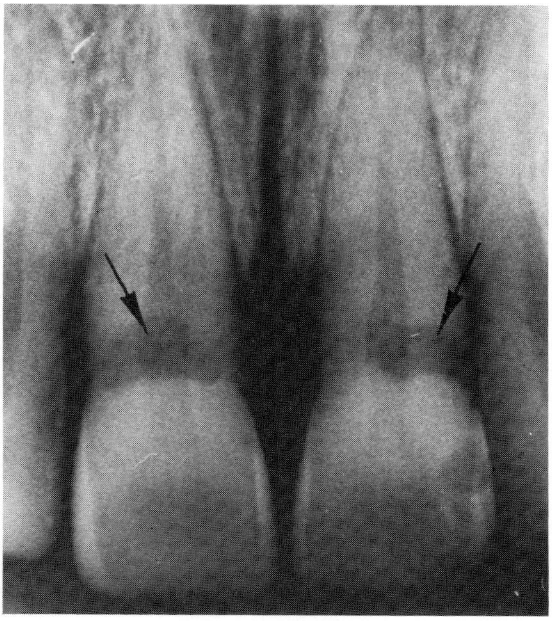

Fig. 3-9. Symmetrical outline forms (arrows) of cervical restorations with synthetic restorative material.

pared to the diffuse borders of the occlusal lesion, is of diagnostic significance. From a radiograph it may be difficult to distinguish a buccal cervical lesion from a lingual cervical lesion, but it can be done easily by clinical examination.

Silicate restorations are radiolucent areas that may be mistaken for cervical (or proximal) carious lesions (Fig. 3-9). They, however, have smooth radiolucent borders and can be detected readily by clinical examination. When these restora-

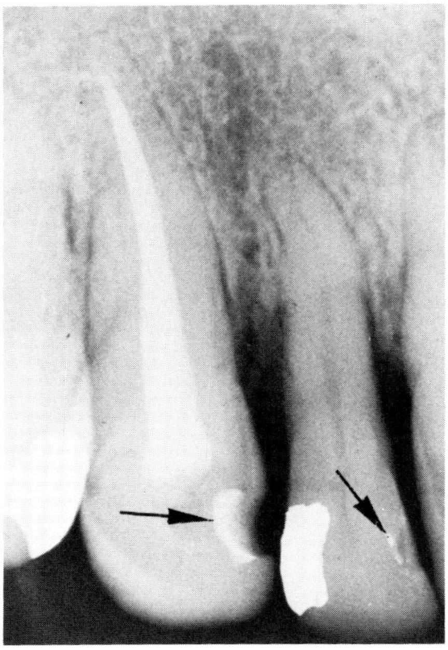

Fig. 3-10. Radiopaque lining is seen under radiolucent silicate restorations.

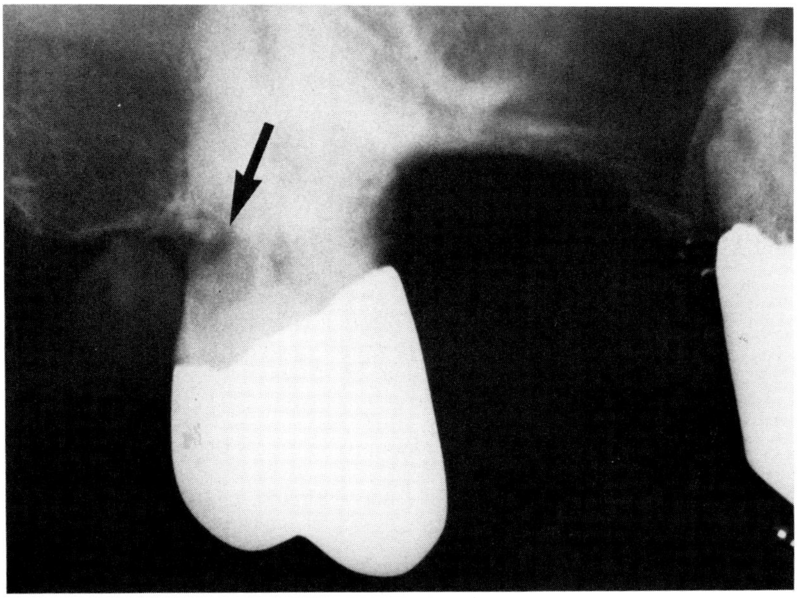

Fig. 3-11. Cementum caries appears as a saucer-shaped radiolucency.

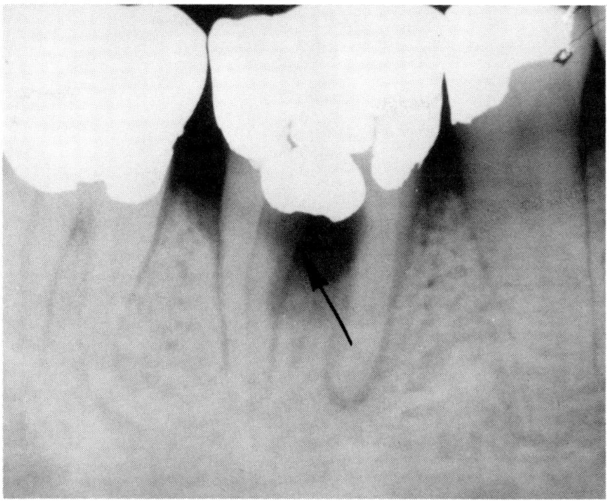

Fig. 3-12. Cementum caries of the bifurcation area of a lower molar. The lesion was associated with a deep periodontal pocket.

tions have a cavity base, it can be detected as a radiopacity underneath the radiolucency (Fig. 3-10).

Cementum caries. Carious lesions of cementum occur in patients with ginvival recession or periodontal pockets (Figs. 3-11 and 3-12). Patients with full coverage of teeth and poor hygiene often show cementum caries. These lesions are easily seen in radiographs (unless they occur under a gold or metallic crown) and present a saucer-shaped appearance (Fig. 3-11).

When a diagnosis of cementum caries is made, however, the phenomenon of *"cervical burnout"* must be kept in mind. This area of relative radiolucency is an artifact and occurs between the part of the root covered by alveolar bone and the enamel-covered crown (Fig. 3-13). The enamel-covered crown and the bone-covered root appear more radiopaque than the portion of root between them. The latter therefore usually shows a triangular radiolucency but sometimes may reveal a radiolucent *zone* in the area. To distinguish a burnout from cementum caries, it is helpful to remember that good alveolar bone is essential to produce the "burnout," whereas cementum decay is usually accompanied by periodontal disease or gingival recession.

Recurrent caries. Recurrent caries appear as radiolucent areas underneath old restorations (Fig. 3-14). Their detection depends on their location and the angulation at which the radiograph is made. When the restorations are large, they are difficult to detect (Fig. 3-15). In these cases clinical examination and clinical symptoms are often the only indications of recurrent lesions.

Indirect pulp-capping shadow. In addition to recurrent caries, a radiolucency beneath a restoration may also signify an area of indirect pulp capping (Fig. 3-16).

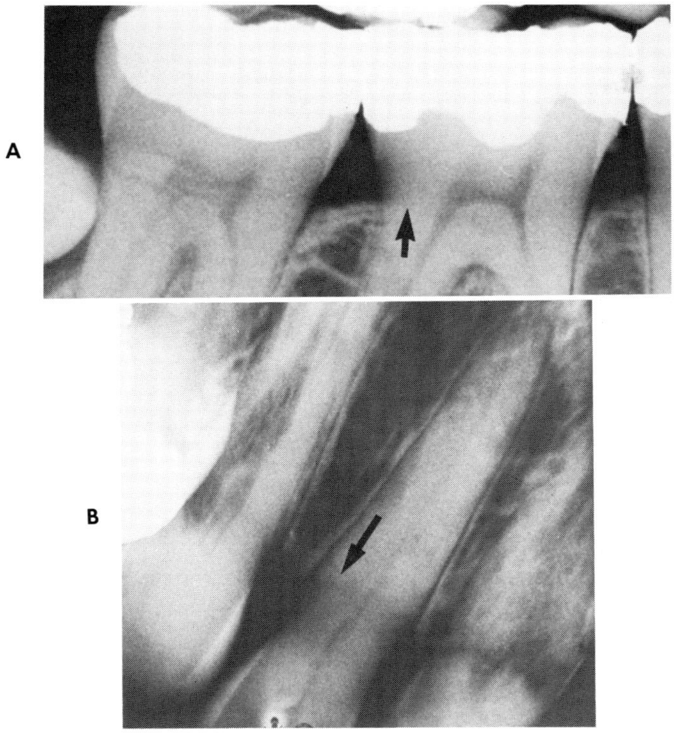

Fig. 3-13. Radiographs of the mandibular molar, **A,** and maxillary incisor, **B,** showing the so-called "burnout" effect. This radiolucent area appears at the neck of the tooth and in that portion of the dentin which is neither covered by enamel nor surrounded by bone. In **B,** due to the elongation of the image, the "burnout" zone is also accentuated.

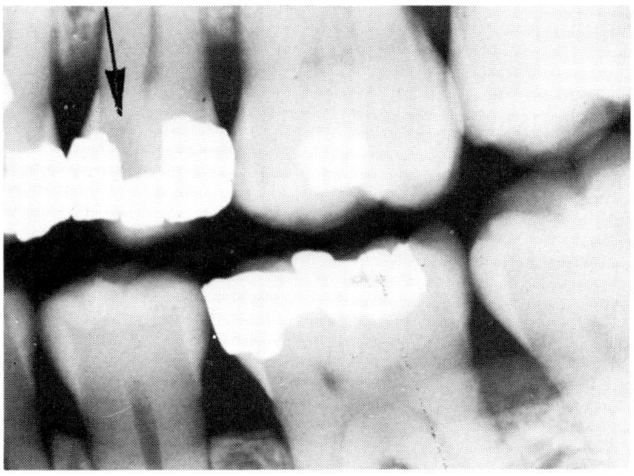

Fig. 3-14. Recurrent carious lesion (arrow) under amalgam restoration.

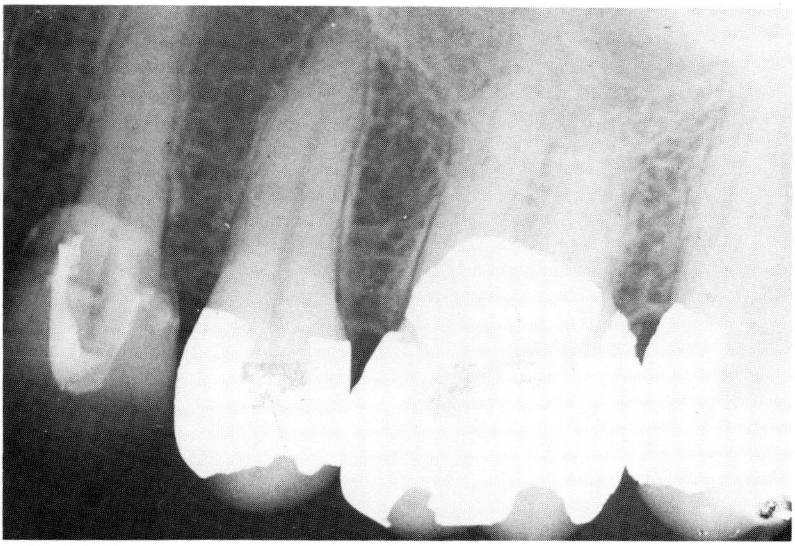

Fig. 3-15. In the presence of many or large restorations, it is difficult to distinguish recurrent lesions. The first molar in this radiograph had clinical symptoms of pulpitis and recurrent caries under the cervical restoration.

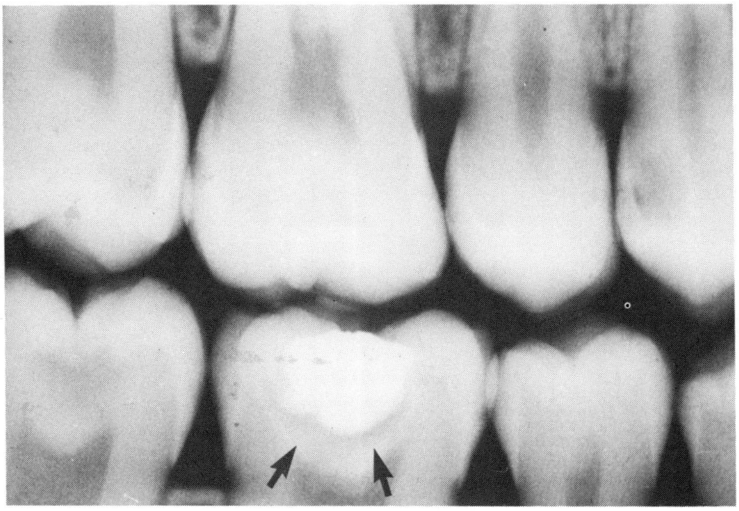

Fig. 3-16. In teeth with indirect pulp capping procedures, a radiolucent area may appear under a restoration (arrow). This radiolucency should not be interpreted as recurrent decay. In some patients it gradually undergoes calcification.

The usual procedure for indirect pulp capping consists of the removal of as much of the carious lesion as possible and the placing of a therapeutic restoration for a few weeks (six to eight). At the end of this time, if the patient has no symptoms, a portion of the temporary restoration is removed and a permanent restoration is placed in the tooth. These teeth have residual carious areas beneath the restorations that may appear as radiolucencies under asymptomatic and clinically good restorations. Such carious areas are sterile, do not progress, and in some cases may undergo calcification. Obviously, such restorations should not be removed. To avoid inadvertent removal of restorations with indirect pulp capping, patients' records should be carefully marked and patients informed of such procedures.

Radiation caries. In patients who receive a therapeutic dosage of radiation for the treatment of malignant tumors of the head and neck areas, a specific form of carious lesions is often observed. These lesions occur in a few weeks to many months after the treatment, begin in the cervical area of teeth, and can lead to the breakdown of the entire crown. Radiographs show extensive cervical decay, and the history of radiation is a valuable aid in diagnosis. The mechanism of this form of caries is unknown. Radiation caries can occur in patients who previous to radiation were caries resistant.

CHAPTER FOUR

RADIOGRAPHIC FEATURES OF PERIODONTAL DISEASES

In this chapter the following aspects of periodontal radiographic interpretation will be considered:

- Periodontal examination
  - Teeth
  - Bone
  - Periodontal space
- Periodontal diagnosis
  - Normal and healthy periodontal tissues
  - Gingivitis
  - Incipient periodontitis
  - Moderate periodontitis
  - Advanced periodontitis
  - Periodontal abscess
  - Combined pulpal-periodontal lesion
  - Occlusal trauma
  - Hyperfunction
  - Orthodontic tooth movement
  - Atrophy of disuse
  - Periodontosis
- Periodontal follow-up

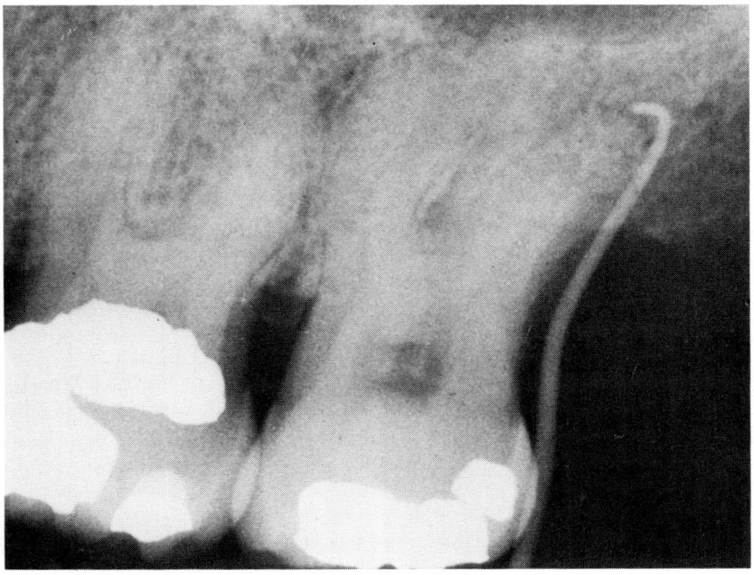

Fig. 4-1. Gutta-percha point placed in distal pocket of maxillary molar indicates an oral communication with the root apex.

A

B

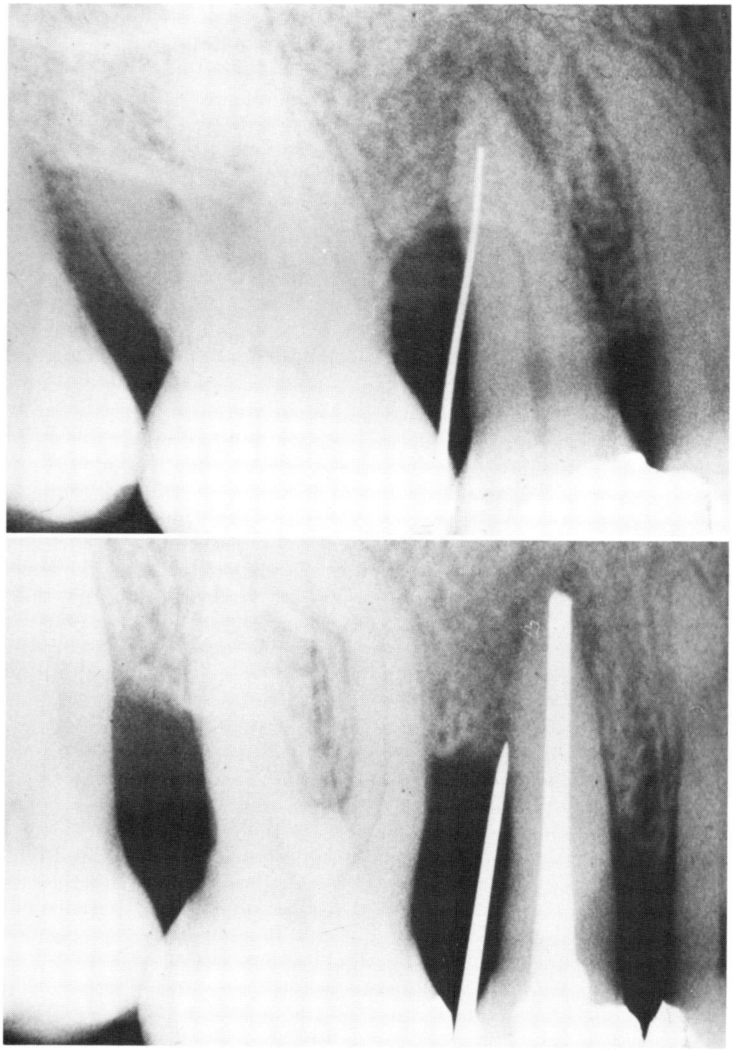

Fig. 4-2. A, Preoperative radiograph. Silver point shows depth of bone loss. **B,** After endodontic and periodontal treatment, evidence of bone regeneration can be demonstrated. (Courtesy Dr. L. Green.)

A

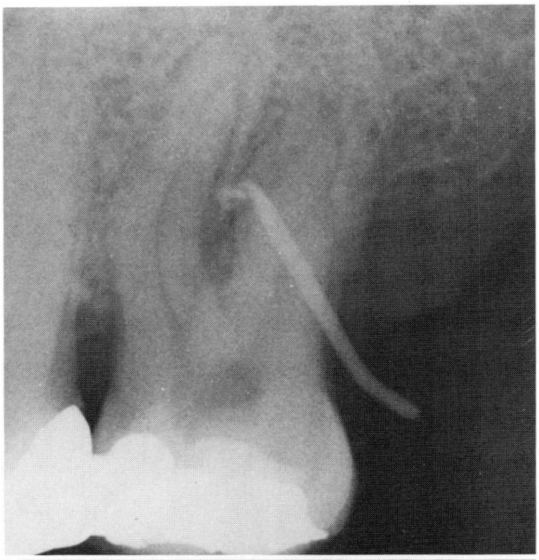

B

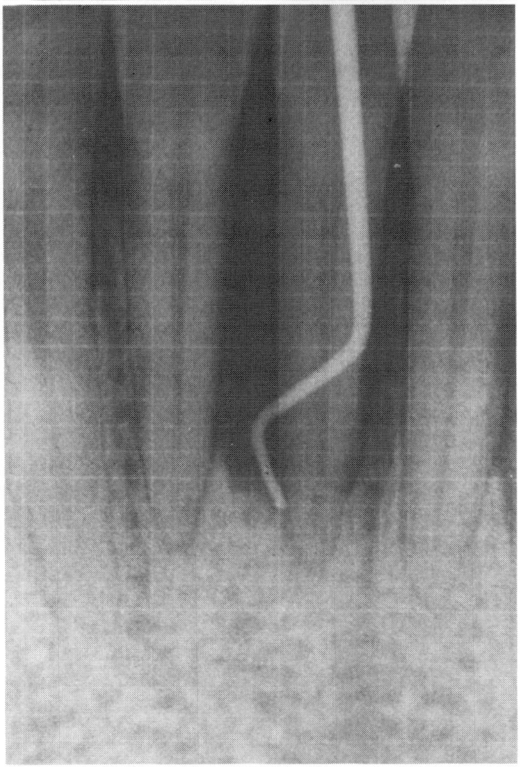

Fig. 4-3. A, Gutta-percha is placed into a distal pocket of a maxillary molar and, due to its flexibility, enters the distal furcation area. **B,** Gutta-percha point is shown following a tortuous pocket. A rigid probe could not be positioned to the same depth. Note the grid on the film for more accurate measurement.

Radiographic analysis is an essential part of periodontal evaluation. For an adequate examination the radiographic survey should at least consist of a full-mouth periapical series and bite-wing radiographs. They should be made by means of the parallel (long-cone) technique. In addition, a panoramic film may be of use in surveying areas other than the periodontium. Since the facial or lingual bone often blocks out portions of a periodontal pocket, the topography of osseous defects is not well visualized on radiographs. Therefore the use of a radiopaque marker in the defect is helpful in obtaining more accurate information on the film (Fig. 4-1). The use of markers is also useful in documenting the changes in pocket depth (Fig. 4-2). There are many types of radiopaque markers that can be used in demonstrating pocket depths. Since many pockets are tortuous, rigid materials are not as useful as gutta-percha points. Gutta-percha points can bend and can therefore give an accurate indication of the pocket topography (Fig. 4-3). Since gutta-percha is not calibrated, it may be used in conjunction with a Fixott-Everett grid, as shown in Fig. 4-3, *B*. The superimposition of a grid on the radiograph can be of value in better quantitating what one sees on the film. The technique has been described in the literature.

PERIODONTAL EXAMINATION

In radiographic examination of the periodontal lesions, special attention is paid to the teeth, the bone, and the periodontal ligament space. Each should be studied carefully.

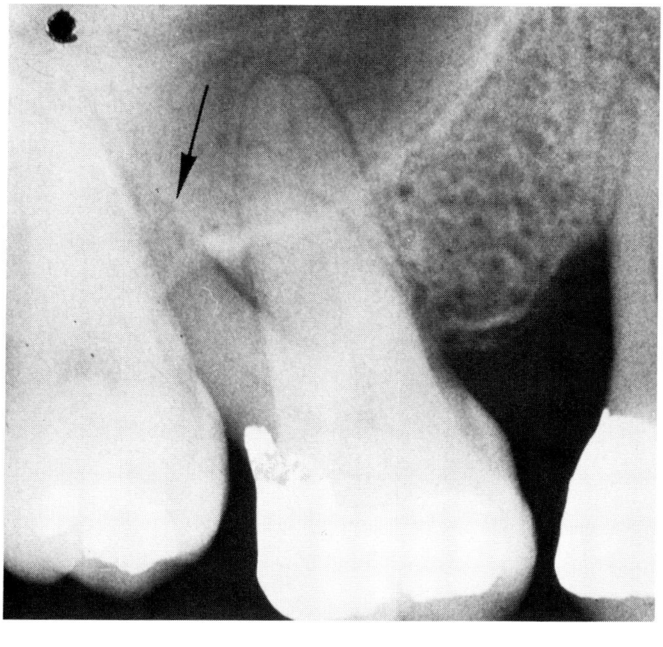

Fig. 4-4. Distofacial root of maxillary molar (arrow), shown in close approximation to adjacent molar. Considerable bone loss is evident.

Teeth. In the examination of the teeth the following aspects are important and can be determined only in the radiographs.

1. Clinical crown-root ratio. In essence, the term clinical crown-root ratio refers to the ratio between the length of the root that is surrounded by bone and the remainder of the tooth.

2. Shape and size of the crown and root. A tooth with a small crown and a long root has a better prognosis than one with a large crown and a short root, and a tapered root has less surface area for bone attachment than a blunt root.

3. Position of roots of multirooted teeth. In multirooted teeth, roots close together present a poorer prognosis than those which are widely separated.

4. Position of a tooth in relation to adjacent teeth. Open contact points or close proximity of adjacent teeth can be seen in the radiographs and are aggravating factors in the developing and progression of periodontal lesions (Fig. 4-4).

5. Presence of calculus on the root (Fig. 4-5).

6. Presence of root resorption areas (internal or external).

7. The contours and status of restorations. Interproximal overhanging margins and poor contours can produce periodontal lesions and are best examined in radiographs (Figs. 4-6 and 4-7).

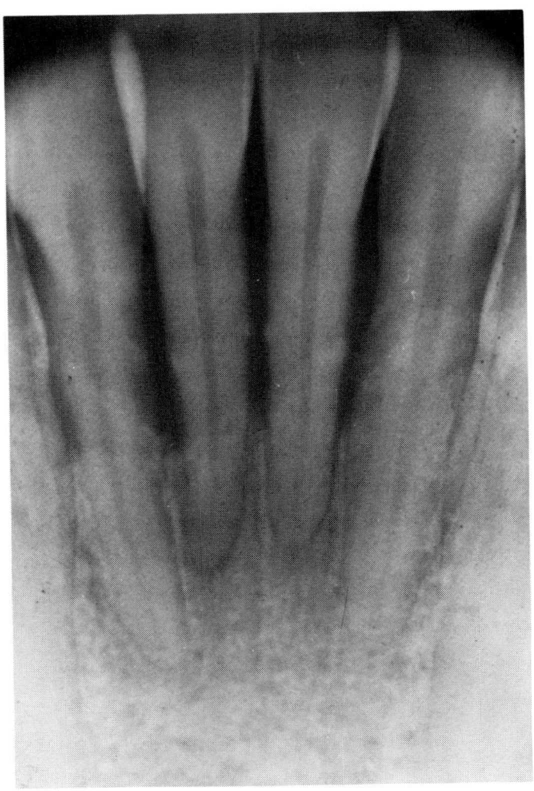

Fig. 4-5. Spurs of calculus can be seen on the interproximal aspects of the mandibular incisor roots.

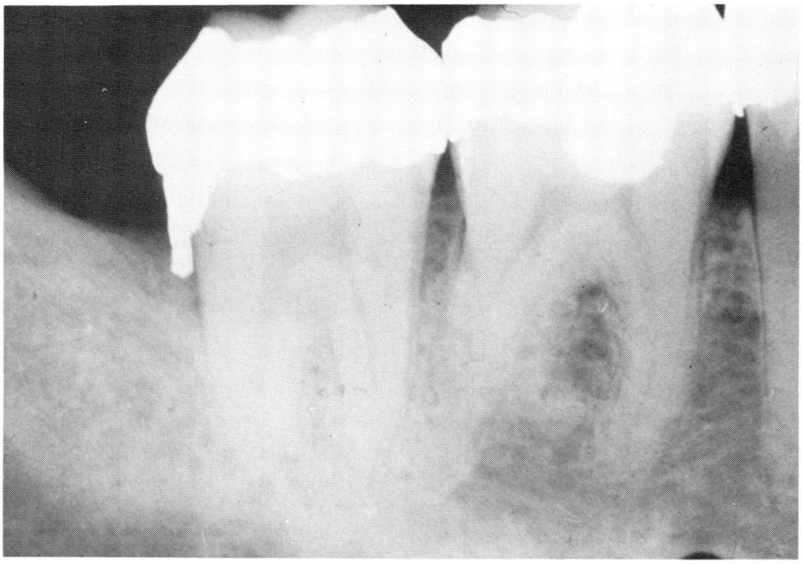

Fig. 4-6. Amalgam overhang on distal aspect of mandibular second molar and its association with a periodontal defect.

8. Fractures of the root. A tooth with a horizontal or vertical fracture can present with periodontal symptoms. Whereas a tooth with a verical fracture down the long axis of the root has a poor prognosis, a tooth with a horizontal fracture can be retained (Fig. 2-14).

9. Foreign bodies and root tips which may produce or aggravate periodontal lesions and can best be seen in radiographs (Fig. 4-8).

Bone. The amount and location of bone around teeth is the most important aspect of radiographic examination in periodontal diagnosis. In the examination of periodontal bone, special attention is paid to the following:

1. Interproximal septum. The interdental bone, under ideal circumstances, is close to the cementoenamel junction and is covered by a radiopaque margin (Fig. 4-9, *A*). In periodontal disease the alveolar crest recedes from the cementoenamel junction, and its coronal margin becomes irregular and loses its radiopaque border (Fig. 4-9, *B*).

2. Interradicular septum. Bone loss in the interradicular septum (Fig. 3-12) indicates periodontal disease.

3. Lamina dura. The significance of the lamina dura was discussed earlier (p. 4 and Fig. 1-4). Whereas its presence indicates good supporting bone, its absence does not always signify pathology.

Periodontal space. The width of the periodontal ligament indicates the relative influence of the occlusal forces and will be discussed elsewhere in this chapter.

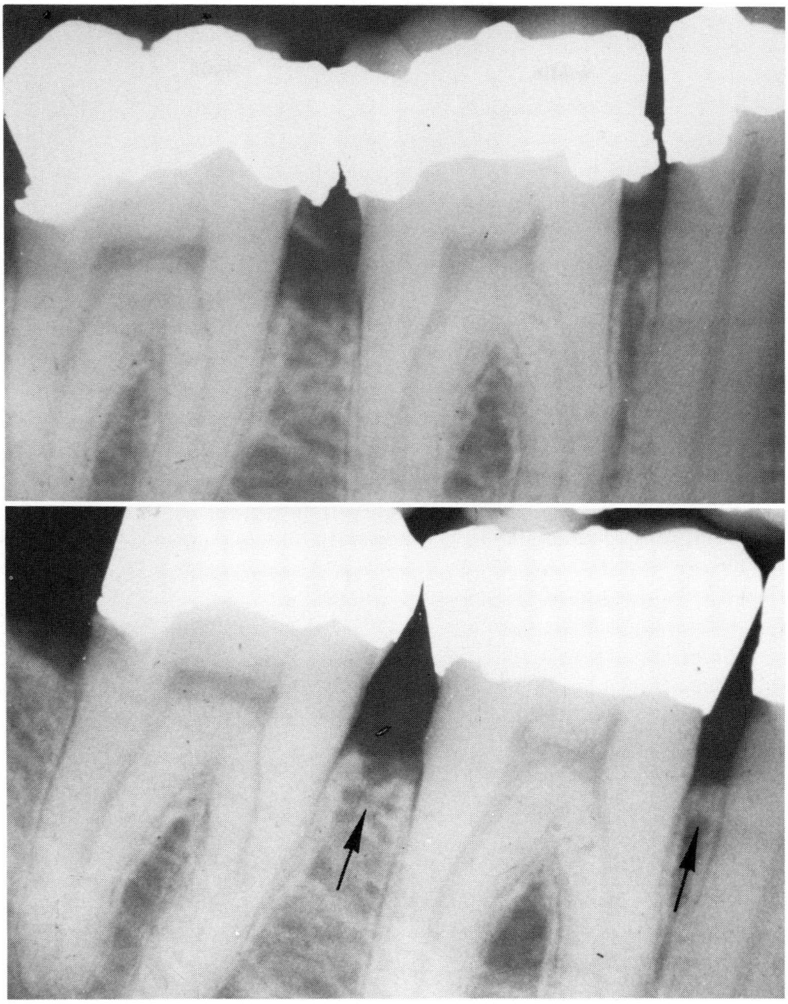

A

B

Fig. 4-7. A, Preoperative radiograph. Poorly contoured amalgam restorations with overhangs, an open contact, and calculus are evident. Note the resorption of the crests of the interproximal septa. **B,** Postoperative radiograph of area shown in **A,** seven months after scaling was done and new restorations were placed. There is evidence of crestal healing (arrows).

PERIODONTAL DIAGNOSIS

Normal and healthy periodontal tissues. The radiograph of normal periodontal tissues shows dense interproximal septa approximating the levels of the cemento-enamel junctions (Fig. 4-10). In addition, an intact, continuous lamina dura surrounds the clinical roots, and the periodontal ligament space is narrow and of uniform width (Fig. 4-11).

In many instances, such as after successful periodontal therapy, the radiographs may not show normal structures, but they may be healthy. Therefore,

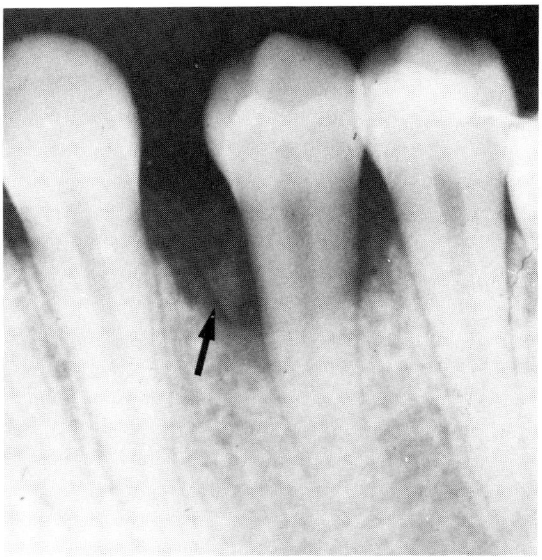

Fig. 4-8. A large periodontal lesion around a mandibular first bicuspid in a 14-year-old girl. Note the retained root tip from a deciduous molar (arrow).

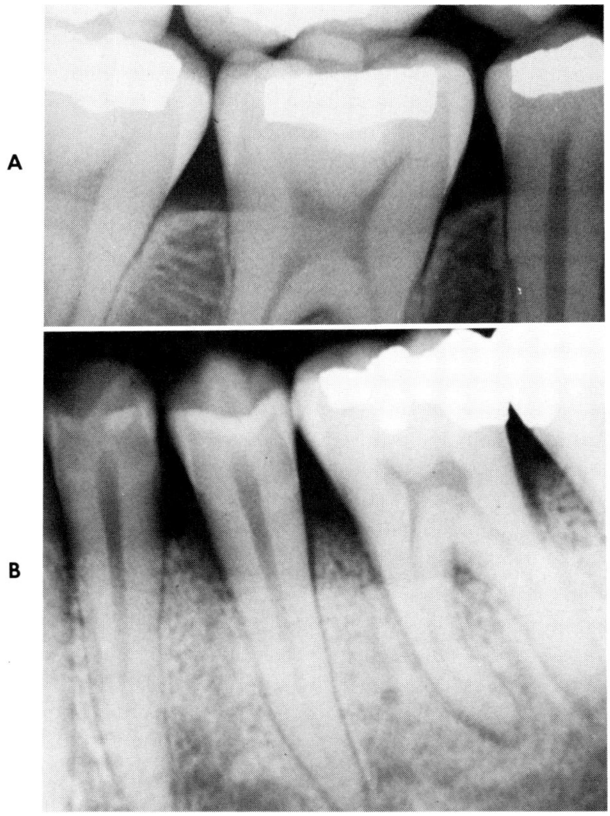

Fig. 4-9. Normal, **A,** and resorbed, **B,** interdental bony septa.

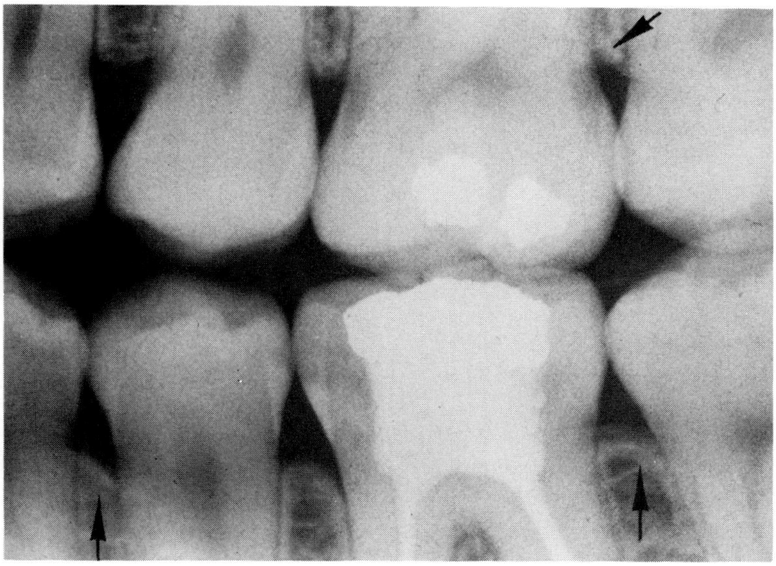

Fig. 4-10. Bite-wing radiograph of normal periodontal tissues. Septa span from cementoenamel junction to cementoenamel junction. Because of the position of teeth, the crestal margin may be slanted (arrows). This does not indicate bone loss and should not be mistaken for pathology.

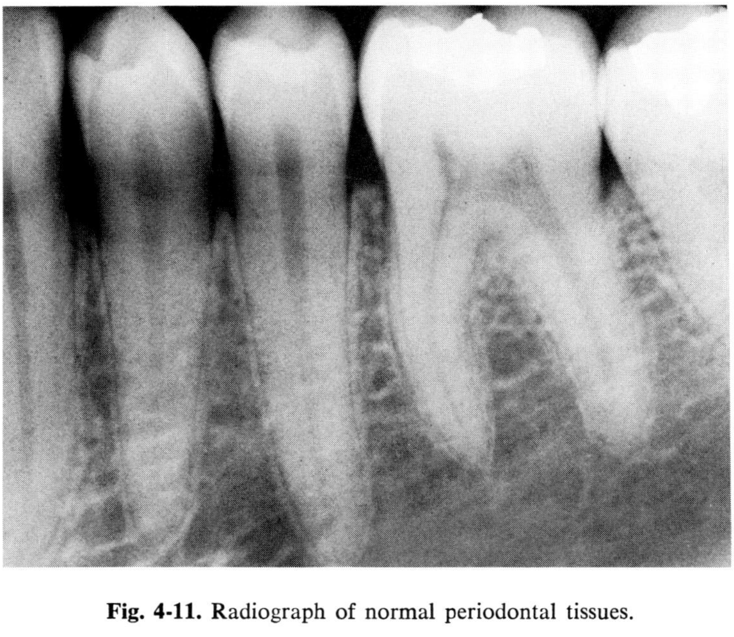

Fig. 4-11. Radiograph of normal periodontal tissues.

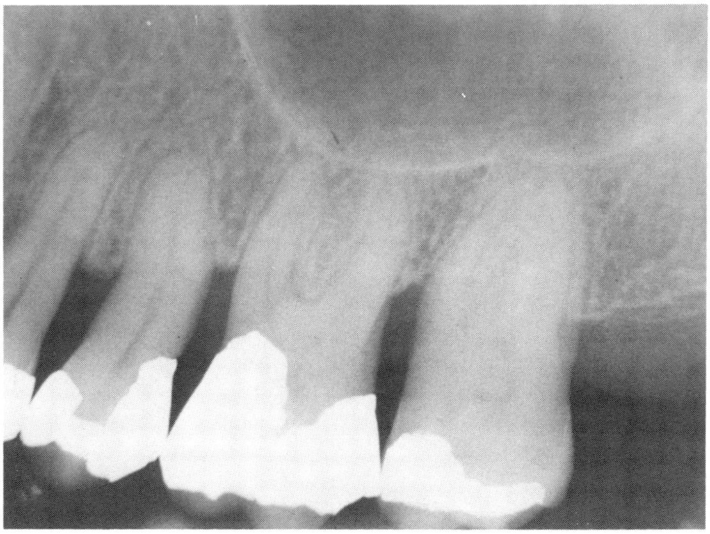

Fig. 4-12. Radiograph taken two years after successful periodontal surgery. Although crestal septa are apically situated, periodontal tissues are healthy. Without clinical examination, however, this radiograph could be easily misinterpreted.

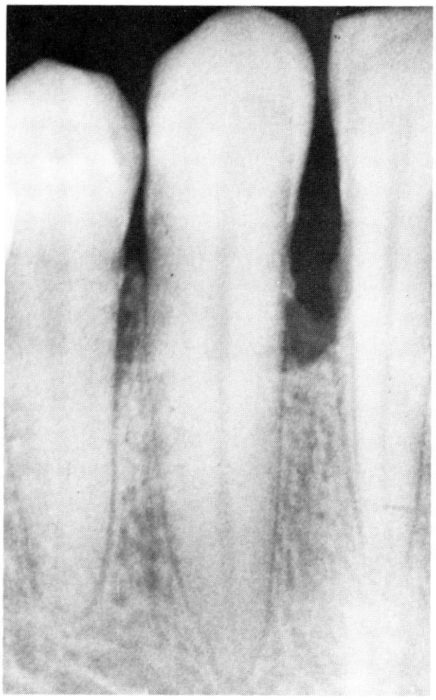

Fig. 4-13. Radiograph showing areas of incipient periodontitis (between cuspid and bicuspid) and moderate periodontitis (between the cuspid and the lateral incisor). Calculus can be seen on the roots of the cuspid and lateral incisor.

the terms "normal" and "healthy" should not be confused. The level of bone may be considerably apical to the cementoenamel junction, the periodontal ligament spaces may appear slightly enlarged, but the patient may have completely healthy tissues (Fig. 4-12).

Gingivitis. Since gingivitis is exclusively a soft tissue lesion, the bone and periodontal ligament are *not* involved. Therefore, on a radiograph one cannot differentiate betwen a normal periodontium and gingivitis.

Incipient periodontitis. The radiograph is of great value in the diagnosis of the initial lesion of periodontitis. In addition to clinical findings of more than normal pocket depth (greater than 3 mm.), hazy or cuplike defects at the crest of the interproximal septa on the radiograph are highly indicative of beginning periodontitis (Figs. 4-9, *B,* and 4-13).

Moderate periodontitis. As progression of the disease occurs, craters, horizontal loss of bone, and vertical osseous defects can result. The interproximal part of the lesion appears as a prominent bony defect (Fig. 4-13). Precise architecture of these defects can be determined by clinical probing, by taking radiographs with "markers," and ultimately by surgical exploration.

Advanced periodontitis. The usual progression of the disease is insidious and painless. When it is allowed to go unabated, considerable bone loss occurs, with resultant mobility and drifting of teeth. Often the molars exhibit bifurcation involvement. Periodontitis at this stage is easily diagnosed in radiographs that show advanced generalized bone loss (Fig. 4-14). The degree of bone loss, however, is more advanced clinically than can be seen in the radiographs.

Periodontal abscess. The periodontal abscess often results from rapidly forming deep pockets. Radiographs show marked bone loss, and clinical examination reveals involvement of the gingiva and the presence of a deep pocket. When the abscess is treated, the regeneration of bone is rapid and can be easily demonstrated in the radiographs (Fig. 4-15).

Combined pulpal-periodontal lesion. Necrotic pulps and periapical lesions

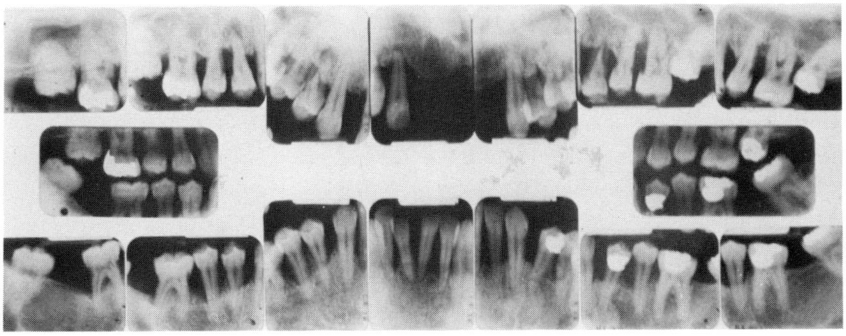

Fig. 4-14. Advanced periodontitis in a 54-year-old male.

A 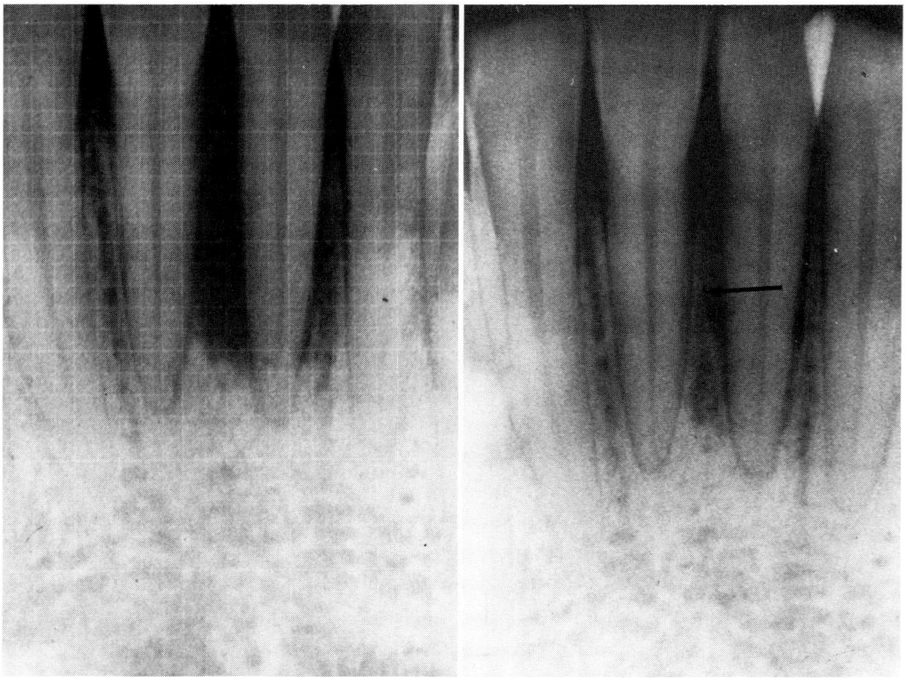 B

Fig. 4-15. A, Acute periodontal abscess between the two mandibular central incisors. **B,** Same case as shown in **A,** six weeks after curettage. Indication of bone repair is evident (arrow).

A 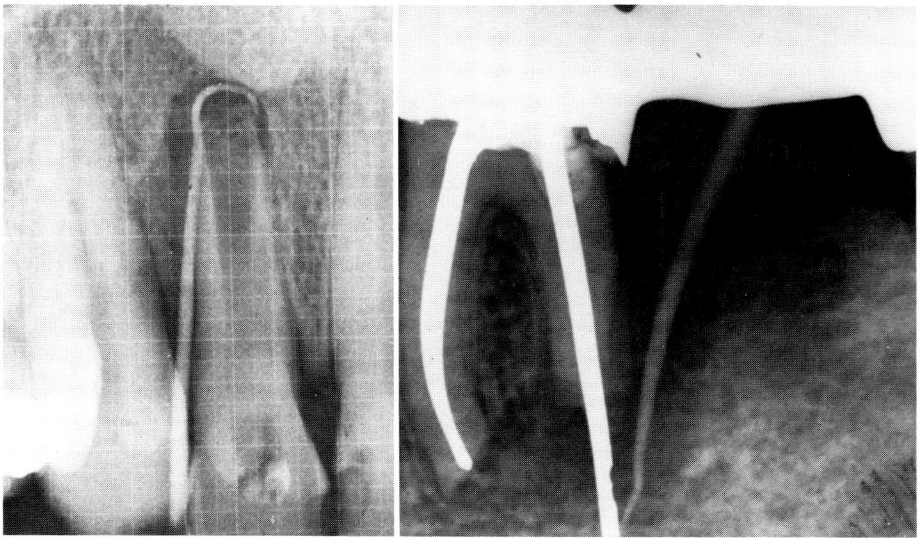 B

Fig. 4-16. Two cases of pulpal-periodontal lesions. **A,** Radiograph of maxillary lateral incisor of a 22-year-old male, showing no apification. A gutta-percha point was inserted through the gingival sulcus to the tooth apex. Endodontic therapy alone resolved the lesion. **B,** A molar with a periapical lesion that communicated with the periodontal pocket.

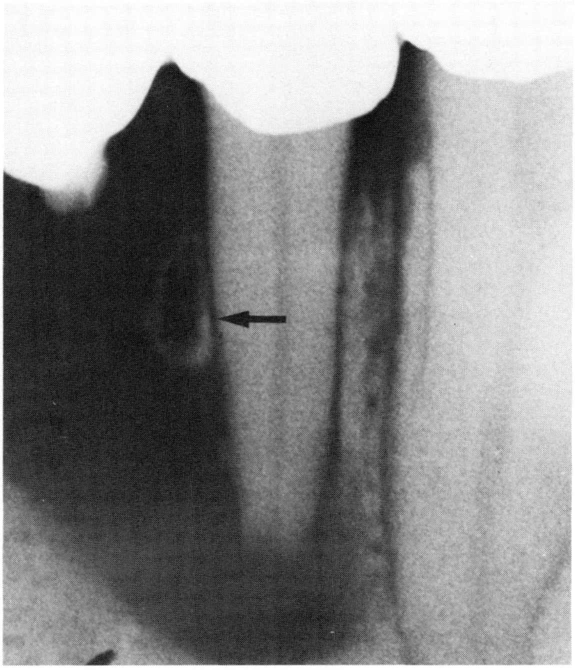

Fig. 4-17. Extensive bone loss in a combined periodontal-pulpal lesion can be seen around the lateral incisor. Note that only a small crestal area of the bone remains on the mesial aspect of the tooth (arrow).

may suppurate and extend to the mucosal surface through a periodontal pocket (Fig. 4-16). They may, in the absence of a pocket, produce destruction of periodontal bone, produce a periodontal lesion, and appear as a periodontal abscess. Clinically, depending on the stage at which a lesion is examined, it may appear as an abscess or only as a deep periodontal lesion without suppuration. Conversely, a deep periodontal pocket may extend to the apex of a tooth and produce pulpitis and pulp necrosis (Fig. 4-1). In the pulpal-periodontal lesions, radiographs show bone destruction from the crest to the apical area (Fig. 4-17). However, it often is difficult to determine whether the periodontal or the pulpal lesion initiated the process.

Occlusal trauma. The uncomplicated lesion of occlusal trauma involves only the tooth, bone, and periodontal ligament and does not elicit any gingival pathology. Clinically, the tooth is mobile; but periodontal pockets and gingival recession are not necessarily present. Thus, the radiograph can be helpful in diagnosis by showing a widened periodontal ligament space, a loss of continuity of the lamina dura, and perhaps hypercementosis (Fig. 4-18). Rarely, root resorption or tooth fractures may also be seen.

Hyperfunction. Teeth in hyperfunction, instead of showing evidence of occlusal trauma may show widening of periodontal space and dense bone trabeculation around the roots (Fig. 4-19).

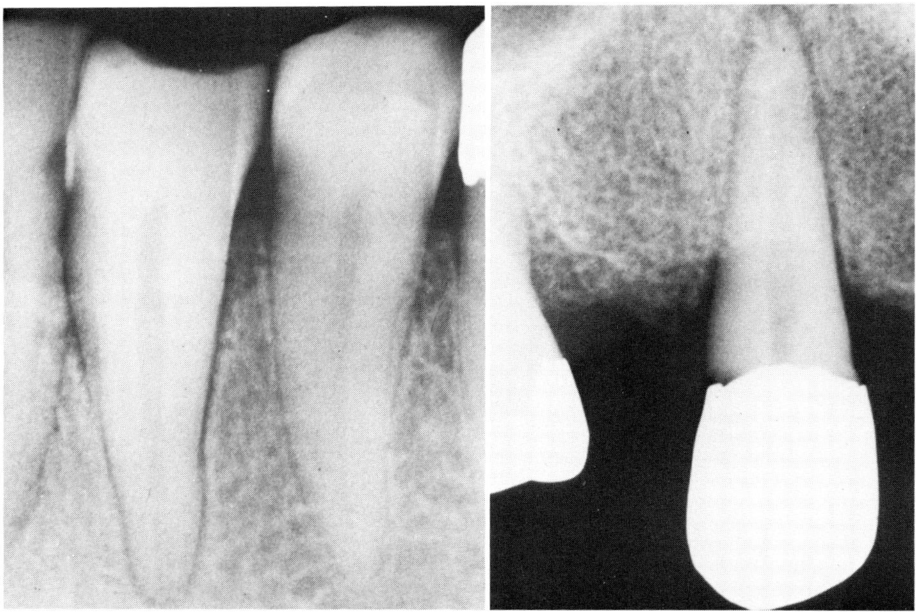

A B

Fig. 4-18. Opposing cuspids (**A**, mandibular; **B**, maxillary) were the only teeth in contact when this patient closed in the retruded position. Both were mobile. Note the enlarged periodontal ligament spaces, lack of a distinct lamina dura, and severe incisal wear on the mandibular tooth. Lesions healed after occlusal adjustment.

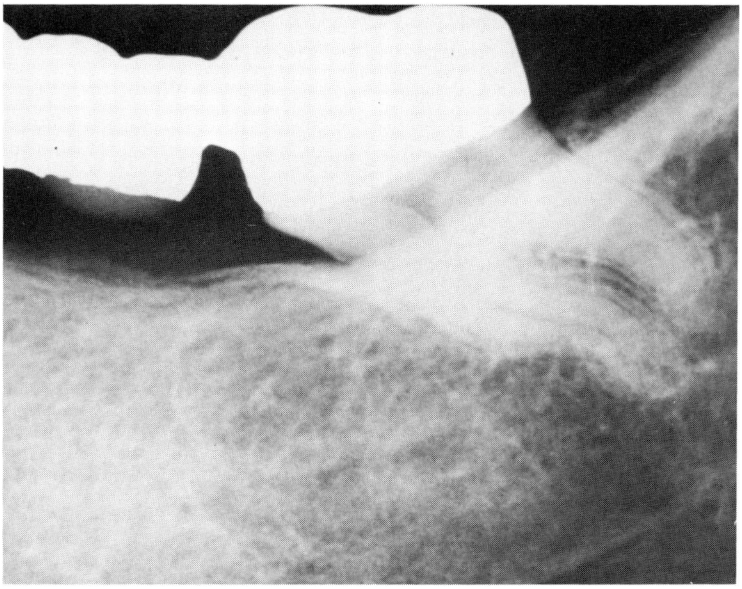

Fig. 4-19. Mandibular molar in hyperfunction. Notice the increase of radiopacity around the roots.

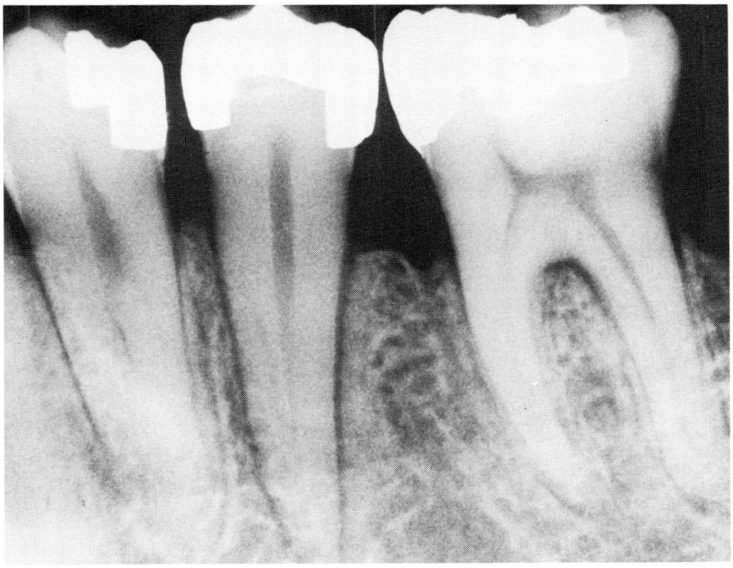

Fig. 4-20. Radiograph taken after orthodontic movement, with enlarged periodontal ligament spaces associated with the premolars. The lack of proximal contacts represents the spaces previously occupied by orthodontic bands.

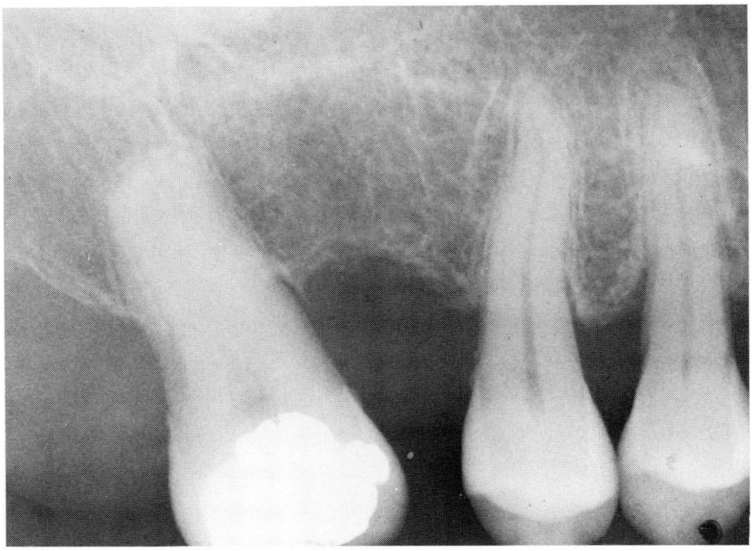

Fig. 4-21. The molar in this radiograph was not in occlusion with a mandibular tooth. The periodontal ligament space is imperceptible, and trabeculation of supporting bone is decreased.

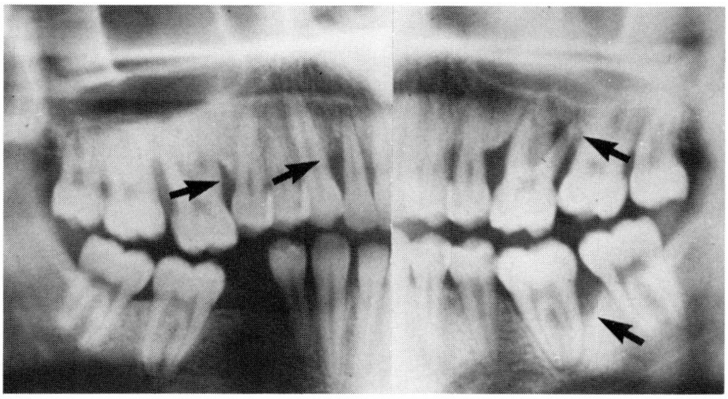

Fig. 4-22. Selective advanced bone loss seen in a young patient with periodontosis (arrows).

Orthodontic tooth movement. Tooth movement by means of removable appliances or fixed-band techniques can produce a radiographic appearance of the periodontium similar to the lesion of occlusal trauma (Fig. 4-20). The history provides the correct diagnosis.

Atrophy of disuse. When a tooth has limited or no function, disuse atrophy of bone occurs. Clinically, the tooth may be slightly mobile. The radiograph shows a very thin, almost nonexistent periodontal ligament space and a lessening of trabeculation around the involved root (Fig. 4-21).

Periodontosis. In periodontosis, a rare disease seen in young patients, characteristic selective bone loss can be seen around the permanent maxillary and mandibular incisors and the first permanent molars. Deep vertical pockets are often present; teeth are mobile and drift from their original position. In such cases the radiographs show selective but advanced bone loss (Fig. 4-22).

PERIODONTAL FOLLOW-UP

The use of the radiograph to obtain a sequential history of disease is a valuable diagnostic procedure. Considerable information can be derived from the old radiographs of a patient. It is often useful to see graphically the progression of a particular lesion for a period of years.

When a patient has completed active periodontal therapy, he is generally placed in a recall system so that the treatment can be continuously evaluated. Radiographs taken at intervals of twelve months are important in management of periodontal patients.

REFERENCES

Bhaskar, S. N., and Orban, B. J.: Experimental occlusal trauma, J. Periodont. **26:** 270, 1955.

Everett, F. G., and Fixott, H. C.: Use of an incorporated grid in the interpretation of dental roentgenograms, Oral Surg. **16:** 1061, 1963.

Hirschfeld, L.: A calibrated silver point for periodontal diagnosis and recording, J. Periodontol. **24:**94, 1953.

Mahan, C. J., and Hurt, W. C.: Retained

deciduous tooth fragments and periodontal lesions: radiographic, clinical and histologic observations, Oral Surg. **35:**708, 1973.

Manson, J. D.: The lamina dura, Oral Surg. **16:**432, 1963.

Prichard, J. F.: The role of the roentgenogram in the diagnosis and prognosis of periodontal disease, Oral Surg. **14:**182, 1961.

Prichard, J. F.: The roentgenographic depiction of periodontal disease, JASPD **3:** 44, 1973.

Rees, T. D., Biggs, N. L., and Collings, C. K.,: Radiographic interpretation of periodontal oral lesions, Oral Surg. **32:** 141, 1971.

Ritchey, B., and Orban, B.: The crests of the interdental septa, J. Periodontol. **24:** 34, 1943.

Suomi, J. D., Plumbo, J., and Barbano, J. P.: A comparative study of radiographs and pocket measurements in periodontal disease evaluation, J. Periodontol. **39:**311, 1968.

Updegrave, W. J.: The paralleling extension-cone technique in intraoral dental radiography, Oral Surg. **4:**1250, 1951.

van der Linden, L. W., and van Aken, J.: The periodontal ligament in the roentgenogram, J. Periodontol. **41:**243, 1970.

Weinmann, J. P.: Variations in the structure of bone and bones and their significance in radiology, Oral Surg. **8:**988, 1955.

PART THREE

JAWS

The major part of radiologic interpretation consists of the analysis of lesions involving the jaws. This aspect of the subject will be discussed in four separate chapters.

CHAPTER FIVE

CLASSIFICATION AND GENERAL PRINCIPLES IN RADIOGRAPHY OF THE JAWS

CLASSIFICATION OF LESIONS

Besides the teeth, radiographic interpretation in dental practice deals with lesions or abnormalities of the maxilla and mandible. Thus, of all lesions biopsied in a dental office, more than 33% are from within the jaws. It is apparent, therefore, that a radiograph is essential to the correct interpretation and therefore to the correct management of oral diseases.

A vast majority of lesions of the jaws occur *within* the jaws—that is, within their outer and inner cortical plates—and are referred to as *central* in location. Some, however, occur on the periosteal surface and are called *peripheral* or *periosteal* in location. In either event, a radiograph of good quality alters the normal pattern of opacities and shadows. Fortunately, in spite of the vast variety of pathology that occurs within the jaws, radiographically it can take only one of three forms. *A lesion may appear either as a radiolucency or a radiopacity, or it may be partly radiolucent and partly radiopaque (mixed)* (Fig. 5-1). Although many lesions are at first radiolucent or radiopaque and throughout their course maintain this feature, there are many others that may change from one group to another. Thus a radiolucent lesion such as a cementoma may gradually become partly radiopaque and finally become completely radiopaque. Similarly, a radiopaque lesion such as condensing osteitis may undergo secondary inflammation and appear as partly radiolucent and partly radiopaque. It is thus apparent that radiologically, the jaw lesions may "migrate" from one group to another. For this reason, in the subsequent discussions some lesions will appear under more than one group.

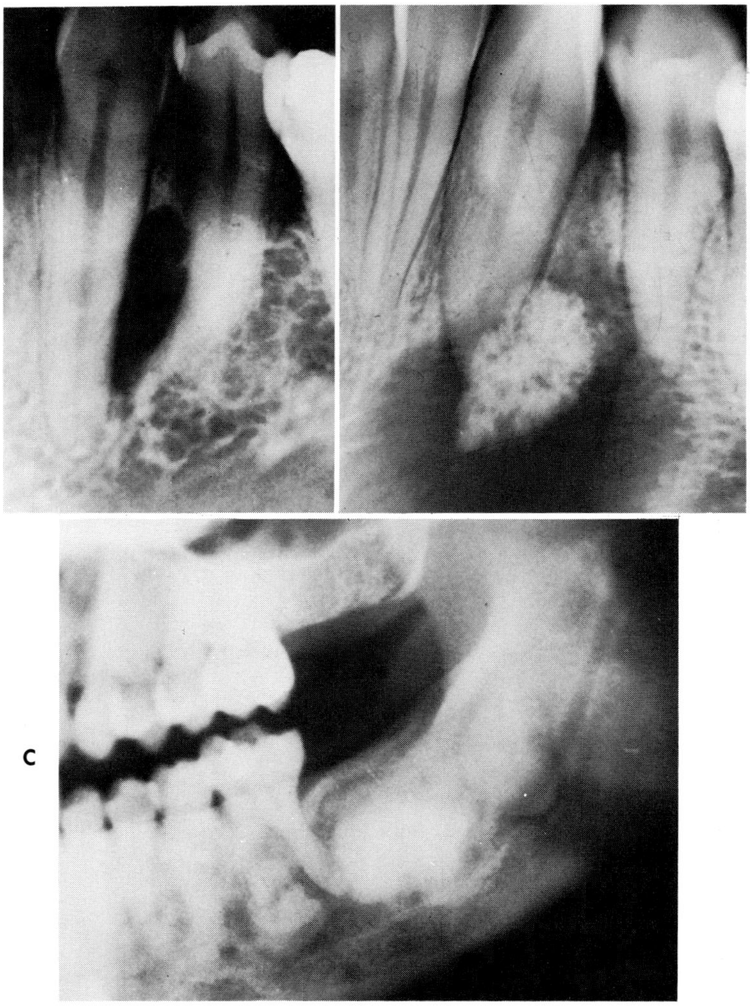

Fig. 5-1. Radiographs showing the three major types of jaw lesions. **A,** Radiolucencies. **B,** Radiopacities. **C,** Lesions that are partly radiolucent and partly radiopaque (mixed).

From a practical, clinical point of view, therefore, the radiographic interpretation of the jaws can be discussed under the following three groups:

1. Radiolucent lesions of the jaws (Chapter 6)
2. Radiopaque lesions of the jaws (Chapter 7)
3. Radiolucent and radiopaque (mixed) lesions of the jaws (Chapter 8)

Although in the following chapters the three major types of jaw lesions (radiolucent, radiopaque, and mixed) are described in detail, it must be emphasized that the radiolucent group occur with far greater frequency than the other two. If one were to exclude periodontal diseases from jaw pathology, it is estimated that about 92% of the jaw lesions appear as radiolucencies, about 7%

as radiopacities, and only about 1% as mixed (radiolucent and radiopaque) lesions.

GENERAL PRINCIPLES OF RADIOGRAPHIC INTERPRETATION

In radiographic interpretation of jaw lesions, the following general principles should be kept in mind:

1. Prior to the establishment of a diagnosis, the *vitality* of the teeth in the area of the lesion must be checked. A radiolucent lesion at the apex of a vital tooth would most likely be a cementoma, whereas one associated with a nonvital tooth could represent one of many lesions.

2. It should be kept in mind that if a tooth tests "nonvital" with the usual vitality tests, the pulp tissue is not necessarily necrotic. The nerve supply to that tooth may have been damaged or severed. A classic demonstration of this phenomenon is seen in cases of physical trauma in which the nerve supply is damaged but the blood supply is left intact. Such teeth test "nonvital" but in reality are vital, that is, their blood supply is normal and the pulp tissue is viable. Thus the nerve may regenerate in a few months, and the teeth may again give a positive vitality test. In cases of trauma, therefore, unless teeth have periapical lesions or symptoms of necrosis of the pulp, endodontic therapy need not be started immediately.

3. The location, duration, and size of the lesion, as well as the age and sex of the patient, often have important diagnostic significance. For example, multiple myeloma occurs most often in older males, whereas a traumatic cyst is seen usually in young patients.

4. The presence of neurologic symptoms such as paresthesia, pain, or paralysis often implies a traumatic or a malignant lesion.

5. Destruction of the cortical plate of bone usually means a rapidly growing lesion. Such lesions are either malignant or represent acute inflammatory diseases (Fig. 5-2).

6. "Expansion" of the cortical plate, without destruction, is usually associated with a slowly growing lesion. Such a process implies that the normal compensatory growth of bone on the periosteal surface keeps pace with the growth of the disease process within the jaw. This occurs in many lesions of the jaws, including cysts as well as odontogenic and nonodontogenic tumors (Fig. 5-3).

7. In the diagnosis of radiolucent lesions, aspiration is a valuable diagnostic aid. Thus aspiration of fluid from a radiolucency of the jaws generally means a cystic lesion, whereas an absence of fluid would imply a solid tumor of some type (Fig. 5-4).

8. Presence or absence of systemic symptoms or lesions in other areas of the skeleton is often important in differential diagnosis. Multiple radiopaque lesions in the jaws, by themselves, would imply a form of condensing osteitis called multiple enostosis. On the other hand, if the same patient also has lesions

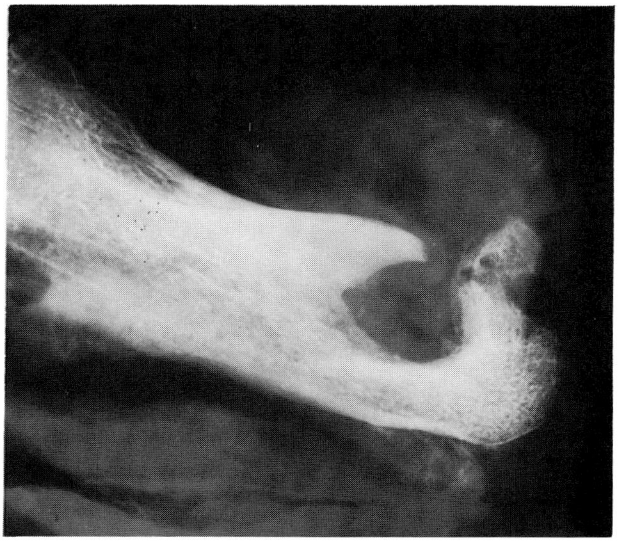

Fig. 5-2. Radiolucent lesion of the mandible that destroyed the cortical plate. This lesion was an osteogenic sarcoma.

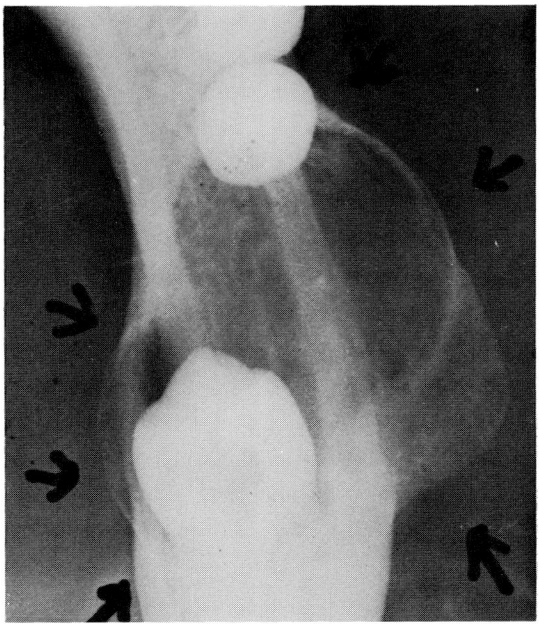

Fig. 5-3. An occlusal radiograph of the mandible, showing a benign central lesion that has "expanded" but has not destroyed the cortex (arrows).

A

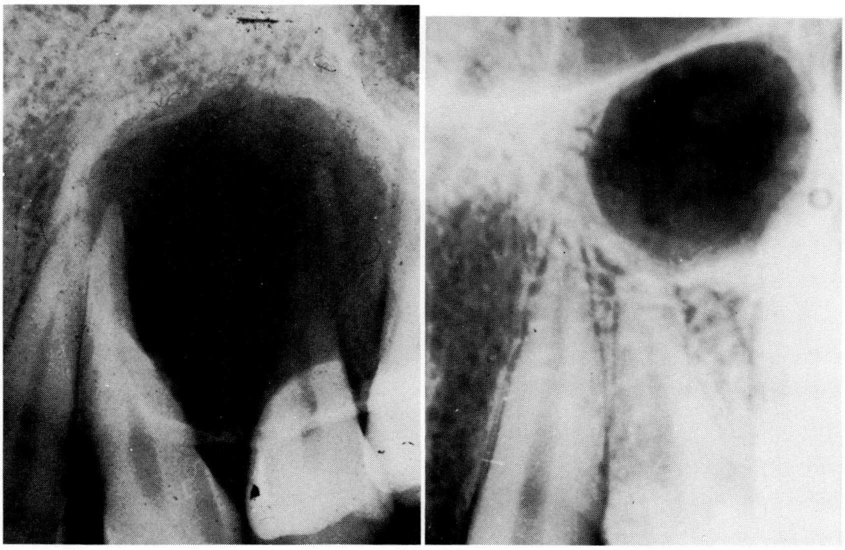

B

Fig. 5-4. Two radiolucencies in the maxilla. **A,** Solid odontogenic tumor in which aspiration was nonproductive. **B,** Cyst that yielded fluid on aspiration.

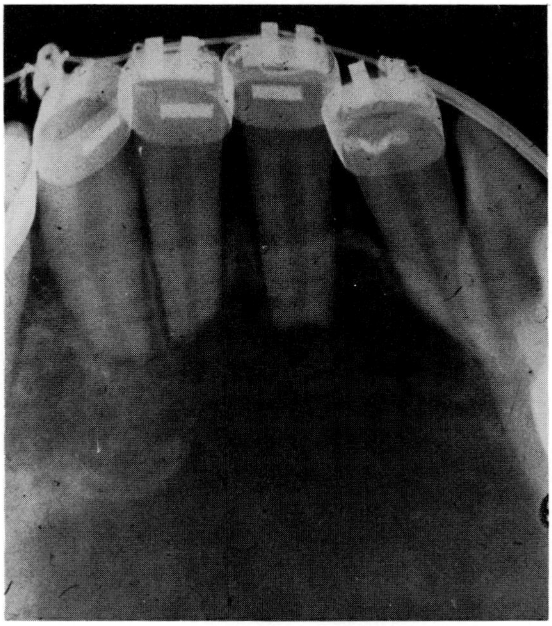

Fig. 5-5. Radiolucent lesion of the mandible that was a benign central connective-tissue tumor and that produced root resorption of the regional teeth.

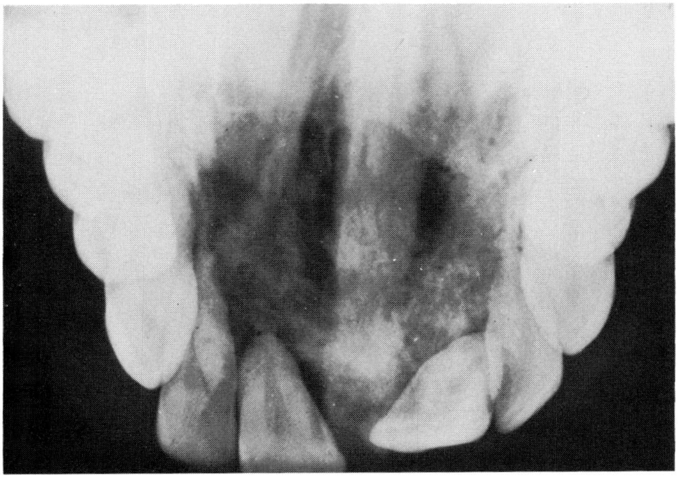

Fig. 5-6. Central malignant tumor of the maxilla (chondrosarcoma) that has produced migration and root resorption of the regional teeth. The lesion appears partly radiolucent and partly radiopaque.

in other parts of the skeleton, Paget's disease is usually suspected. One or more radiolucencies in the jaws of a patient with a history of malignant disease should arouse a suspicion of possible metastasis.

9. Resorption of roots associated with a lesion usually means a slow connective tissue growth (Fig. 5-5). There are, however, exceptions to this rule, and epithelial lesions, even cysts, as well as rapidly growing lesions such as malignant tumors, may produce root resorption (Fig. 5-6).

10. Migration of teeth usually occurs in slowly growing lesions (Fig. 5-7).

11. Loosening of teeth in the area of the lesion usually indicates rapid growth.

12. A radiolucency completely surrounding the roots of teeth implies rapid growth. Eosinophilic granuloma, osteomyelitis, abscess, and carcinoma invading bone are examples of such diseases (Fig. 5-8).

13. A radiograph showing a lesion with a distinct border signifies slow growth, and an indistinct, irregular border in a radiograph means an infiltrating, rapidly growing lesion (Fig. 5-9). Lesions of slow growth destroy bone completely in an area and occupy that space. For this reason, their boundaries are often well defined. Rapidly growing lesions, however, infiltrate and extend into the surrounding bone without destroying all the trabeculae in the area. Their boundaries, therefore, are ill defined.

14. The appearance of the oral mucosa covering a radiographically apparent lesion often has diagnostic significance. Ulceration overlying a central jaw lesion implies rapid growth and should be viewed with concern.

15. Whenever the location, outline, or other features of a lesion are not dis-

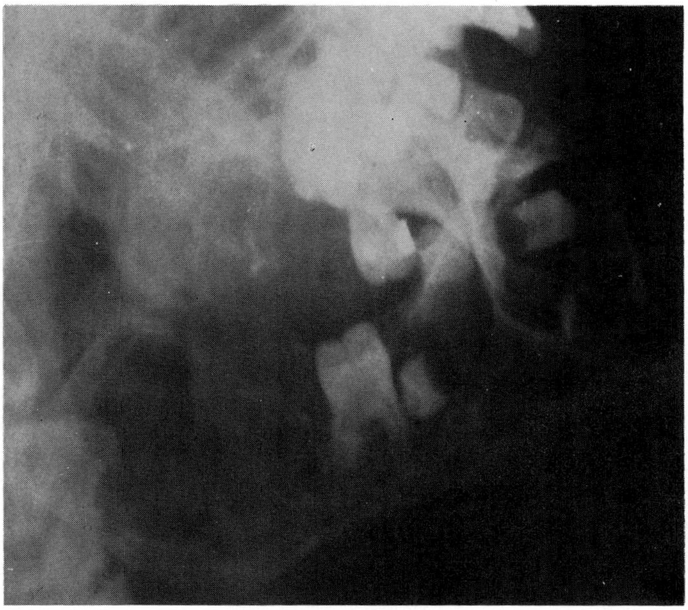

Fig. 5-7. Central radiolucent lesion of the mandible (cherubism) that has produced migration of many teeth.

tinct in a radiograph, or when the clinical features are not compatible with the radiographic appearance, additional radiographs taken at varied angulations should be examined.

16. There are three types of bone tissue in man: mature, immature, and bundle bone (Fig. 5-10). The *mature bone* tissue is seen in the normal adult skeleton, and most of the bone after the first year of life is of this type (Fig. 5-10, *A*). This bone is radiopaque.

Bundle bone is seen in those areas of the skeleton which give attachment to ligaments and tendons. Into this type of bone tissue are anchored parts of the ligament or tendon fibers, and it contains a greater amount of calcium salts per unit area than the mature bone. Bundle bone, therefore, is more radiopaque than the mature bone. In the jaws, the lamina dura is composed of this type of bone tissue (Fig. 5-10, *B*). The *immature bone* tissue is seen in the fetus and occurs up to about the first year of life (Fig. 5-10, *C*). A fetus may have all the bones in the process of development, but in radiographs only some of them may be identified. In the adult, immature bone is seen in bone repair (such as healing extraction sockets or bone fractures) or in areas of pathology (such as tumors). Bone tissue, therefore, is not always radiopaque (Fig. 5-11).

17. Lesions may be larger or smaller than their apparent size in radiographs. Thus an ameloblastoma may extend far beyond the radiolucency it creates, and a radicular cyst almost always occupies only a portion of the radiolucent shadow

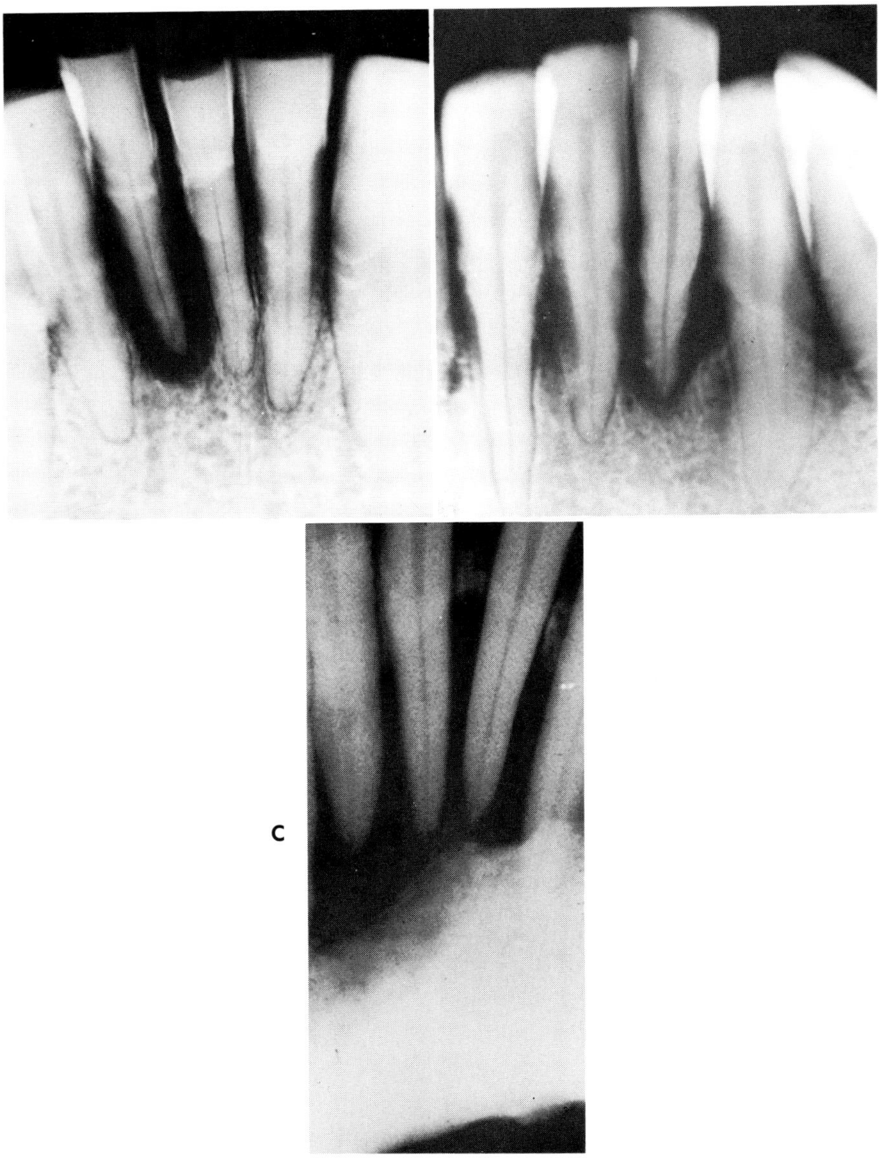

Fig. 5-8. Three radiolucent lesions that completely surround roots of teeth. **A,** Metastatic carcinoma. **B,** Advanced periodontitis and abscess. **C,** Eosinophilic granuloma.

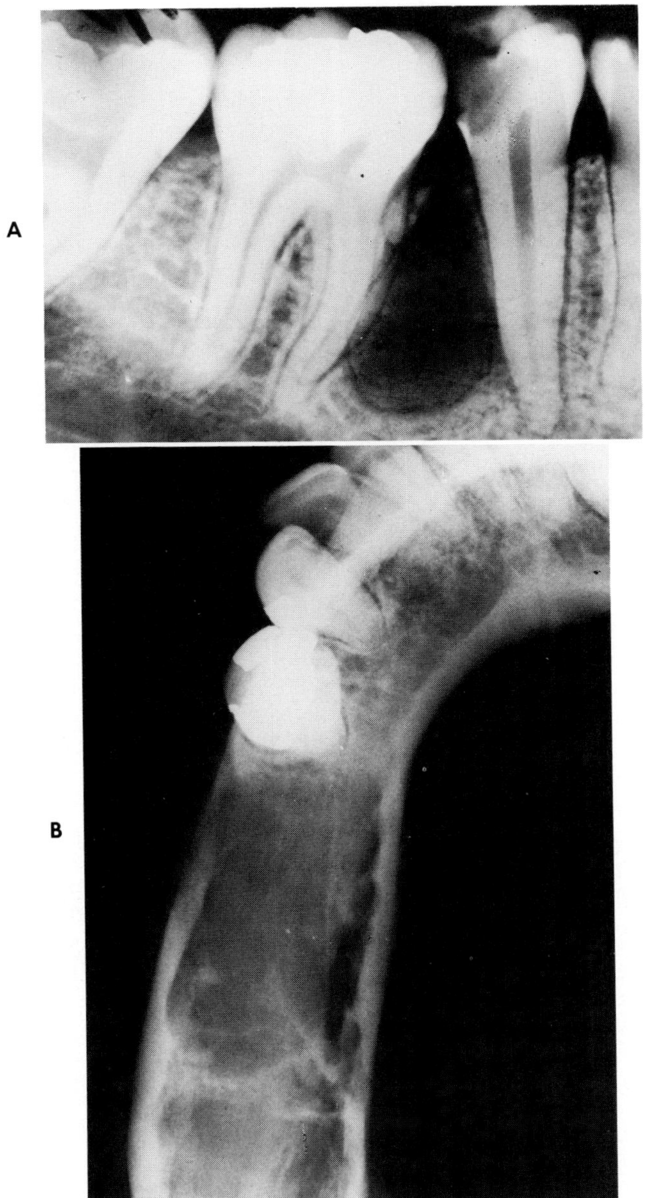

Continued.

Fig. 5-9. A, Well-circumscribed, slow-growing radiolucency of the mandible (benign cyst). **B** and **C,** Rapidly growing, ill-defined radiolucent lesion of the mandible (reticulum cell sarcoma).

C

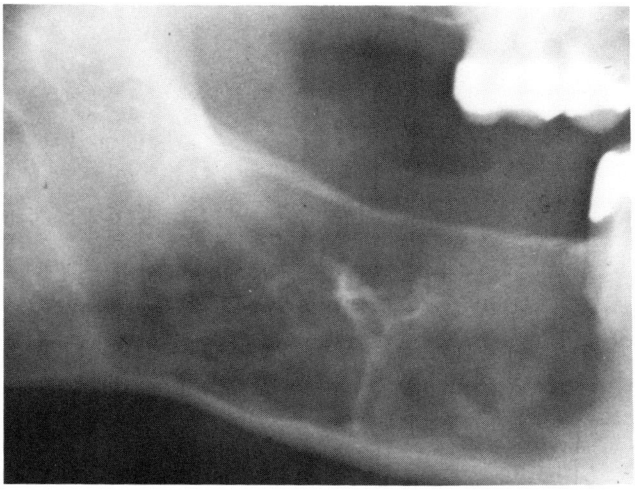

Fig. 5-9, cont'd. For legend see p. 97.

A

B

C

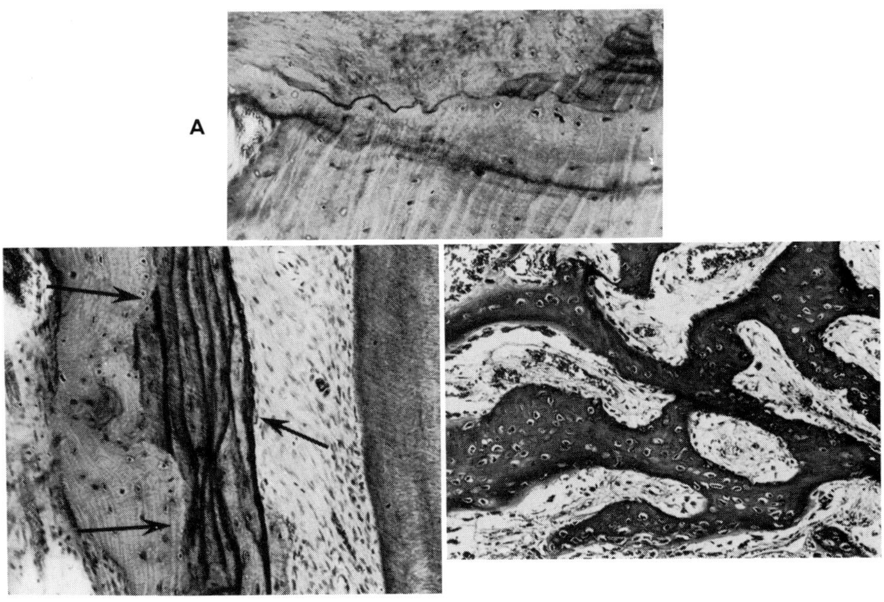

Fig. 5-10. Photomicrographs of bone tissue. **A,** Mature bone tissue. **B,** Bundle bone (arrows). **C,** Immature bone tissue. In **B** the periodontal ligament and the root surface can be seen in the right half of the figure. Bundle bone is the dark area outlined by arrows and it represents the lamina dura seen in the radiographs.

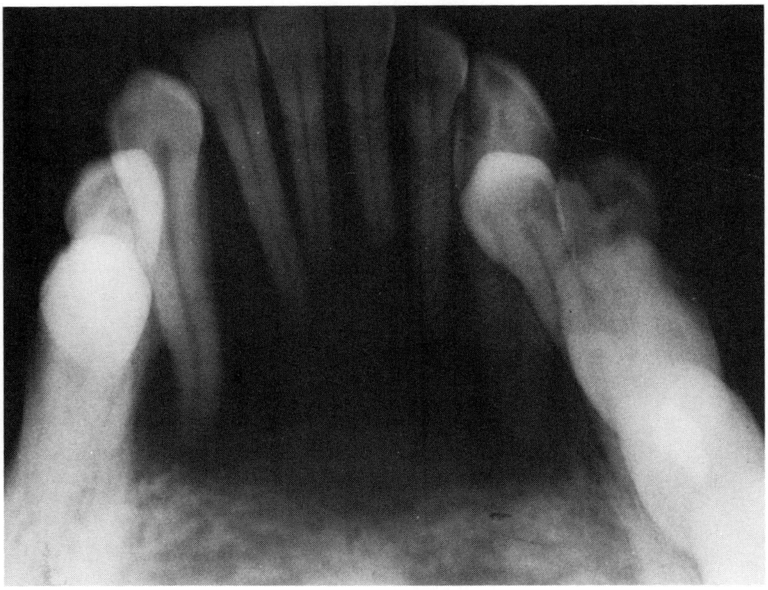

Fig. 5-11. An osteogenic sarcoma that appears as a large radiolucency. Microscopic examination of this lesion showed many fine foci and trabeculae of immature bone.

associated with it. In the latter case the remainder of the area is filled with granulation tissue.

REFERENCES

Bhaskar, S. N.: Synopsis of oral pathology, ed. 4, St. Louis, 1973, The C. V. Mosby Co.

Bhaskar, S. N., and Rappaport, H.: The dental "vitality" tests and pulp status, 1973, J. Am. Dent. Assoc. **86:**409, 1973.

Weinmann, J. P., and Sicher, H.: Bone and bones, ed. 2, St. Louis, 1955, The C. V. Mosby Co.

CHAPTER SIX

RADIOLUCENT LESIONS OF THE JAWS

The radiolucent lesions of the jaws comprise about 92% of all jaw lesions (excluding periodontal diseases). They are, therefore, the most important segment of radiologic interpretation. About 85% of them occur at the apical area of teeth. From a diagnostic point of view the radiolucent lesions can be divided into the following subgroups:

- Lesions at apex of tooth (85% of central jaw lesions)
  - Radiolucency at apex of nonvital tooth
    - Dental granuloma
    - Radicular cyst
    - Abscess
  - Radiolucency in extraction site
    - Residual cyst
  - Radiolucency at apex of vital tooth
    - Cementoma (stage I)
  - Radiolucency at apex of endodontically treated tooth
    - Radicular cyst
  - Radiolucency associated with root canal filling and apical surgery
    - Apical scar
  - Rare apical lesions
    - Cholesteatoma
    - Foreign body reactions
    - Central giant cell reparative granuloma
  - Healing of apical lesions
- Lesions in midline of maxilla (7% of central jaw lesions)
  - Nasoalveolar cyst (nasolabial cyst)
  - Globulomaxillary cyst
  - Median alveolar cyst
  - Nasopalatine cysts
    - Incisive canal cyst
    - Cyst of palatine papilla
  - Median palatine cyst
  - Rare midline lesions
- Lesions in place of missing tooth
  - Primordial cyst

- Ameloblastoma
- Rare odontogenic lesion

Lesions around crown of impacted tooth
- Dentigerous cyst
- Odontogenic fibroma (and odontogenic myxoma)
- Eruption cyst
- Ameloblastoma
- Adenoameloblastoma

Soap bubble-like radiolucencies
- Central giant cell reparative granuloma
- Aneurysmal bone cyst
- Ameloblastoma
- Rare lesions
  - Cherubism
  - Myxoma
  - Multilocular follicular cyst

Multiple but separate radiolucent lesions
- Cementoma (stage I)
- Histiocytosis X
- Hyperparathyroidism
- Cherubism
- Multiple myeloma
- Metastatic tumors

Lesions that destroy the cortical plate
- Primary malignant tumors of the jaws
- Metastatic tumors to the jaws
- Osteomyelitis

Miscellaneous and rare lesions
- Traumatic cyst
- Idiopathic bone cavity
- Gingival cyst
- Lateral periodontal cyst
- Physiologic osteoporosis
- Hematopoietic marrow
- Periodontal disease
- Median mandibular cyst
- Central hemangioma
- Mandibular cleft
- Salivary gland tissue and tumors
- Fractures

} 7% of central jaw lesions

LESIONS AT APEX OF TOOTH

About 85% of *all* jaw lesions occur in the apical area of teeth. This group is therefore the largest and most important in radiologic diagnosis. When a radiograph shows a radiolucency at the apex of a tooth, information about the vitality of the regional teeth is of the utmost diagnostic importance. In addition, certain *rare lesions* occur in this area. The clinician should also be aware of the changes in the apical radiolucencies that follow endodontic therapy. All these aspects of the apical lesions will therefore be considered in this section.

To distinguish the *common* apical lesions from each other, certain features are of great significance. These features, as well as their interpretation, are given in Table 1.

Table 1. Diagnostic features of common apical lesions

DIAGNOSTIC FEATURE	DIAGNOSIS
Radiolucency at apex of nonvital tooth	Dental granuloma, radicular cyst, or abscess
Radiolucency in extraction site	Residual cyst
Radiolucency at apex of vital tooth	Cementoma, stage I
Radiolucency at apex of endodontically treated tooth	Radicular cyst
Radiolucency associated with the root canal filling and apical surgery	Apical scar

These lesions will now be discussed in more detail.

Radiolucency at apex of nonvital tooth. If the tooth is nonvital, the apical radiolucency indicates a *dental granuloma,* a *radicular cyst,* or an *abscess* (Table 1). If the lesion is associated with a draining fistula or fluctuation, the diagnosis of abscess is easily made. Otherwise, on a radiologic basis, it is impossible to distinguish the three types of lesions (Figs. 6-1 to 6-3). The only exception to this rule are radiolucencies that are greater than 200 $mm.^2$, and in such cases the lesions have been consistently shown to be radicular cysts.

Since endodontic therapy is indicated in all the lesions of this group, a distinction between them is not necessary. Statistically, about 48% of apical radiolucencies are dental granulomas, 43% are radicular cysts, and 1.1% represent dental abscess. (This does not include the large fluctuant and easily identified dentoalveolar abscesses.) In a differential diagnosis of the three lesions of this group, the presence of a distinct border, a radiopaque margin, or other frequently quoted criteria are of no diagnostic significance. In the examination of a periapical lesion the vitality test is, of course, of great importance. In addition, however, the examination of the periodontal tissues should not be overlooked. There are instances in which an *apparent* lesion of this group represents, in reality, the apical extension of a deep periodontal pocket (Fig. 6-4). In these cases, teeth are usually vital, and a radiograph taken with a gutta-percha point in the pocket establishes the diagnosis. On occasion, however, a deep periodontal lesion may be accompanied by pulp disease (pulpitis or necrosis) and a periapical lesion. Such a condition is called *combined lesion.*

As a matter of therapeutic interest, it should be mentioned that radicular cyst occupies only a small portion of the radiolucency associated with these lesions (Fig. 6-5). The radiolucent area surrounding the cystic portion is composed only of granulation tissue (dark area in Fig. 6-5). In surgical treatment of these lesions, therefore, it is not necessary to accomplish extensive curettage of the bony defect.

Radiolucency in extraction site. Persistent radiolucency in an area where a tooth has previously been extracted represents a *residual cyst* (Fig. 6-6). Be-

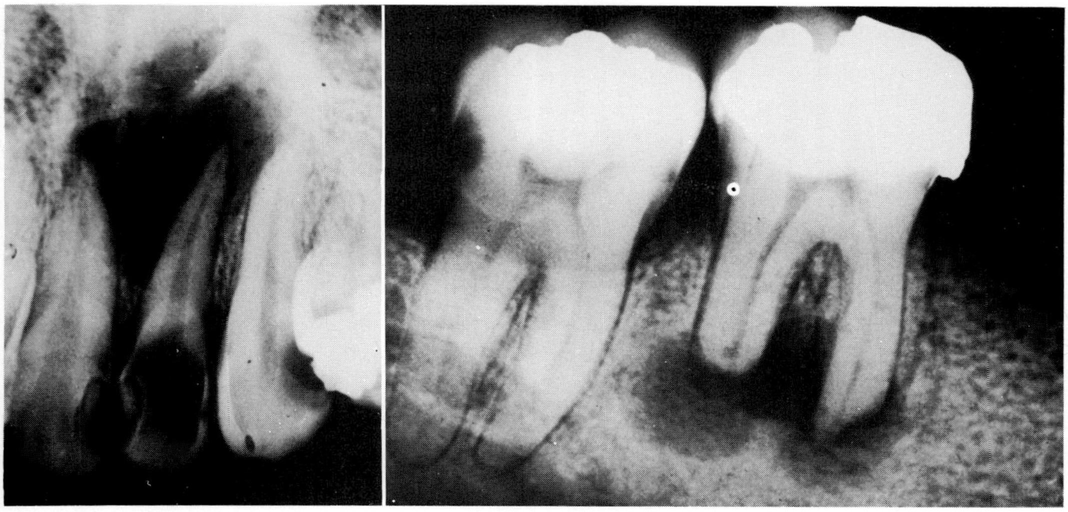

Fig. 6-1. Two periapical radiographs of dental granuloma.

A

B

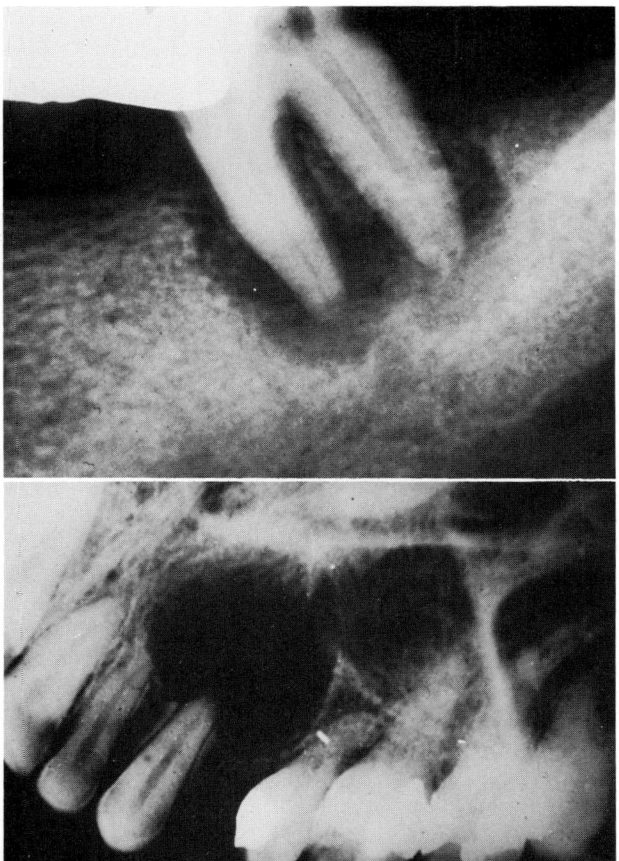

Fig. 6-2. Radiographs of two radicular cysts. In **A** the cyst is not well circumscribed, whereas in **B** the well-defined radiolucency at the apex of the cuspid is partly superimposed on the radiolucency of the maxillary sinus.

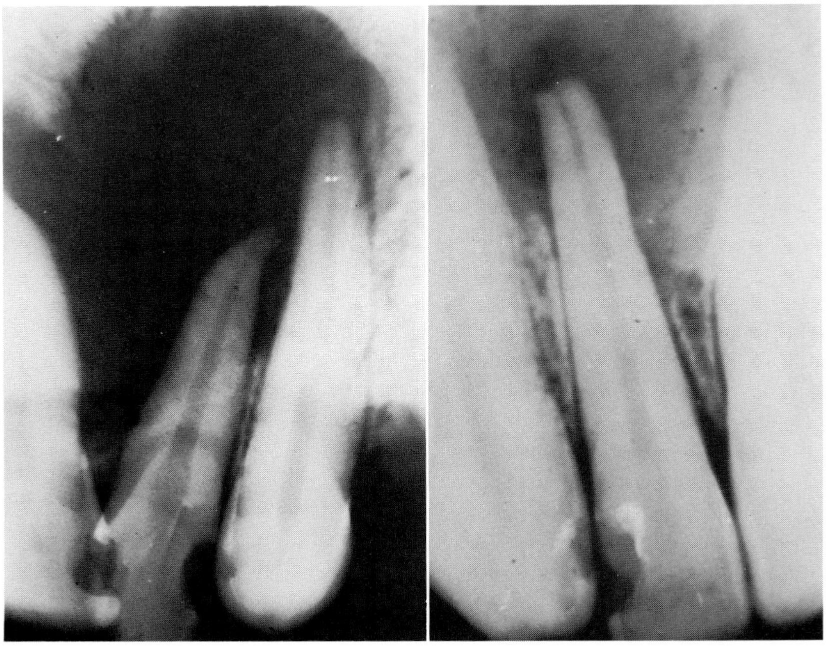

Fig. 6-3. Radiographs of two periapical abscesses. In apical lesions associated with nonvital teeth it is not possible to distinguish the granuloma and the cyst from the abscess.

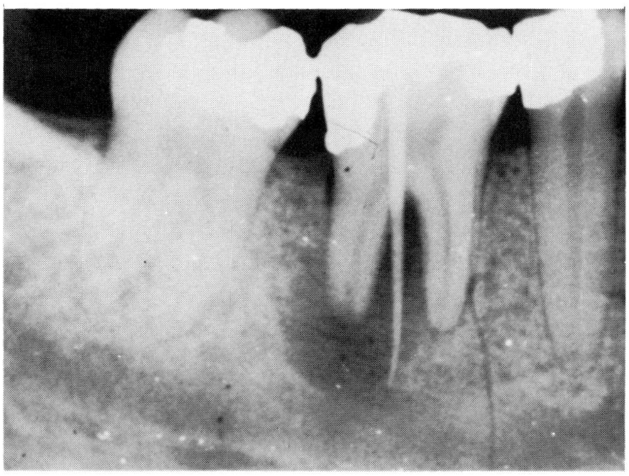

Fig. 6-4. Radiograph of the lower first molar area, showing an apical radiolucency that was of periodontal rather than pulpal origin. A gutta-percha point is seen in the periodontal pocket.

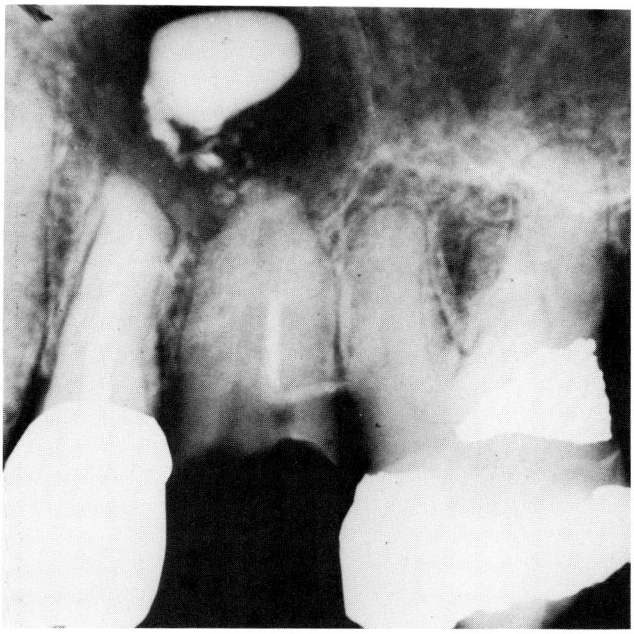

Fig. 6-5. Radicular cyst injected with Lipiodol. The cystic area occupies only a portion of the radiolucency.

A

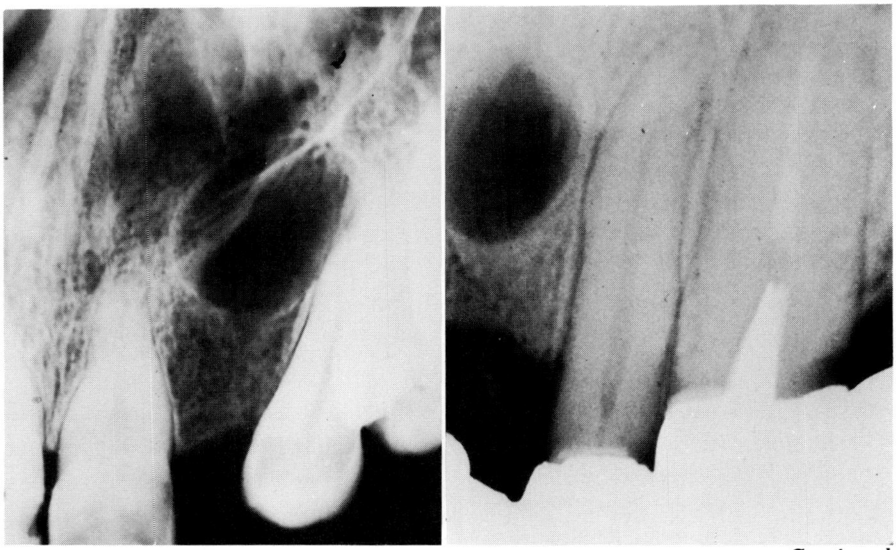

B

Continued.

Fig. 6-6. Radiolucent areas in extraction sites represent residual cysts.

C

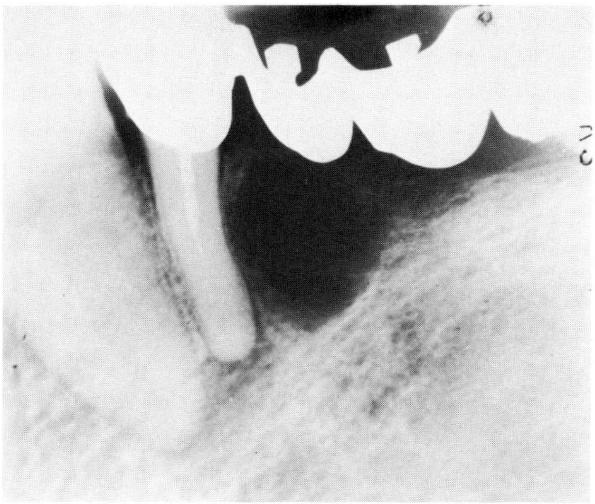

Fig. 6-6, cont'd. For legend see p. 105.

cause of hemorrhage and trauma associated with surgical extraction, many radicular cysts undergo spontaneous resolution. In some cases, however, this does not occur, and such lesions persist as residual cysts. They account for about 3.5% of lesions of the apical area, and they require surgical enucleation. On rare occasions a persistent radiolucency at an extraction site may represent an apical scar (p. 108).

Radiolucency at apex of vital tooth. When the tooth is vital, an apical radiolucency indicates a *cementoma* in stage I (Fig. 6-7). These lesions are often multiple, occur in the lower anterior region, involve females ten times as often as males, and comprise about 1.7% of all apical radiolucencies. They undergo gradual transition to radiopacity (stage II) and in about 6 years become completely radiopaque (stage III). Cementoma requires no treatment.

Radiolucency at apex of endodontically treated tooth. When a radiolucency exists at the apex of a tooth that has previously been treated (root canal filling) but in which (1) the radiolucency continues to enlarge, (2) there are symptoms of pain, (3) there is a draining fistula, or (4) in spite of a waiting period of 6 months or more the apical radiolucency shows no sign of regression, the lesion can be assumed to represent a *radicular cyst* (Figs. 6-8 and 6-9). In such cases apicoectomy or apical curettage is the treatment of choice.

When a root canal filling is obviously defective, such as a grossly underfilled canal, the apical radiolucency could represent either a *radicular cyst* or a *dental granuloma.* The operator has the choice of reopening and refilling the root canal or performing an apicoectomy and a retrograde filling.

Radiolucency associated with root canal filling and apical surgery. An apical radiolucency that fits this description and in which there is neither a

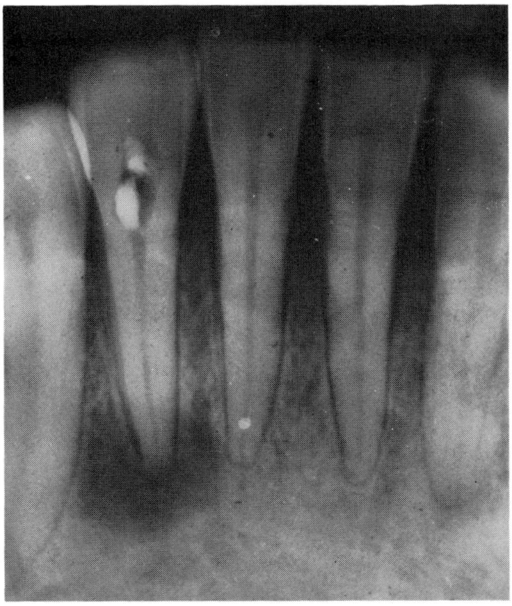

Fig. 6-7. Cementoma (stage I) occurs at the apices of vital teeth. Root canal therapy was started in this case because of inaccurate diagnosis.

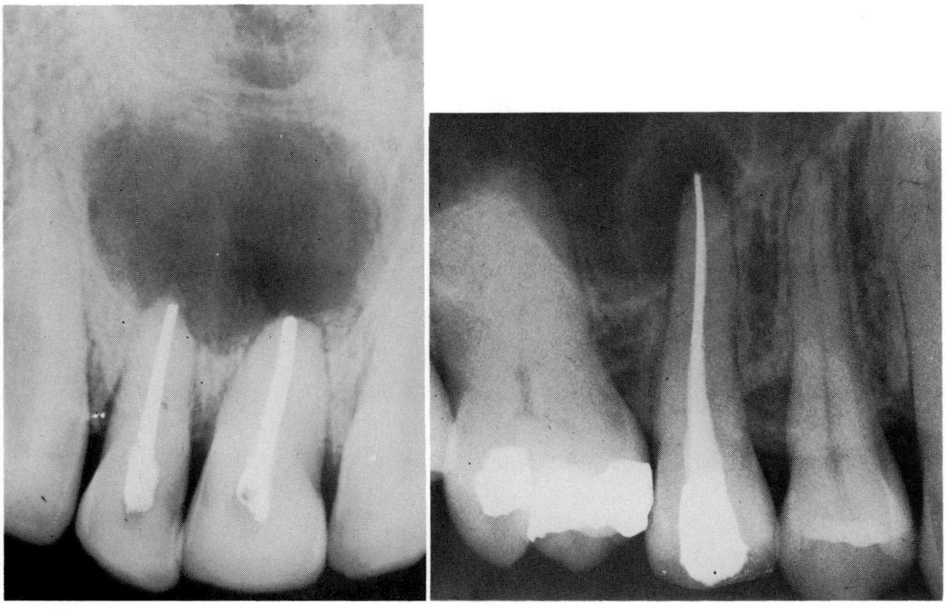

Fig. 6-8. Apical radiolucencies that persisted after adequate root canal fillings. Both these cases represent radicular cysts.

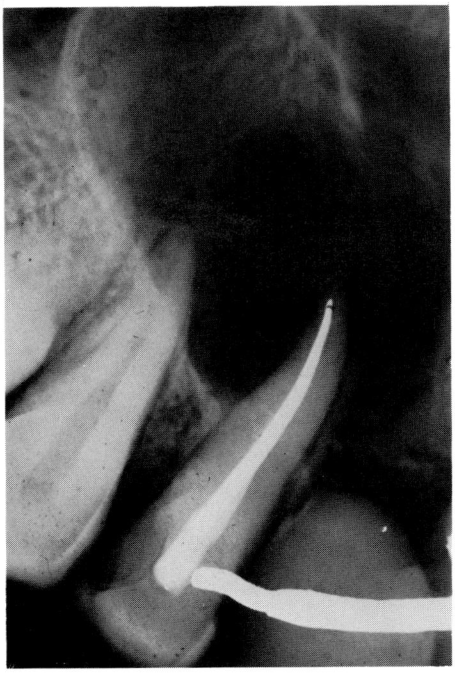

Fig. 6-9. Radiolucent area in the apical region of an endodontically treated tooth that proved to be a radicular cyst.

draining fistula nor any other local symptoms of pain represents an *apical scar* (Figs. 6-10 and 6-11). This lesion is self-limiting, and therefore the radiolucent zone *does not increase in size*. It consists of dense connective tissue that has no evidence of pathology but lacks the ability to form bone. The apical scar is often associated with a perforation of the buccal and/or the lingual (or palatal) cortical plate. It usually occurs in the maxillary and mandibular anterior teeth but can occur anywhere else in the jaws. Although in radiographs one can make the diagnosis of an apical scar only when an *asymptomatic* endodontically treated tooth has a previous history of apicoectomy or apical curettage, apical scars can and do occur in teeth where there is no history of apical surgery. In such cases, however, one cannot make an unequivocal diagnosis from the radiograph alone. The chance always exists that it could represent a dormant, or quiescent, radicular cyst or dental granluoma. If, however, apical surgery has previously been accomplished, the possibility of a granuloma or cyst is eliminated, and the clinician can make a definite diagnosis from the radiograph alone.

Apical scars do not always disappear after tooth extraction, and they may follow a tooth extraction. For this reason this type of radiolucency can occur in an edentulous site.

Apical scar constitutes about 3% of apical radiolucencies and requires no treatment.

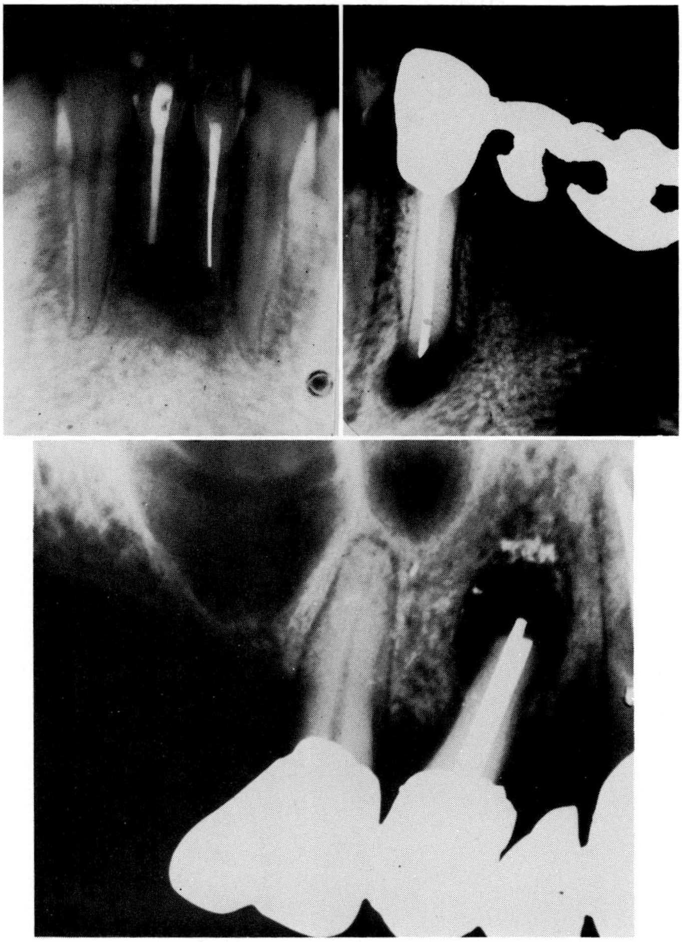

Fig. 6-10. Three teeth showing apical scars. These lesions were asymptomatic.

Rare apical lesions. On extremely rare occasions certain other lesions may occur at the apex of a tooth, but they can be diagnosed only on microscopic examination. They comprise less than 1% of apical radiolucencies, and their diagnosis should not be made from the radiographic examination alone. *Cholesteatoma* is a dental granuloma with numerous cholesterol crystals, and in radiographs it is indistinguishable from the dental granuloma, radicular cyst, or abscess (Fig. 6-12). Its treatment consists of endodontic therapy, but this procedure alone cannot lead to the disappearance of cholesterol deposits, and in spite of an apparently good root canal filling the apical radiolucency persists. The lesion is then treated surgically, and if the material is examined microscopically, the true nature of the radiolucency is revealed.

Radiolucent *foreign bodies* such as paper points, cotton, medicaments, or other materials may be left in the apical areas during endodontic therapy. They

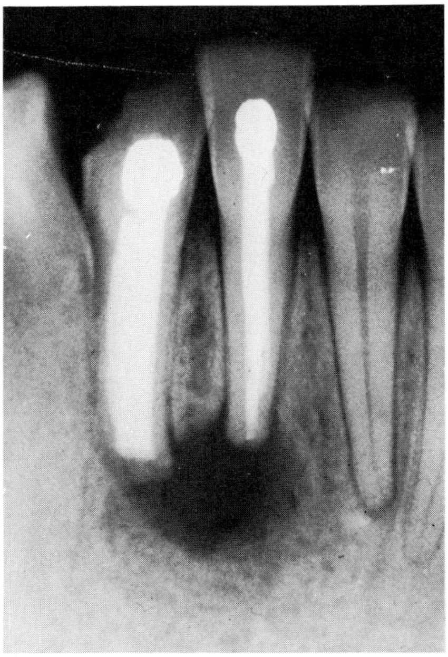

Fig. 6-11. Apical scar associated with two lower anterior teeth. These teeth had been subjected to three apical surgical procedures each. In the lateral incisor the root canal fillings had been removed and the canal refilled on two occasions.

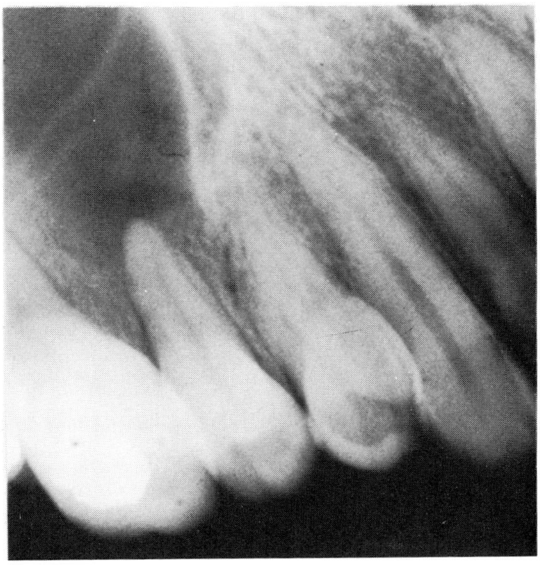

Fig. 6-12. Apical radiolucency associated with a nonvital second bicuspid. On histologic study it proved to be a cholesteatoma.

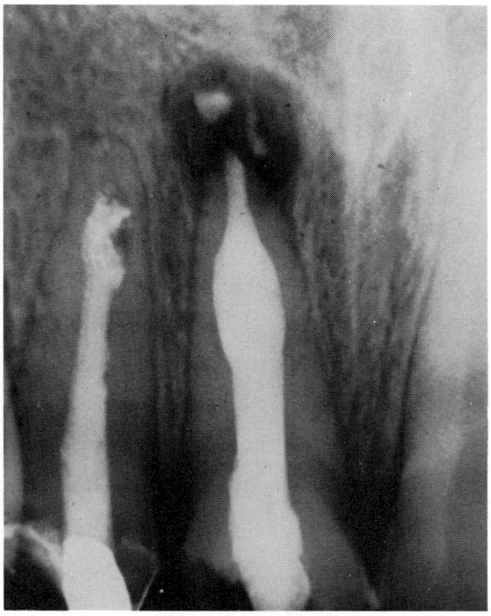

Fig. 6-13. Apical radiolucency representing scar tissue and foreign body reaction to a fragment of gutta-percha (seen as a radiopaque area in the radiolucency).

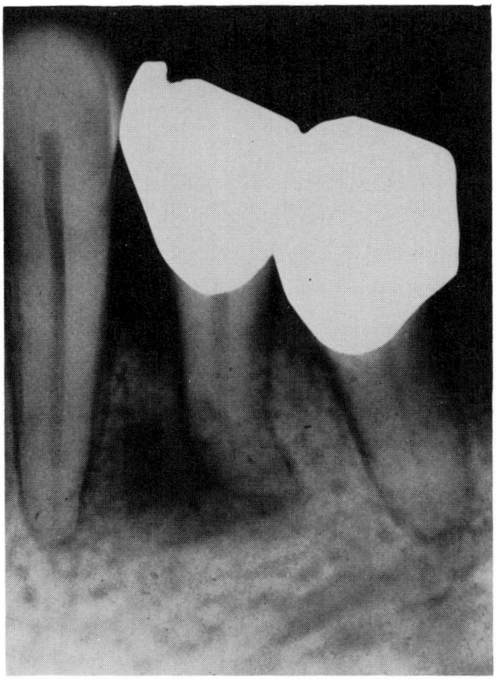

Fig. 6-14. Apical radiolucency associated with a vital lower bicuspid. It represented a central giant cell reparative granuloma.

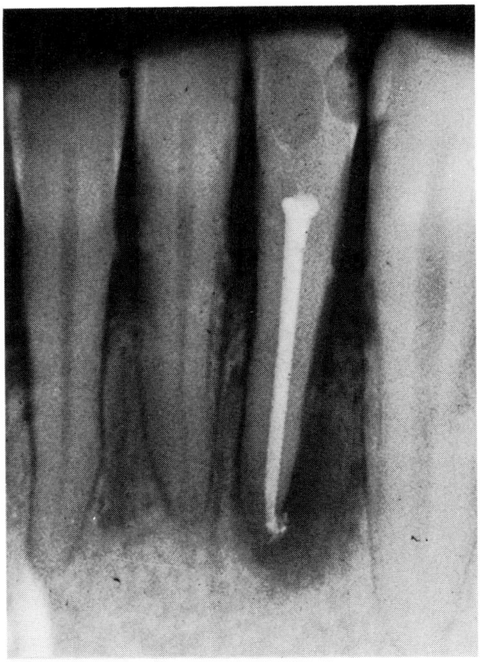

Fig. 6-15. Healing dental granuloma. Healing begins in the periphery and proceeds inward.

produce radiolucent *foreign body reactions* (Fig. 6-13). On extremely rare occasions a radiolucent lesion of the jaw, called *central giant cell reparative granuloma,* has been described in the apical area of a single tooth (Fig. 6-14). However, it is a rare phenomenon and has no clinical significance. The teeth in the region of this lesion are vital.

Healing of apical lesions. After endodontic therapy the dentist observes the outcome by checking the clinical symptoms and by examining periodic periapical radiographs. Interpretation of the posttreatment radiographs is therefore important. Both microscopically and in radiographs the formation of new bone first begins on the periphery of the radiolucent zones (Fig. 6-15). Although new bone formation has been shown microscopically to begin about four days after successful endodontic therapy, radiographs may not show any change in the size of the radiolucency for at least 3 or 4 weeks. On the other hand, if the apical repair occurs primarily with the formation of immature bone, the radiolucency may show no change for many months. After endodontic therapy it is necessary, therefore, to bear in mind the fact that if the apical radiolucency *does not increase in size* and the tooth remains asymptomatic, the healing process may well be progressing satisfactorily.

LESIONS IN MIDLINE OF MAXILLA

For radiologic purposes, the midline of the maxilla is defined as a Y-shaped line that extends from between the lateral incisor and cuspid on either side to the

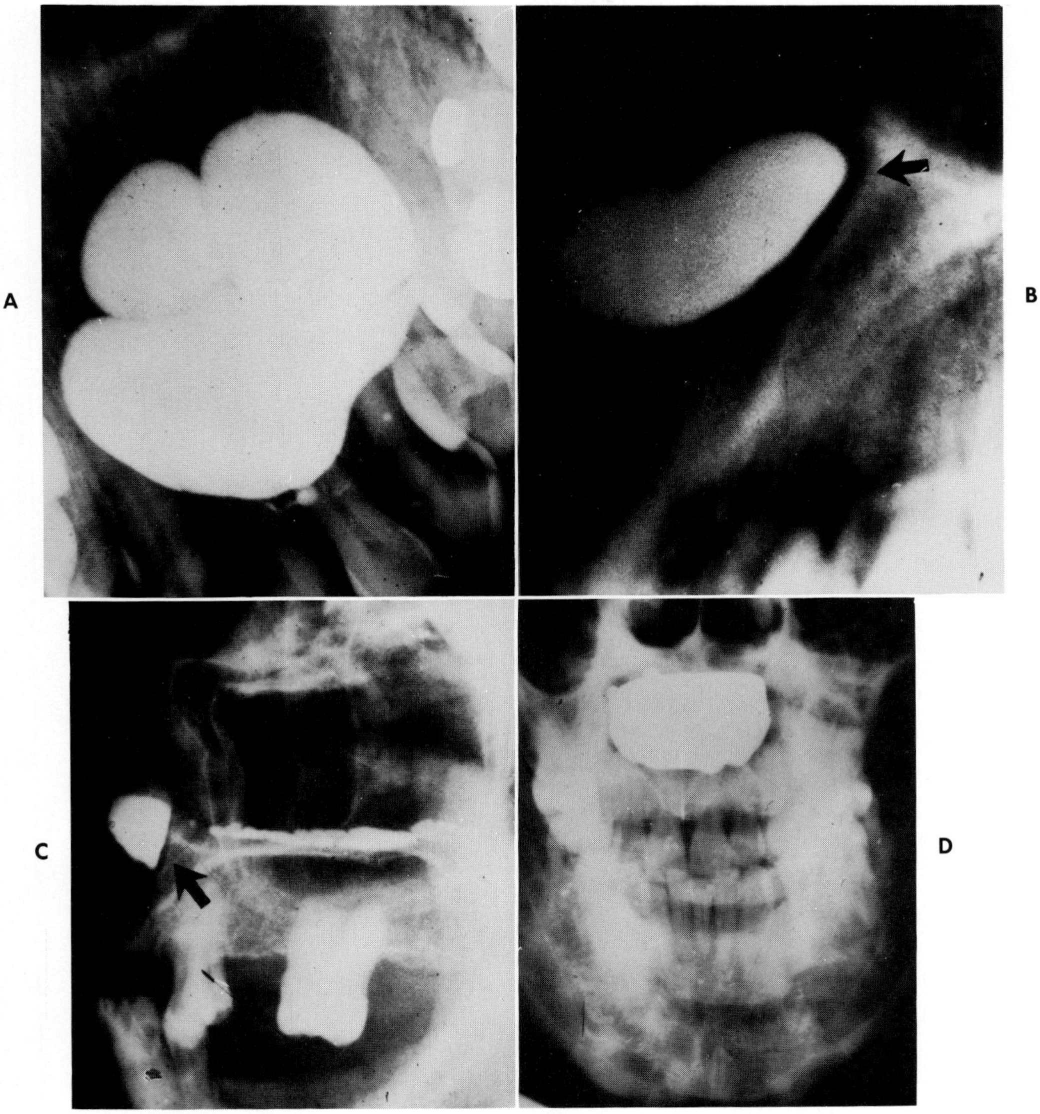

Fig. 6-16. Radiographs of three cases of nasolabial cyst, taken after the lesions were injected with Lipiodol. Without the radiopaque material there was no evidence of any abnormality. **A** and **B,** Occlusal and lateral views of the same case. **C** and **D,** Lateral and anteroposterior views of two nasolabial cysts. Note that in **B** the lesion appears to produce a slight depression on the outer aspect of the maxilla (arrow).

incisive papilla, and from there backward along the midline to the posterior end of the hard palate. The name, clinical features, and radiographic diagnosis of lesions along this line are discussed below.

Nasoalveolar cyst (nasolabial cyst). Located in the vestibule of the upper lateral and cuspid area, the nasoalveolar cyst, which is a soft tissue lesion, may not produce any radiolucency at all. In such cases, aspiration and/or radiographs taken with radiopaque contrast media establish the diagnosis (Fig. 6-16). On the other hand, it may destroy bone from the periosteal side, produce a de-

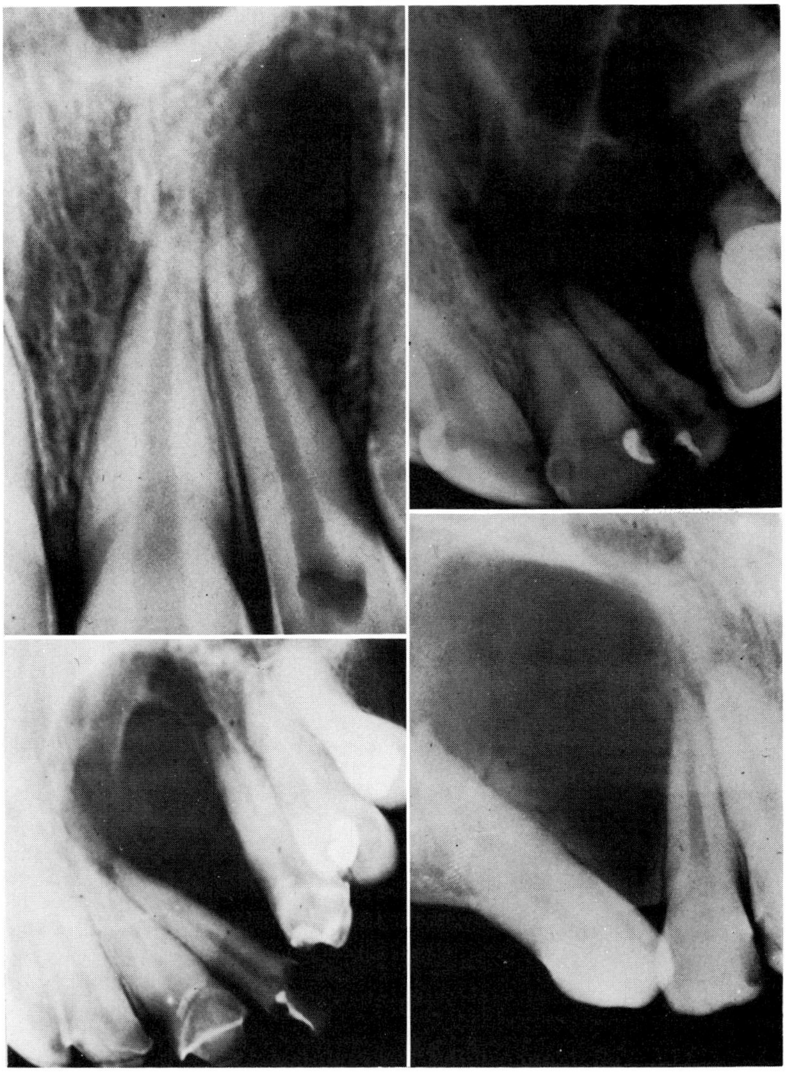

Fig. 6-17. Four cases of globulomaxillary cyst. All teeth in the area were vital. Location and pear-shaped outline are diagnostic.

pression on the buccal surface of the maxilla, and appear as a radiolucent defect. This is also seen best in the lateral radiographs when the cyst is partially filled with a contrast medium (Fig. 6-16, *B*). All teeth in the area are vital, and clinically one can see the involvement of the lip and the floor of the nose. It comprises about 3% of maxillary midline radiolucencies and is treated by excision.

Globulomaxillary cyst. About 21% of radiolucencies of the midline of the maxilla represent globulomaxillary cyst. It is always located between the lateral and the cuspid, the teeth are vital, and there may be palpable enlargements in the area. The radiograph often shows as an inverted, pear-shaped radiolucency that extends between the roots of the cuspid and the lateral (Fig. 6-17). The roots of the teeth are usually pushed apart, and it is treated by excision.

Median alveolar cyst. The extremely rare radiolucency representing a median alveolar cyst is located between the maxillary central incisors. Teeth are vital. It is believed by some that this lesion does not exist as an entity but merely represents an incisive canal cyst (Fig. 6-18).

Nasopalatine cysts. Incisive canal cyst and cyst of palatine papilla, the most common radiolucent lesions of this group, are referred to as the nasopalatine cysts and comprise about 66% of all radiolucent lesions of the midline of the maxilla. Located in the midline, between central incisors, the *incisive canal cyst* is a heart-

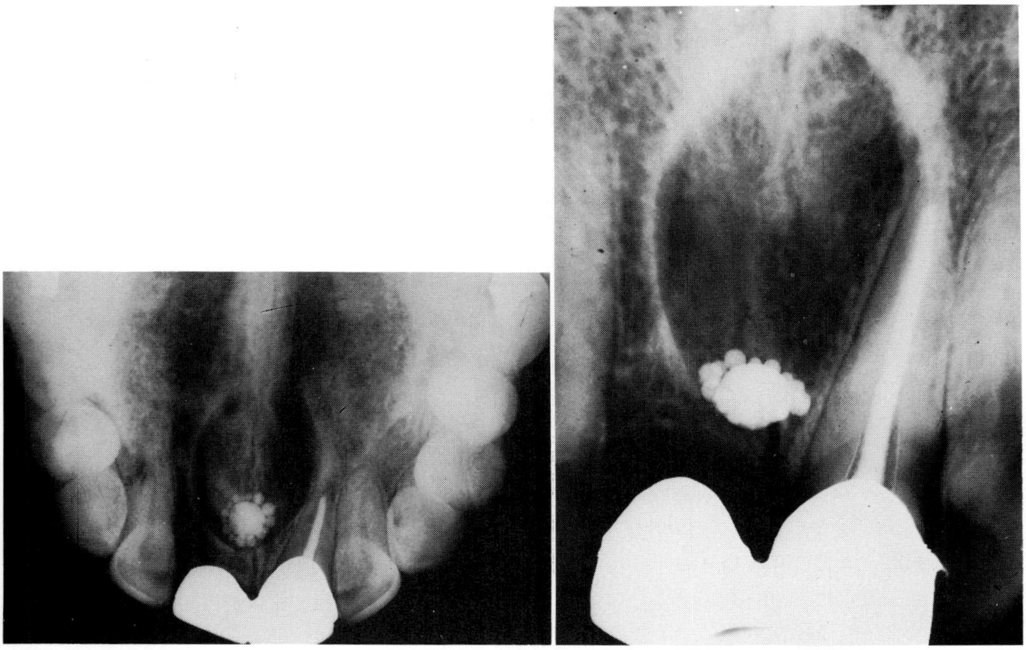

Fig. 6-18. Radiographs showing a so-called median alveolar cyst. In the two views the radiopaque area is a small amount of Lipiodol that was injected to demonstrate the lower border of the cyst.

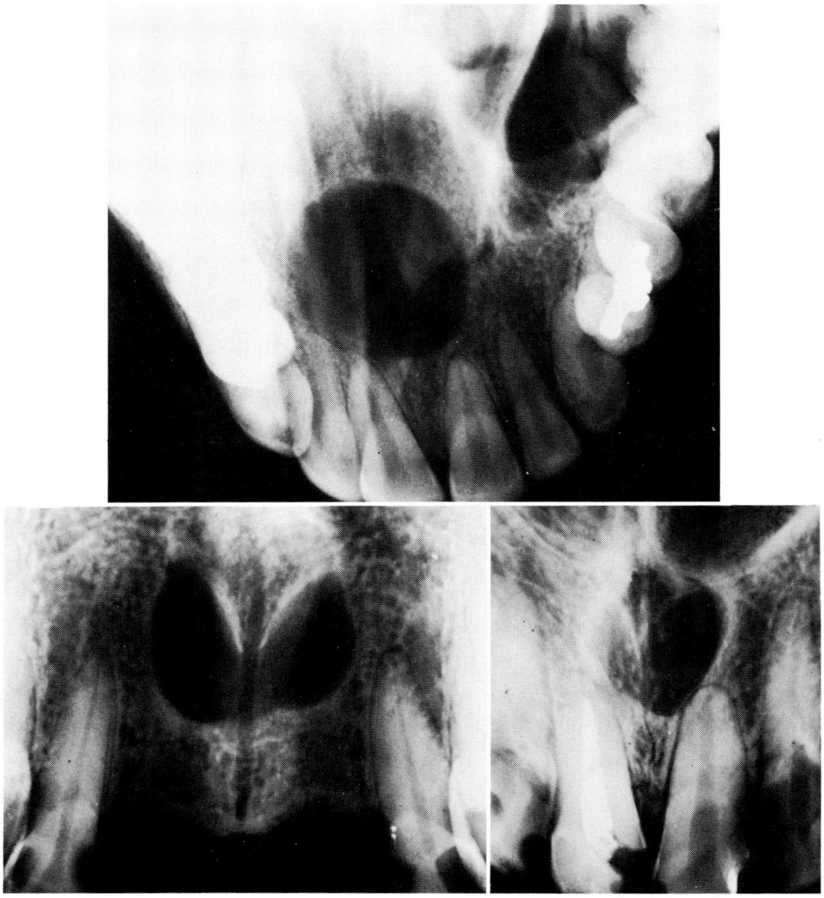

Fig. 6-19. Three cases of incisive canal cyst. Note that in the intraoral apical views the nasal spine is usually superimposed on the radiolucency, giving it a heart-shaped appearance.

shaped radiolucency (Fig. 6-19). The heart-shaped appearance is produced by the superimposition of the nasal spine over the radiolucency of the cyst. In occlusal views both the nasal spine and the septum are superimposed on the cyst. The teeth are vital. This lesion is located higher than the so-called medial alveolar cyst. Since the incisive canal appears as a radiolucency in radiographs, it is often difficult to distinguish between a large incisive canal and a small incisive canal cyst. This distinction can be made, however, by attempting aspiration of the area. If fluid can be aspirated, the radiolucency can be assumed to represent a cyst.

The *cyst of the palatine papilla* occurs in soft tissue over the incisive canal and may produce no radiolucent defect. On the other hand, it may produce a "cupping" of the underlying bone, and in radiographs it is indistinguishable from the cyst of the incisive canal. Nasopalatine cysts are treated by excision.

Table 2. Diagnostic features of radiolucencies in midline of maxilla

LOCATION	RADIOLOGIC AND CLINICAL ASPECTS	DIAGNOSIS
Vestibule of lateral and cuspid area	All teeth vital; radiolucency occurs only if this soft tissue cyst produces bone resorption from periosteal side; about 3% of midline radiolucencies	Nasolabial cyst or nasoalveolar cyst
Between cuspid and lateral incisor	Teeth vital; radiolucency often "inverted pear" shaped; about 21% of midline radiolucencies	Globulomaxillary cyst
Between central incisors	Teeth vital; lesion not heart-shaped; incisive canal and papilla not involved	Median alveolar cyst
Between central incisors (area of incisive canal)	Heart-shaped radiolucency; teeth vital; most common radiolucency of midline of maxilla; comprises about 66% of such lesions	Incisive canal cyst or cyst of palatine papilla (nasopalatine cysts)
Posterior to incisive papilla	Swelling and radiolucency in midline of hard palate; only about 9% of lesions of midline	Median palatine cyst

Median palatine cyst. About 9% of midline radiolucencies of the maxilla occur posterior to the incisive papilla in the midline of the hard palate and represent the *median palatine cyst.* Teeth in the area are vital, and excision is the treatment of choice.

Rare midline lesions. Salivary gland tumors of the palate can, on rare occasions, produce radiolucent defects in the midline of the maxilla.

The diagnostic features of radiolucencies in the midline of the maxilla are summarized in Table 2.

LESIONS IN PLACE OF MISSING TOOTH

When a tooth (usually permanent) is missing in the arch and its place is occupied by a radiolucency, the following possibilities exist:

1. Primordial cyst
2. Ameloblastoma
3. Rare odontogenic lesion

When a radiolucency exists in place of a tooth that failed to develop, it most likely represents a primordial cyst (Fig. 6-20). The possibility of ameloblastoma or an odontogenic tumor is far less likely, and biopsy is the only means of definitive diagnosis. In all these cases the regional teeth are vital. If they are not, one cannot exclude the possibility of radicular cyst. The primordial cyst may arise in the presence of the normal complement of teeth (Figs. 6-21 and 6-22). Such cysts originate from the enamel organ of supernumerary teeth. The treatment of all these lesions is surgical excision.

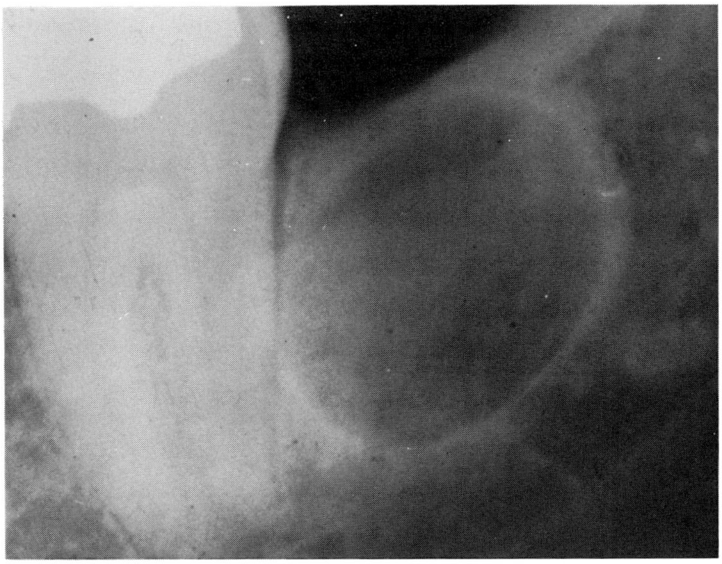

Fig. 6-20. Radiolucent area in place of a missing third molar. Lesion represents a primordial cyst.

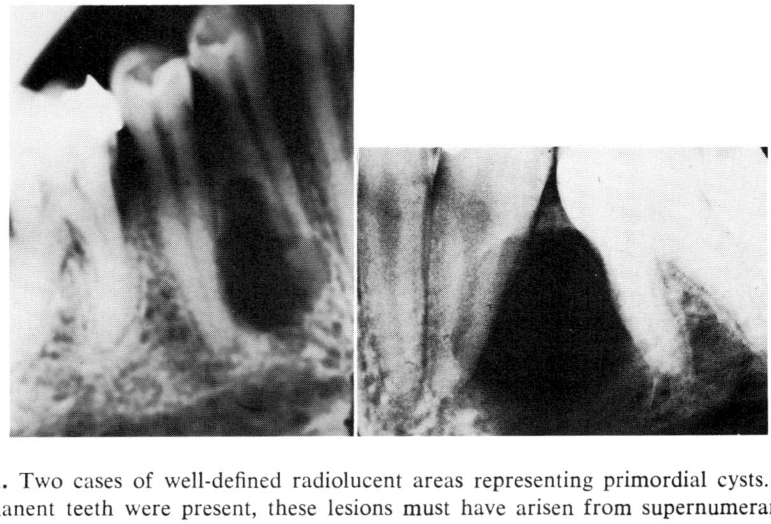

Fig. 6-21. Two cases of well-defined radiolucent areas representing primordial cysts. Since all the permanent teeth were present, these lesions must have arisen from supernumerary, or accessory, tooth germs.

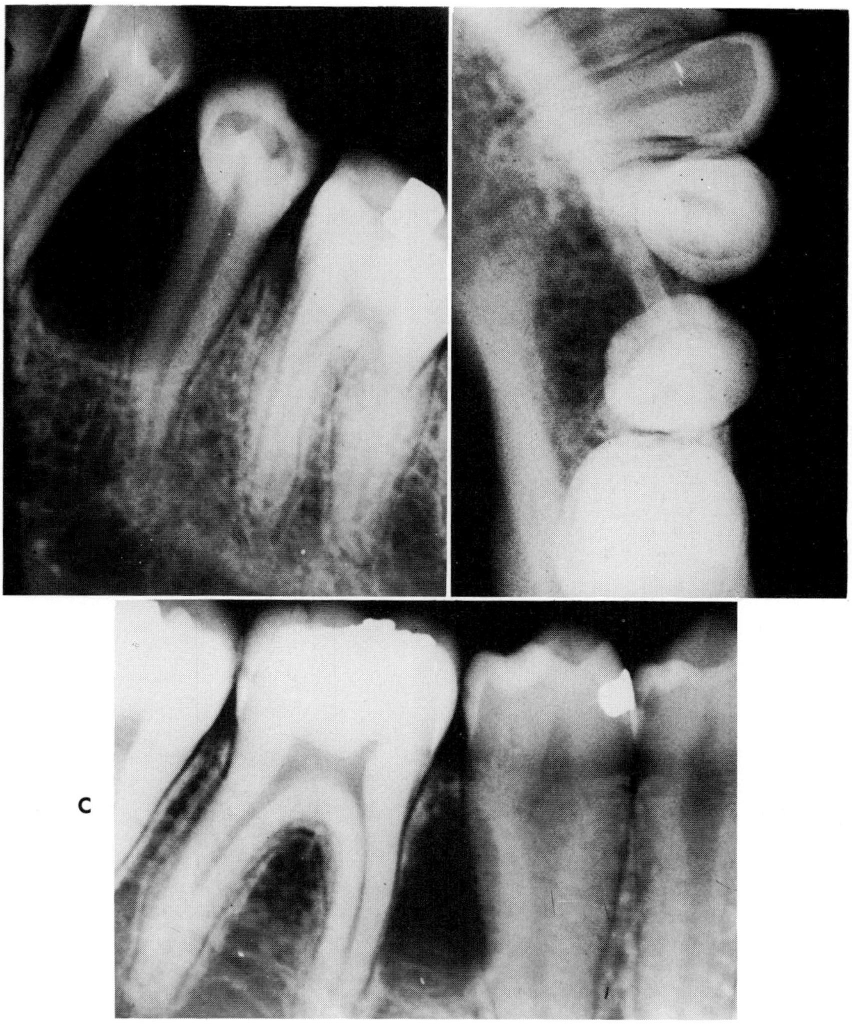

Fig. 6-22. Two primordial cysts. **A** and **B** represent the intraoral and occlusal radiographs of the same case. These radiolucencies are of long duration and are clearly outlined. The second case is shown in **C.**

LESIONS AROUND CROWN OF IMPACTED TOOTH

A radiolucency around the crown of an unerupted tooth represents one of the following lesions:

1. Dentigerous cyst
2. Odontogenic fibroma (and odontogenic myxoma)
3. Eruption cyst
4. Ameloblastoma
5. Adenoameloblastoma

A

B

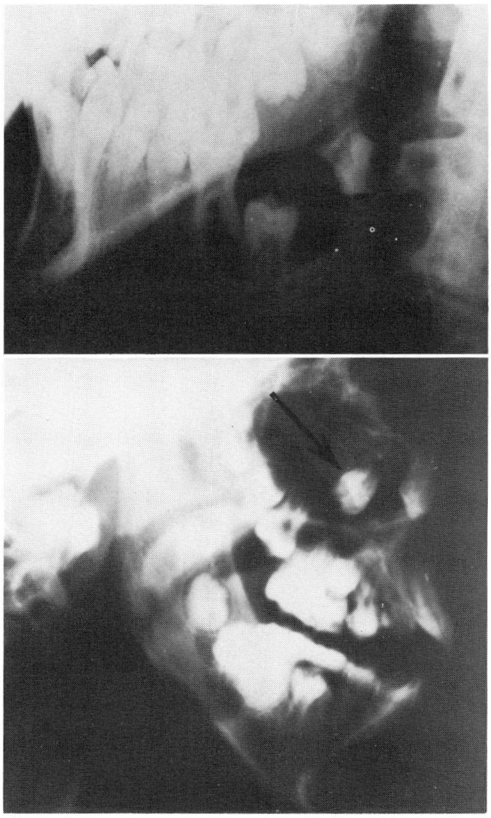

Fig. 6-23. Radiolucencies around impacted crowns usually represent dentigerous cysts. In **B** the dentigerous cyst has led to the migration of the molar into the maxillary sinus (arrow).

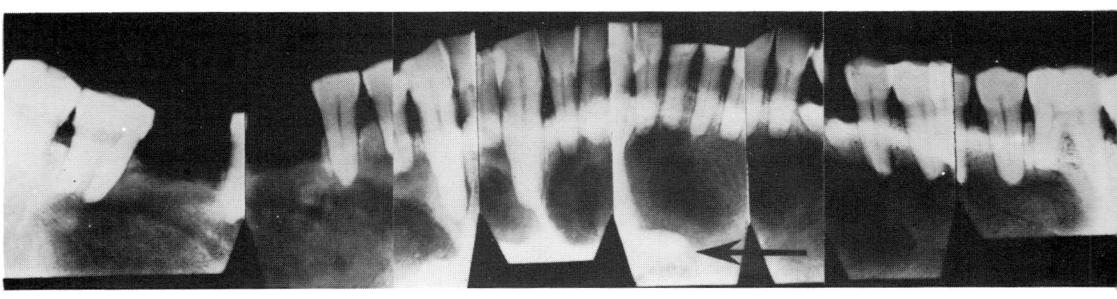

Fig. 6-24. Intraoral apical radiographs of the mandible, showing a large dentigerous cyst associated with an impacted tooth (arrow). Lesion extends from the right to the left first molar teeth.

A 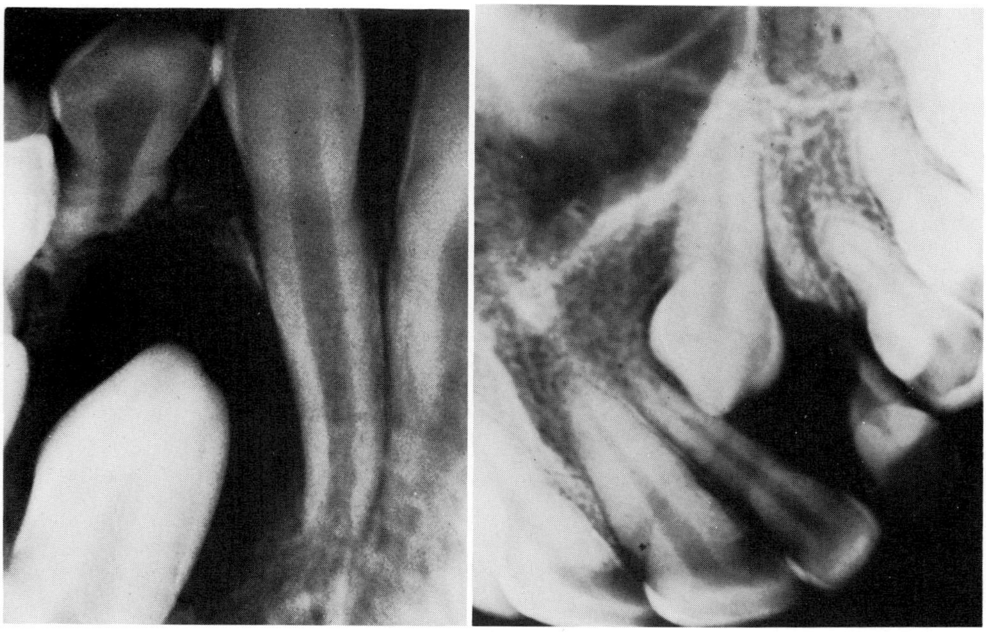 B

Fig. 6-25. A, Odontogenic fibroma. **B,** Odontogenic myxoma.

Dentigerous cyst and odontogenic fibroma. More than 95% of radiolucencies around an impacted tooth represent the dentigerous cyst and the odontogenic fibroma (Figs. 6-23 to 6-25). Distinction between these two can be made only at surgical exploration. The dentigerous cyst is a cystic, fluid-containing lesion, whereas the odontogenic fibroma is a benign tumor that presents as a solid mass. These two lesions are identical in the radiographs, and in the past, many radiolucent lesions that represented odontogenic fibroma were misinterpreted as dentigerous cysts. Both of these conditions may lead to the "expansion" of the jaw, but it usually indicates a dentigerous cyst. In these cases the cortical plate is always unbroken (Fig. 6-26). The *odontogenic myxoma* is only a variant of the odontogenic fibroma and can be distinguished from it only histologically (Fig. 6-25). Its radiographic appearance is identical to that of the dentigerous cyst and the odontogenic fibroma.

On rare occasions a dentigerous cyst may be located to one side of an impacted or erupted crown, and for these cases the term *lateral dentigerous cyst* is often used (Fig. 6-27).

Eruption cyst. Many radiographs show an erupting tooth surrounded by a radiolucency that may or may not show cortical bone on the oral surface (Fig. 6-28). Such a radiolucency represents an eruption cyst. In reality, however, an eruption cyst is a dentigerous cyst that begins to develop during the active eruptive phase of a tooth and is carried by the eruption into the soft tissues of the alveolar crest (Fig. 6-29).

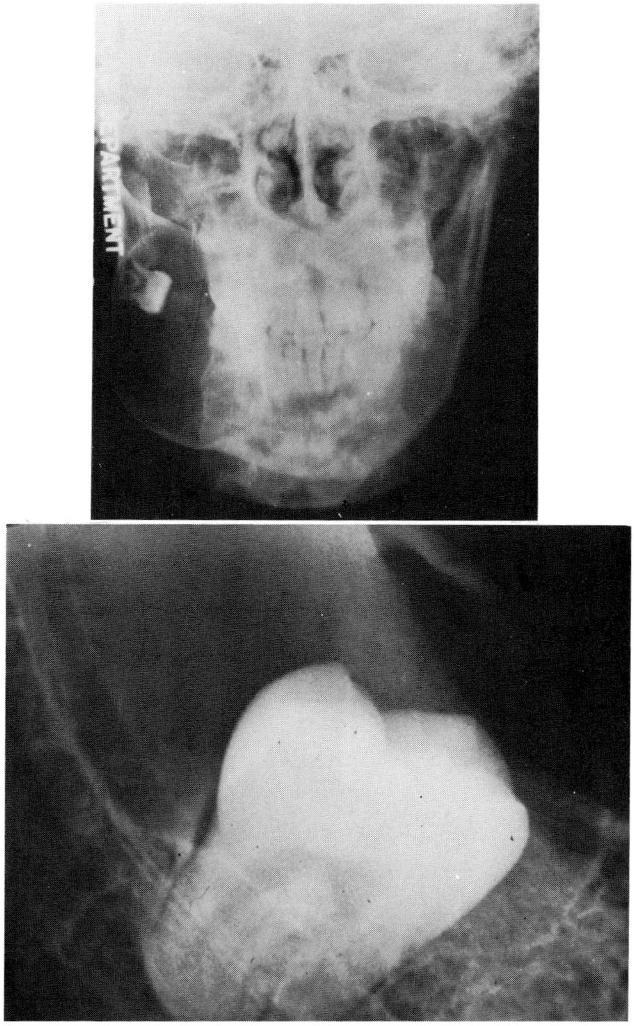

Fig. 6-26. Two dentigerous cysts with "expansion" of the cortical plate. Note that the cortex is not eroded or destroyed.

Ameloblastoma and adenoameloblastoma. The ameloblastoma and the adenoameloblastoma are far less common lesions of this group. The possibility of an ameloblastoma is usually considered only in radiolucencies around the crowns of mandibular molars (Fig. 6-30). Patients are usually, but not always, older than 30 years. The adenoameloblastoma, also a rare member of this group, occurs in patients who are younger than 20 years of age and most often involves the cuspid area of the maxilla (Fig. 6-31). It can, however, occur elsewhere (Fig. 6-32). The diagnosis of ameloblastoma, when there is a unicystic radiolucency around an impacted crown, or of adenoameloblastoma is made only on histologic

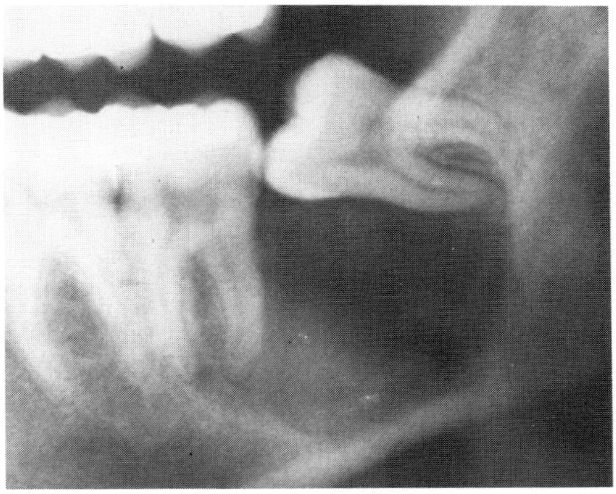

Fig. 6-27. Lateral dentigerous cyst develops or migrates to the lateral side of the crown.

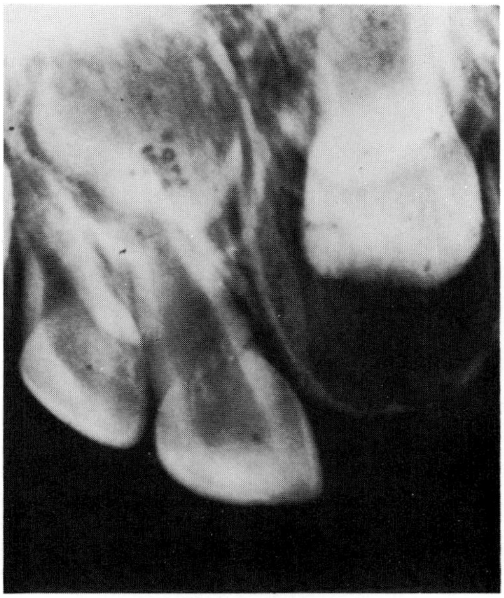

Fig. 6-28. Radiolucency around the crown of an erupting central incisor. This type of a dentigerous cyst is called an eruption cyst.

A B C D

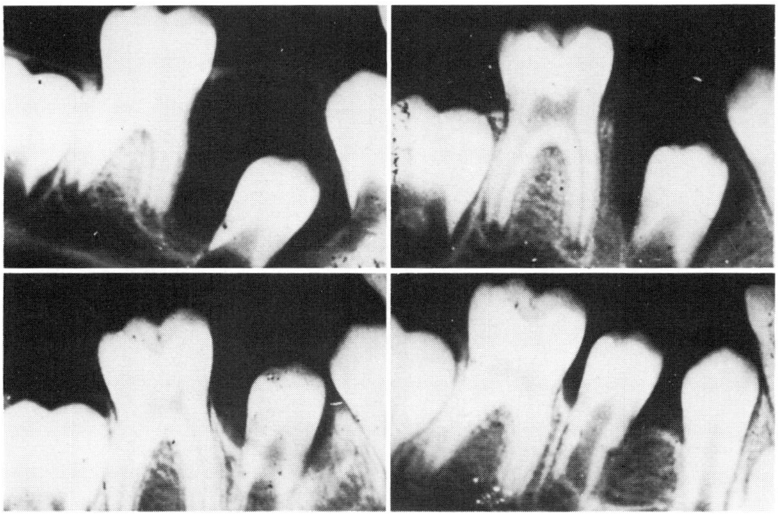

Fig. 6-29. Series of radiographs taken of a radiolucency around a developing second mandibular cuspid, **A.** As the tooth continued to develop and erupt, the dentigerous cyst became an eruption cyst, **B** and **C,** and finally disappeared in oral cavity, **D.**

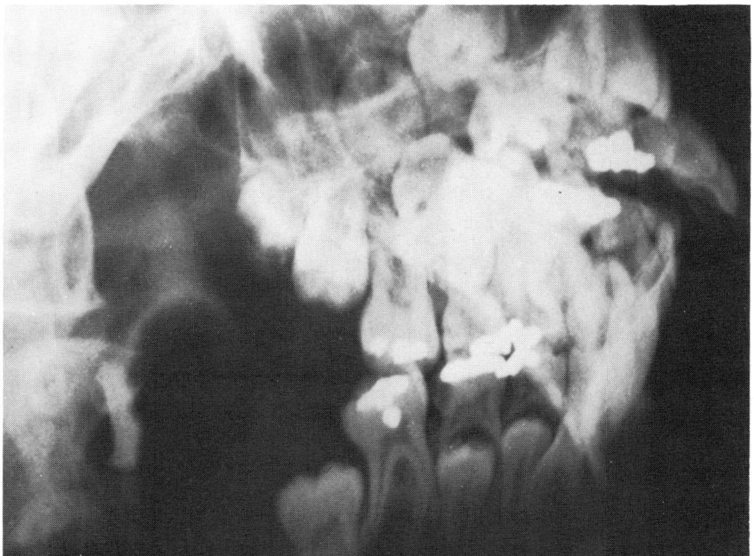

Fig. 6-30. Radiolucency around the crown of an impacted second lower molar. This radiolucency represented an ameloblastoma. Such a lesion in a young patient is rare.

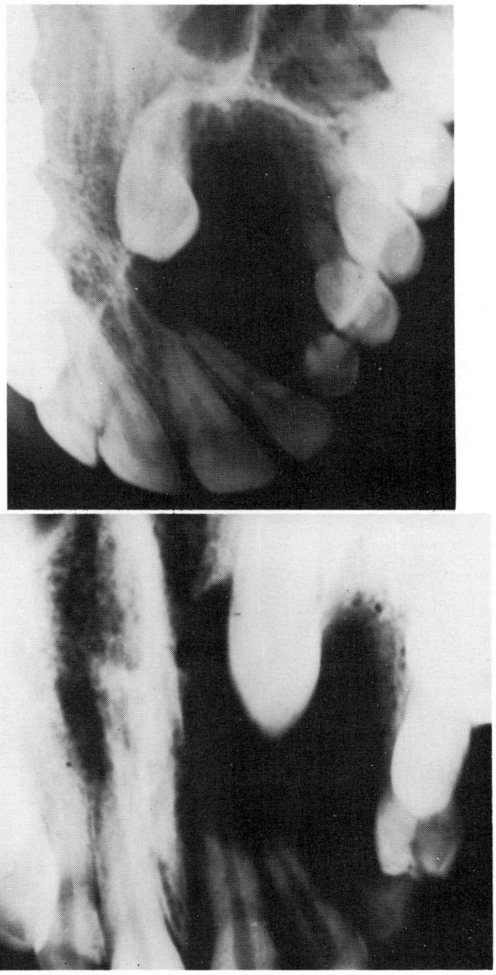

Fig. 6-31. Two cases of radiolucencies around crowns of impacted maxillary cuspids, representing adenoameloblastoma.

examination. Radiologically, these lesions are usually mistaken for a dentigerous cyst or an odontogenic fibroma.

SOAP BUBBLE–LIKE RADIOLUCENCIES

A soap bubble–like lesion appears as multiple radiolucent foci located at the same area. The soap bubble appearance is caused by the presence of radiopaque septa in the radiolucent area. Since these lesions do not destroy all bony trabeculae in their path of growth, radiopaque lines can be seen. Furthermore, since the lesions grow in different directions and at different rates, the radiolucencies have a scalloped outline.

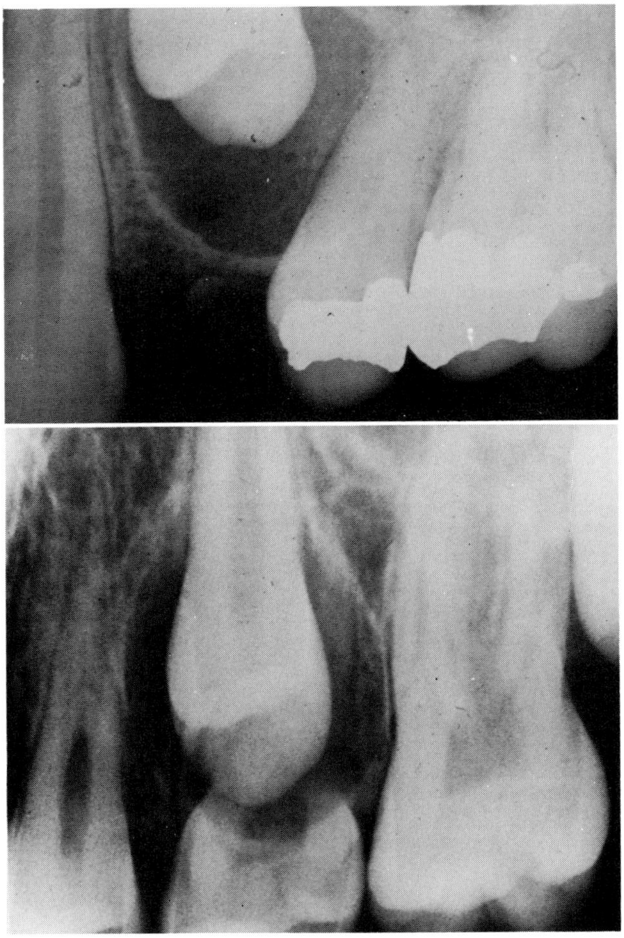

Fig. 6-32. Radiolucent lesions around crowns of impacted bicuspid teeth. Both radiographs show adenoameloblastoma.

To this group belong the following:

1. Central giant cell reparative granuloma
2. Aneurysmal bone cyst
3. Ameloblastoma
4. Rare lesions (cherubism, myxoma, and multilocular follicular cyst)

All these conditions are benign and are of long duration. The regional teeth are vital. They all tend to produce enlargement (expansion) of the jaw. The major clinical features of these radiolucencies are discussed below. Although these features often assist the dentist in making a correct diagnosis from the radiograph alone, in most cases surgical intervention is unavoidable, and a definitive diagnosis is subsequently established on tissue examination.

Central giant cell reparative granuloma. This lesion occurs usually in patients under 20 years of age, is more common in females, and presents an expansile

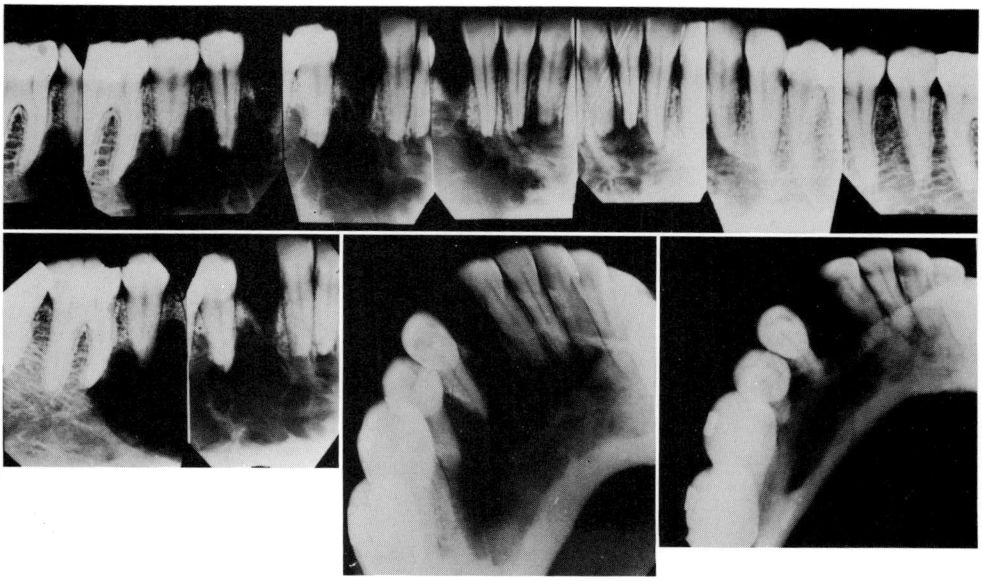

Fig. 6-33. Soap bubble–like radiolucency in the mandible. Lateral incisor was extracted prior to making a correct diagnosis. Lesion was in a patient 21 years old and represented a central giant cell reparative granuloma (intraoral and extraoral views).

soap bubble appearance (Figs. 6-33 to 6-35). There is often a history of trauma. The teeth are always vital, but some cases show root resorption. The lesion is often expansile, but there are usually no symptoms. Treatment consists of local curettage.

Aneurysmal bone cyst. The aneurysmal bone cyst is only a variant of the central giant cell reparative granuloma and can be distinguished from it only by histologic examination. In all other aspects it is identical to the central giant cell reparative granuloma (Fig. 6-36).

Ameloblastoma. About 80% of ameloblastomas occur in the bicuspid and molar area of the mandible. Although radiographically the lesion may be unicystic (p. 122), usually it presents as a soap bubble–like lesion (Figs. 6-37 and 6-38). It is often expansile, and it occurs more often in the male and usually in persons older than 30 years of age. Teeth in the area are vital. Tooth migration is common, but root resorption is rare. In some borderline cases differential diagnosis from the central giant cell reparative granuloma is not possible, and biopsy is the only way to distinguish them.

Rare lesions. In the presence of a soap bubble-like lesion, the three conditions just described should be the first to be considered in a differential diagnosis. There are, however, some rare lesions of the jaws that also present a soap bubble appearance: cherubism, myxoma, and multilocular follicular cyst.

Cherubism is usually a bilateral lesion that presents a soap bubble appearance.

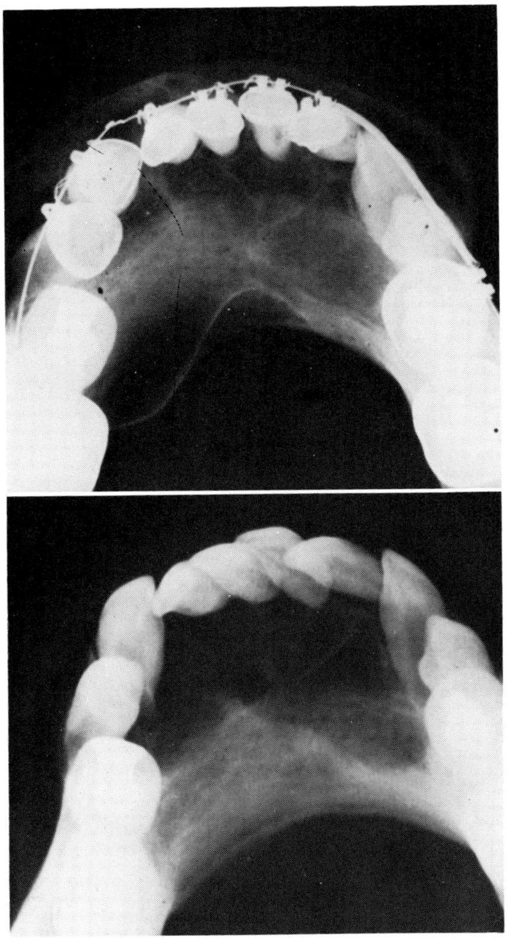

Fig. 6-34. Central giant cell reparative granuloma of the mandible in a young patient. Note the soap bubble, expansile radiolucency and the migration of teeth.

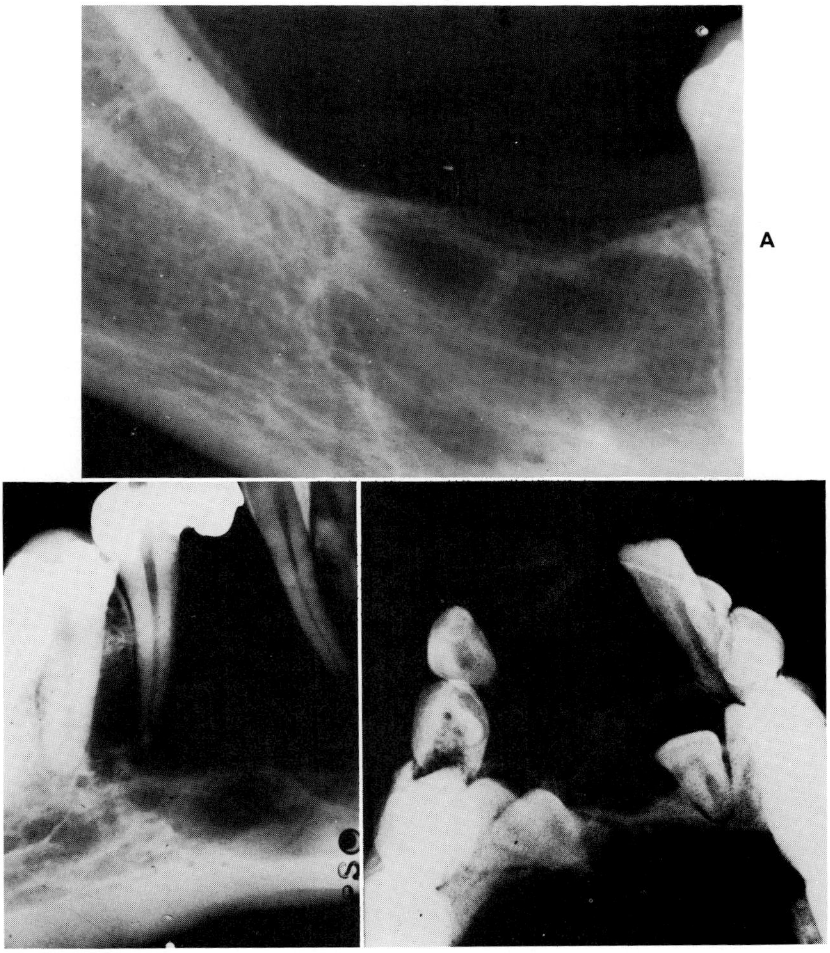

Fig. 6-35. Three cases of central giant cell reparative granuloma. **A,** Soap bubble radiolucency is characteristic. Migration of teeth can be frequently seen in intraoral, **B,** and occlusal, **C,** radiographs.

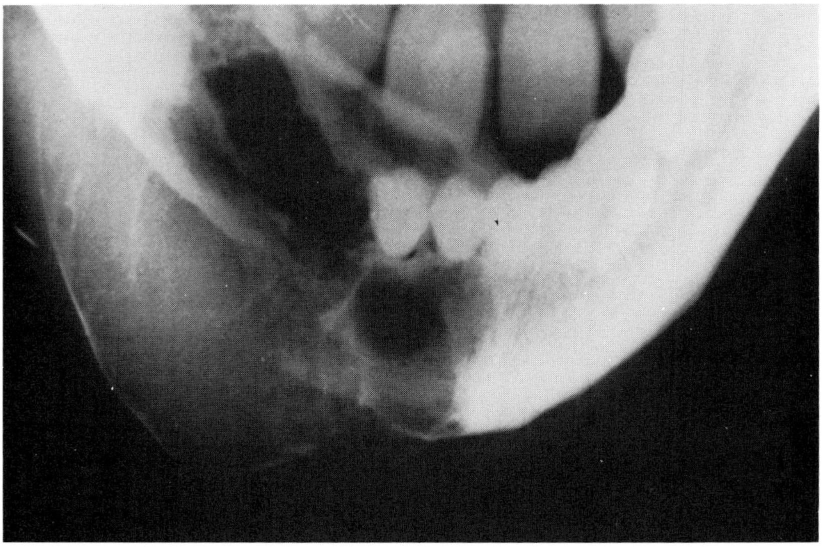

Fig. 6-36. Occlusal radiograph of an aneurysmal bone cyst of the mandible. Soap bubble radiolucency is the usual feature of this lesion.

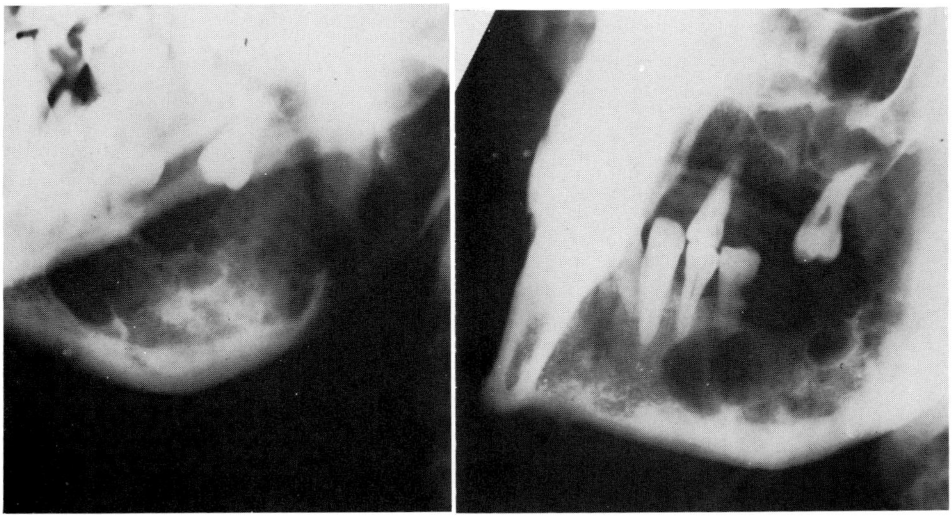

Fig. 6-37. Soap bubble radiolucency of the molar area of the mandible that revealed an ameloblastoma on biopsy.

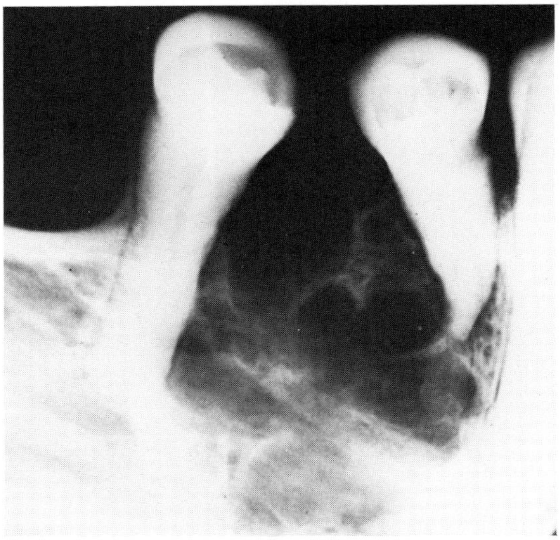

Fig. 6-38. Radiograph of an ameloblastoma, showing a soap bubble–like radiolucency. Multilocular cyst has an identical radiographic appearance.

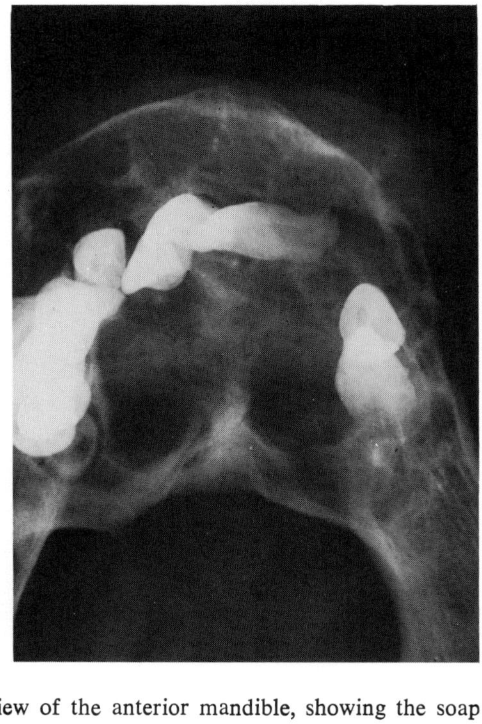

Fig. 6-39. Occlusal view of the anterior mandible, showing the soap bubble-like radiolucency of cherubism.

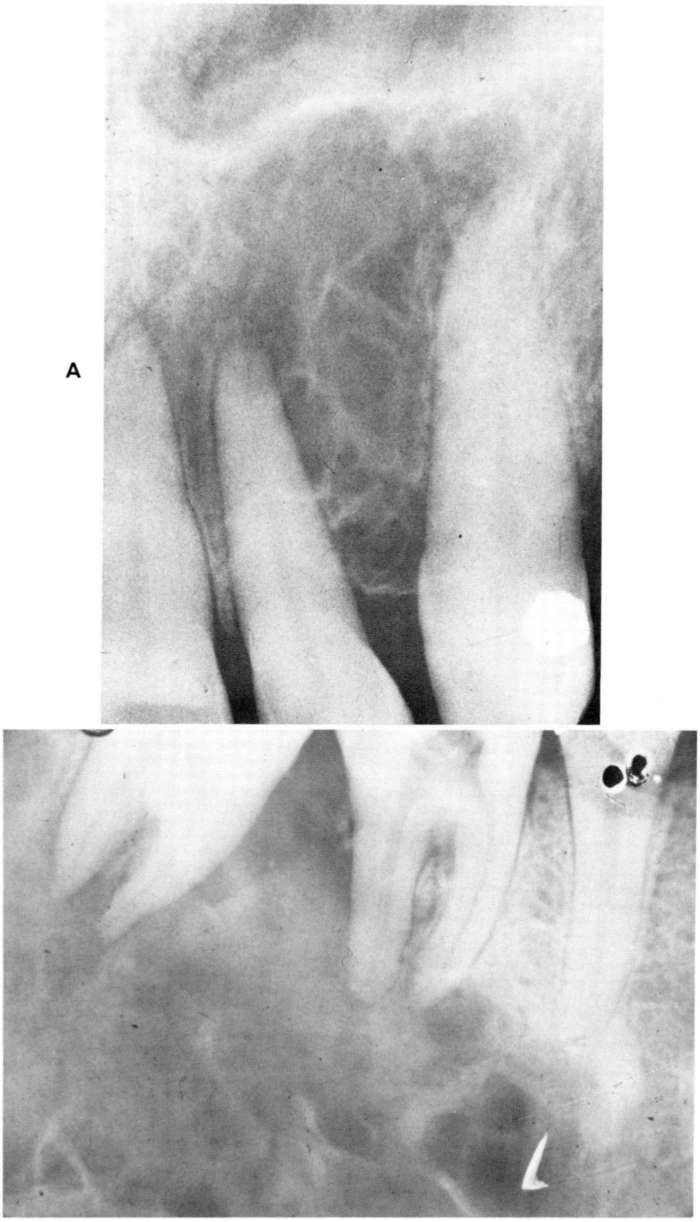

Fig. 6-40. Two cases of rare myxoma of the jaws. **A,** Maxilla and, **B,** mandible. In **A** the entire lesion can be seen, but **B** shows only a part of the tumor. These cases can be diagnosed only by histologic examination.

Table 3. Diagnostic features of soap bubble type of radiographic lesions of the jaws

LESION	CLINICAL FEATURES
Central giant cell reparative granuloma—and aneurysmal bone cyst	Patient under 20 years; more common in female; history of trauma
Ameloblastoma	Patient over 30 years; more common in male; posterior part of mandible favored site
Cherubism	Occurs in children of either sex; long duration; hereditary; migration of teeth; lesions may involve both jaws; no pain or symptoms
Myxoma	Extremely rare; migration and loosening of teeth common
Multilocular follicular cyst	Indistinguishable from ameloblastoma but very rare

It will be discussed with multiple but separate radiolucent lesions. Sometimes, when discovered early, however, it may be seen only in one area of the jaws (Fig. 6-39). The condition is hereditary, involves a number of members of the family, begins in early years (3 to 5 years of age), and therefore can be distinguished from other members of this group with ease. Migration of erupted and unerupted teeth is common, but loosening and exfoliation are rare (Fig. 6-39). Cherubism requires no treatment.

Myxoma is a very rare central tumor of the jaw. It has a multilocular or reticulated appearance (Fig. 6-40) and produces enlargement of the jaw as well as migration and loosening of teeth. Its definitive diagnosis is made only on histopathologic examination, and its treatment is wide local excision. Because of its rarity, one cannot make a presumptive diagnosis of myxoma from a radiographic examination.

The *multilocular follicular cyst* is a very rare form of follicular cyst that occurs in the mandibular molar area and may be associated with other developmental disturbances such as sebaceous cysts.

Table 3 gives a brief summary of the diagnostic features of soap bubble–like lesions of the jaws.

MULTIPLE BUT SEPARATE RADIOLUCENT LESIONS

Multiple but separate radiolucent lesions are rare, but when they occur, they represent one of the following:

1. Cementoma (stage I)
2. Histiocytosis X
3. Hyperparathyroidism
4. Cherubism
5. Multiple myeloma
6. Metastatic tumors

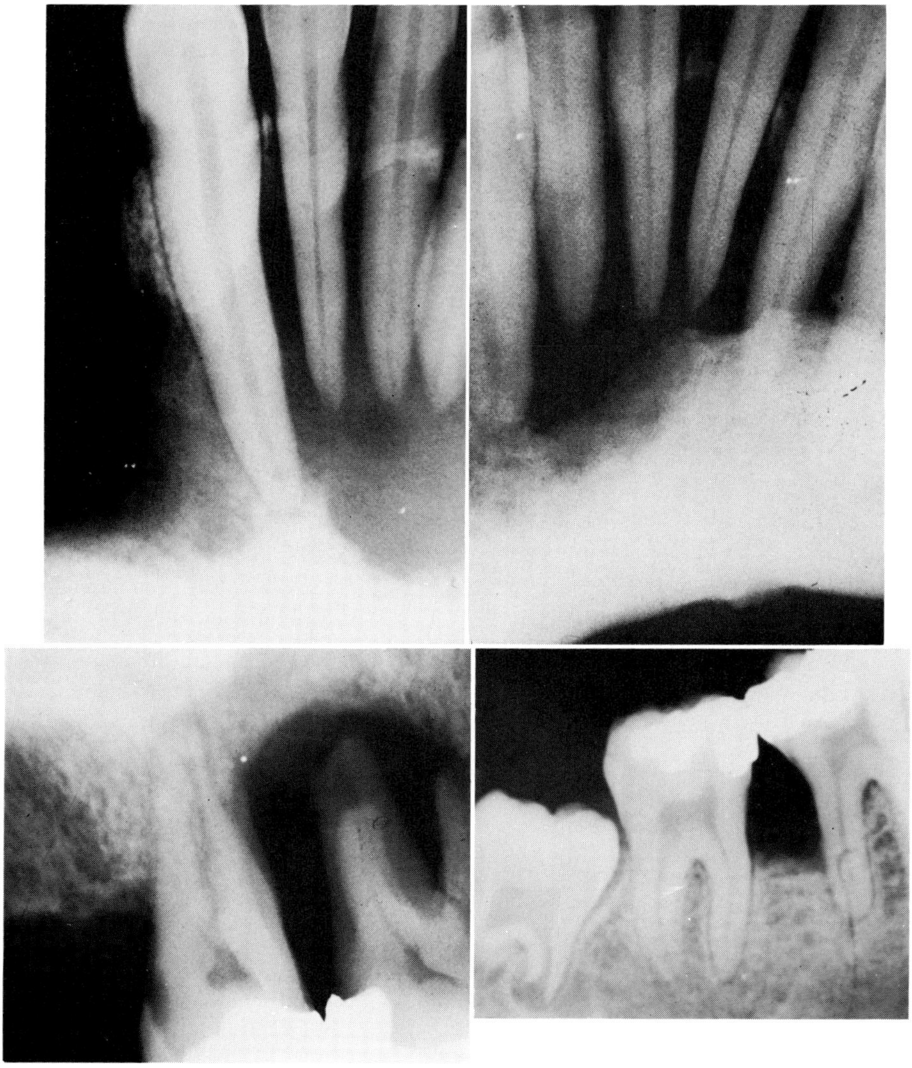

Fig. 6-41. Four radiographs of the maxillary and mandibular teeth, showing multiple radiolucent foci of eosinophilic granuloma in the same patient. Teeth in the area of the lesion appear to "hang in air."

The essential diagnostic features of these lesions are discussed below and are summarized in Table 4, p. 148.

Cementoma (stage I). This lesion was described previously (p. 106). Usually it occurs in multiple apical sites as discrete radiolucent lesions. Its location at the apices of teeth and the fact that all teeth are vital are important diagnostic features.

Histiocytosis X. The term histiocytosis X applies to three related diseases which, in ascending order of severity, are *eosinophilic granuloma, Hand-Schüller-Christian disease,* and *Letterer-Siwe disease.* Whereas the eosinophilic granuloma occurs in the second or third decade of life, Hand-Schüller-Christian disease occurs in the first decade, and Letterer-Siwe disease usually occurs before 2 years of age. The most important feature of histiocytosis X is that the jaws usually show multiple radiolucent foci that are independent of each other and that may be the first evidence of the disease (Figs. 6-41 to 6-44). Radiographs are almost diagnostic and are similar in the three diseases. Intraoral radiographs show

Text continued on p. 140.

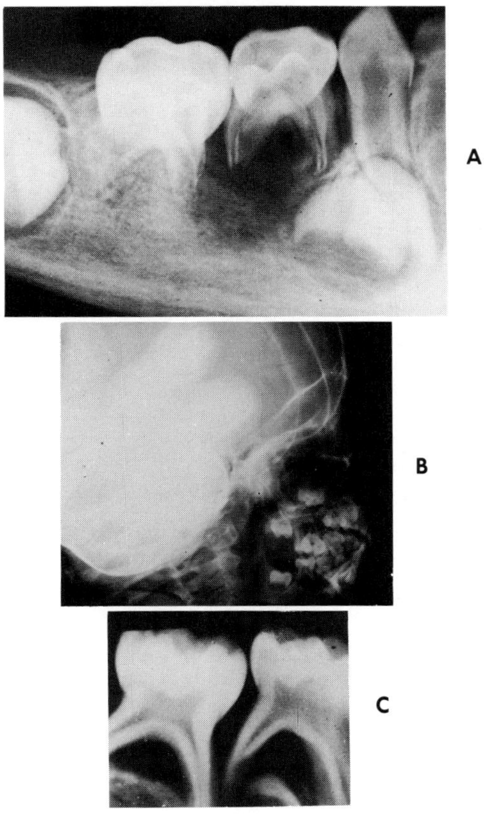

Fig. 6-42. Radiolucencies of eosinophilic granuloma in two cases. **A,** Single lesion of eosinophilic granuloma. **C,** Enlargement of an area of **B,** showing the teeth with "hanging in air" appearance. Patient shown in **B** had multiple radiolucencies.

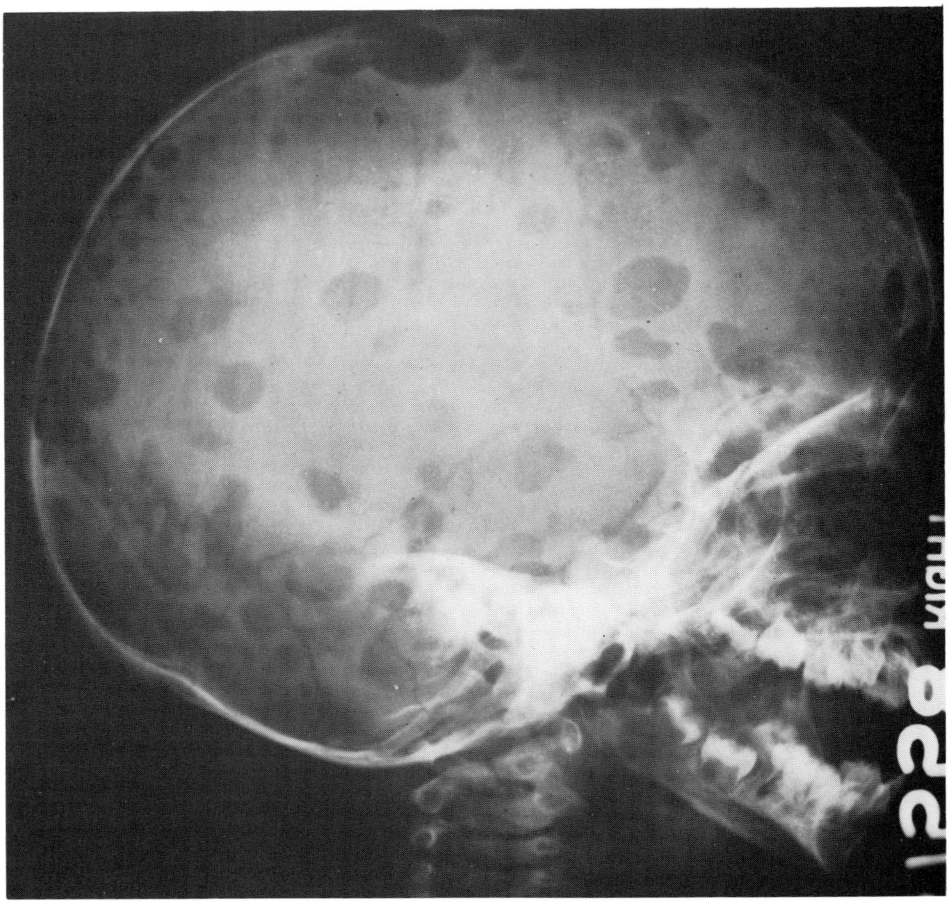

Fig. 6-43. Multiple radiolucencies in the skull and mandible of a child with Hand-Schüller-Christian disease.

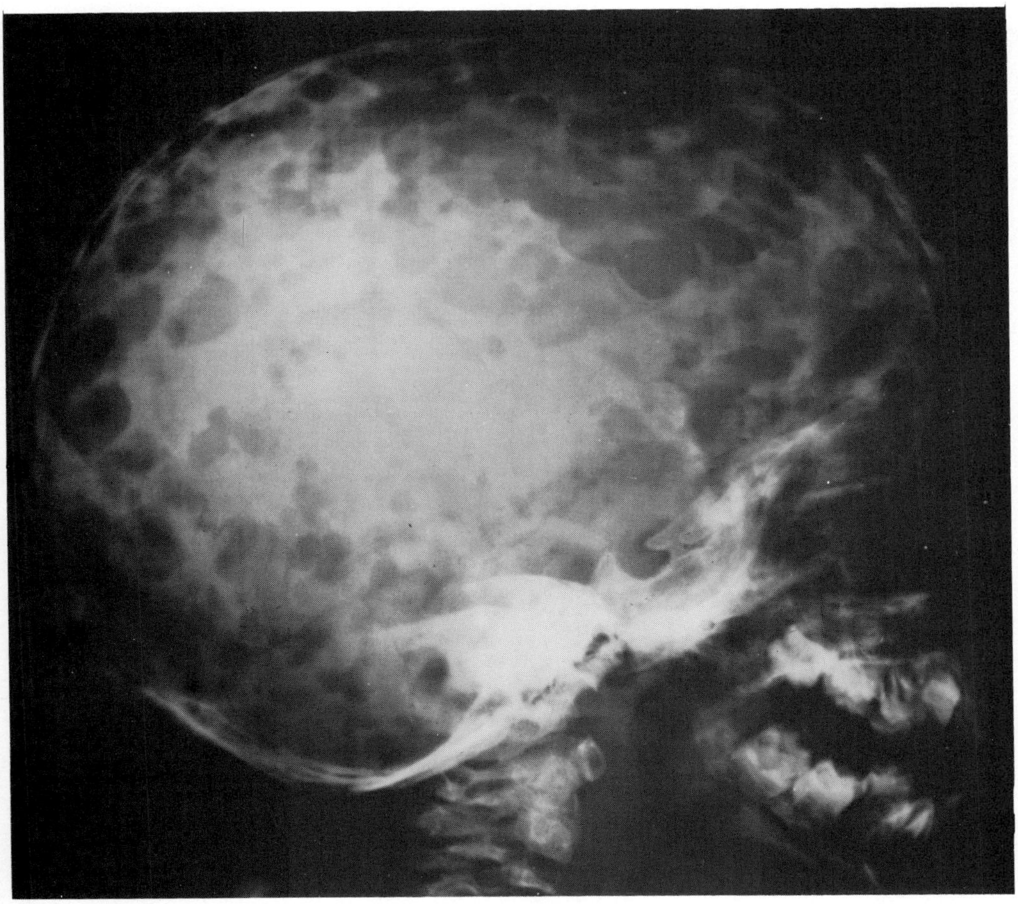

Fig. 6-44. Multiple radiolucencies in the skull and jaws of a child with Letterer-Siwe disease. Because of the irregular dark areas and the white contrasting areas of the unaffected bone, the term "geographic skull" is applied to this appearance.

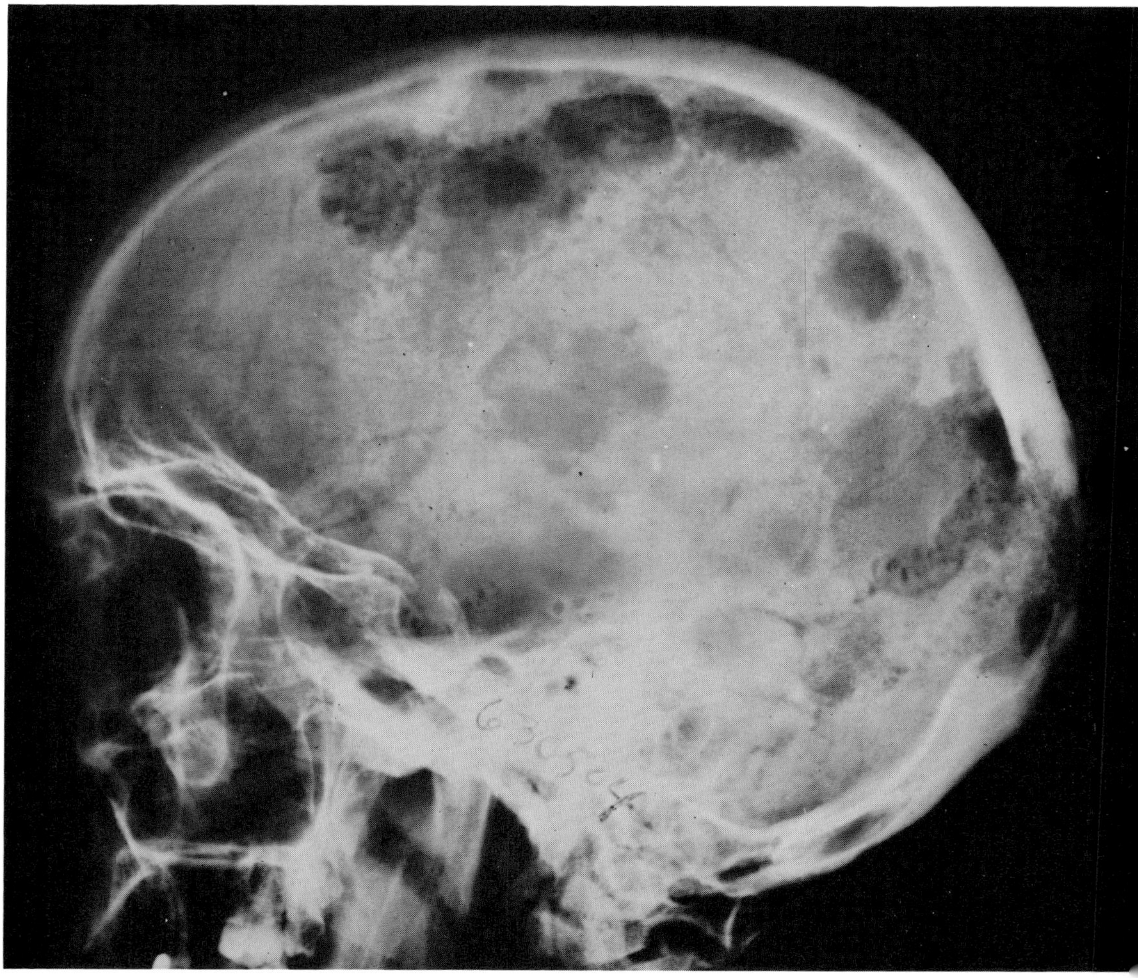

Fig. 6-45. Radiolucencies in the skull of a patient with Hand-Schüller-Christian disease.

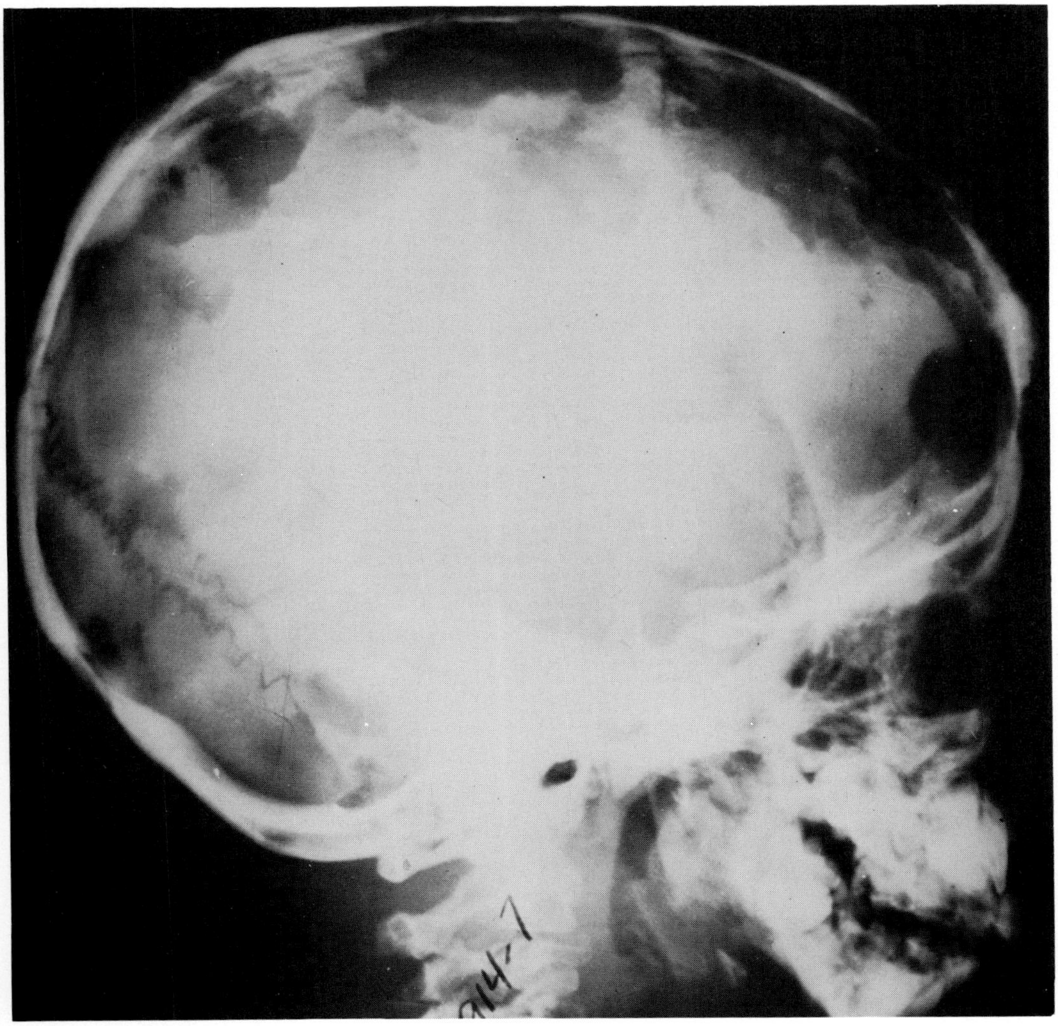

Fig. 6-46. Radiolucencies in the skull of a child with Letterer-Siwe disease. Lesions have irregular outlines and are progressive. The radiographic appearance is sometimes referred to as geographic skull.

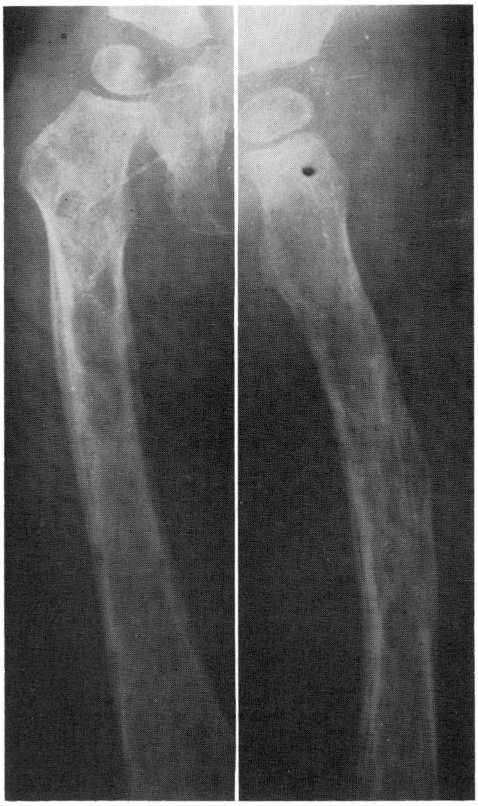

Fig. 6-47. Multiple radiolucencies in the right and left femurs of a patient with Hand-Schüller-Christian disease.

multiple radiolucent areas usually involving interdental and interradicular bone, so that teeth seem to "hang in air" (Figs. 6-41 and 6-42). Although some radiographs show a single lesion, multiple foci develop rapidly. Exfoliation of teeth and tooth germs and ulceration of the overlying mucosa are frequently seen. Radiographs of other bones of the skeleton also show multiple radiolucencies (Figs. 6-43 to 6-48). In late stages of these three diseases, the lateral radiographs of the skull show many progressively enlarging irregular areas of radiolucency (Figs. 6-43 to 6-46). The contrast between the multiple dark, irregular lesions and the light, normal portions of the skull gives it the appearance of a geographic map, and the term *geographic skull* is sometimes used to describe it (Figs. 6-44 to 6-46). Treatment varies with the type of disease and consists of surgical excision or radiation (eosinophilic granuloma), administration of cortisone, and palliative or symptomatic therapy.

Hyperparathyroidism. Hyperparathyroidism may not produce any radiographically visible changes in the jaws. On the other hand, it may manifest itself

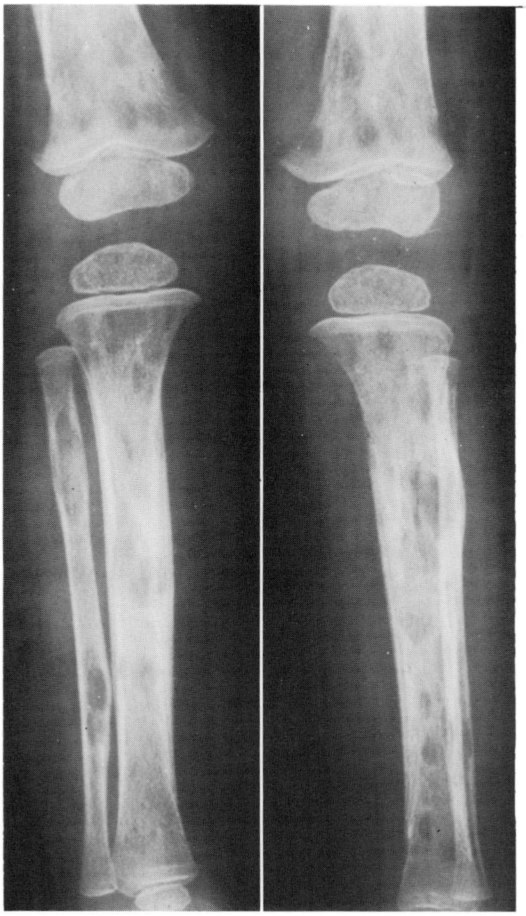

Fig. 6-48. Multiple radiolucencies in the right and left tibias and fibulas of a patient with Letterer-Siwe disease.

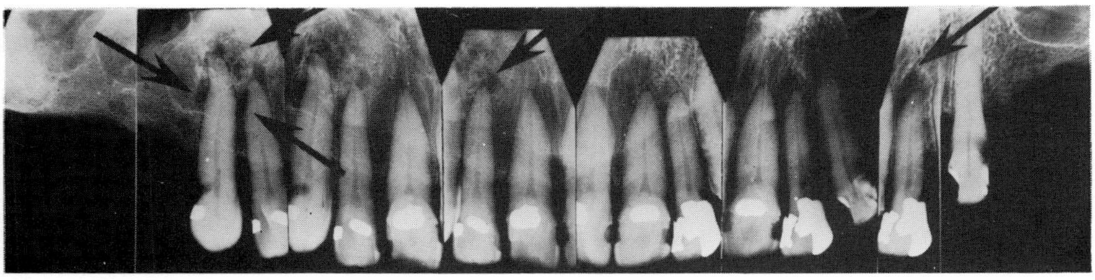

Fig. 6-49. Multiple radiolucencies (arrows) in the maxilla of a patient with hyperparathyroidism.

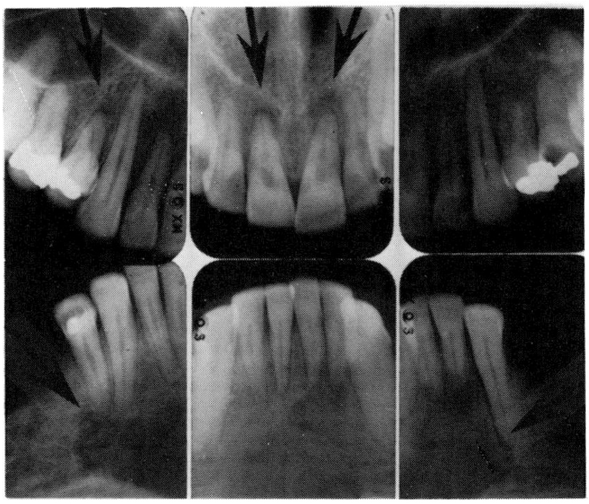

Fig. 6-50. Radiographs of the maxilla and mandible of a patient with hyperparathyroidism. Mandible shows a large single radiolucency (arrows), whereas in the maxilla, multiple small radiolucencies are seen (arrows).

A

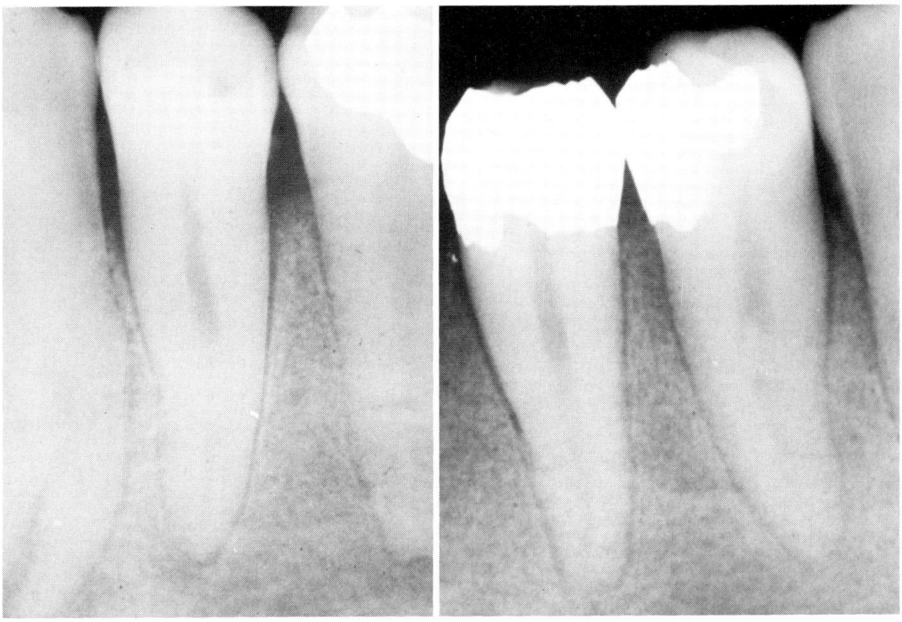

B

Fig. 6-51. **A** and **B,** Hyperparathyroidism in which the bone has a "ground glass" appearance and there is a loss of lamina dura. **C** and **D,** A normal mandible.

as multiple radiolucencies in the mandible or the maxilla (Fig. 6-49), as a single radiolucency (Fig. 6-50), or as a generalized loss of the normal trabecular pattern, as seen in Fig. 6-51. In the last-mentioned form, as the normal bone trabeculae are destroyed, they are replaced by many fine, poorly calcified, but closely spaced bone spicules that give the radiograph a "ground glass" appearance. This last feature, when present, is believed to be characteristic of hyperparathyroidism. In some cases the lamina dura is missing or interrupted (Fig. 6-51). This disease is more common in females, and patients with hyperparathyroidism are usually middle-aged and show evidence of weakness, fatigue, kidney disease, fractures, and presence of radiolucent lesions elsewhere in the skeleton. It must be borne in mind, however, that a case of hyperparathyroidism may show little or no

C

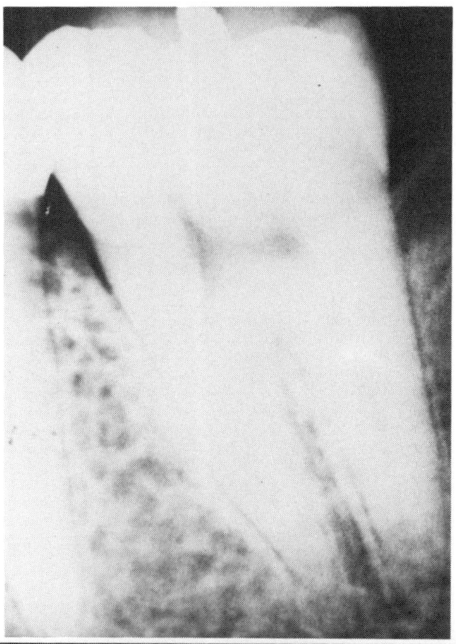

D

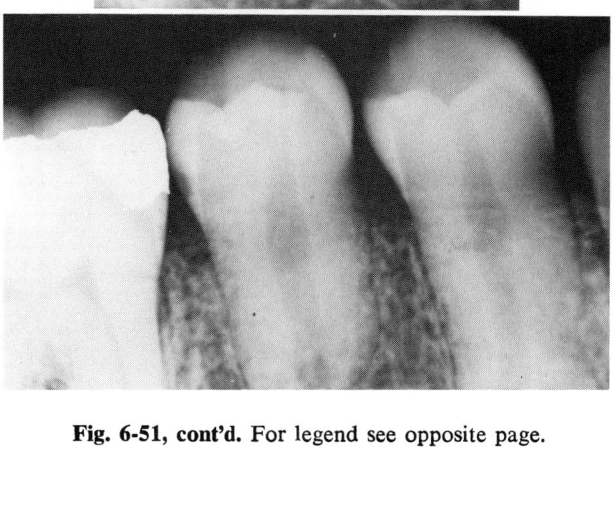

Fig. 6-51, cont'd. For legend see opposite page.

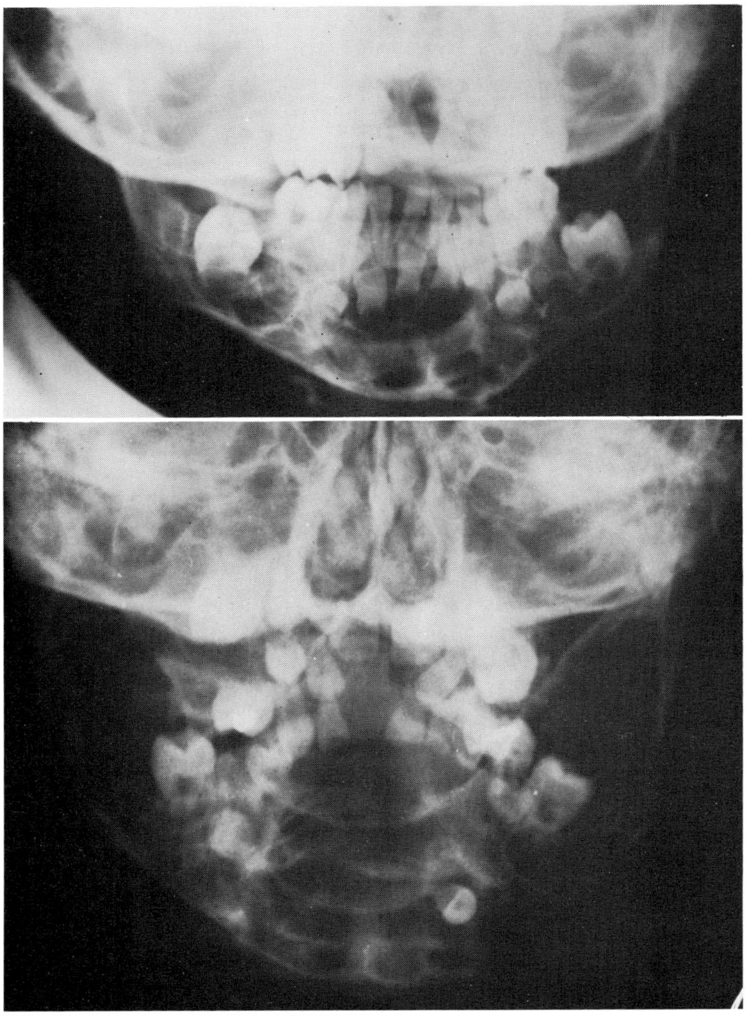

Fig. 6-52. Anteroposterior extraoral views of the skull of a patient, taken about two years apart, showing multiple radiolucencies of the mandible in cherubism.

evidence of change in the radiographs of the jaws, or if present, it may be classified as no more than "osteoporosis." In the presence of multiple radiolucencies in the jaws, however, the evidence of systemic symptoms described above and an elevation of serum calcium and alkaline phosphatase would indicate hyperparathyroidism.

Cherubism. In a classic case of cherubism, there are bilateral, exansile, multiple, soap bubble–like radiolucencies in the mandible (Figs. 6-52 to 6-54). In earlier stages, however, there may be only a single soap bubble–like area of radiolucency (Fig. 6-39). The radiolucent lesions produce migration of teeth and tooth germs, but teeth do not exfoliate or become loosened, and the patient has no systemic

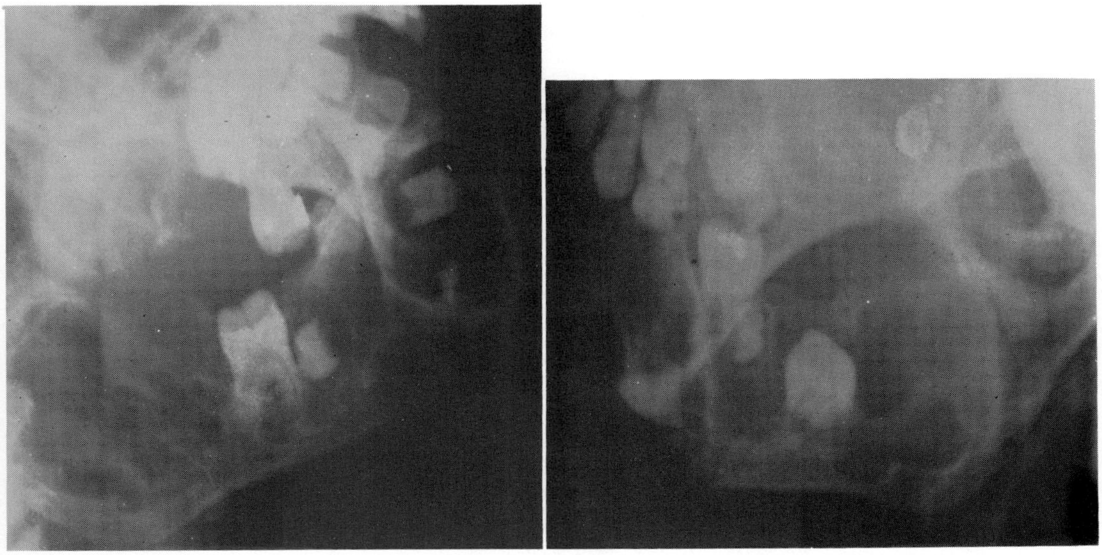

Fig. 6-53. Lateral extraoral radiographs of the right and left portions of the mandible in a patient with cherubism. Note multiple radiolucencies and displacement of teeth.

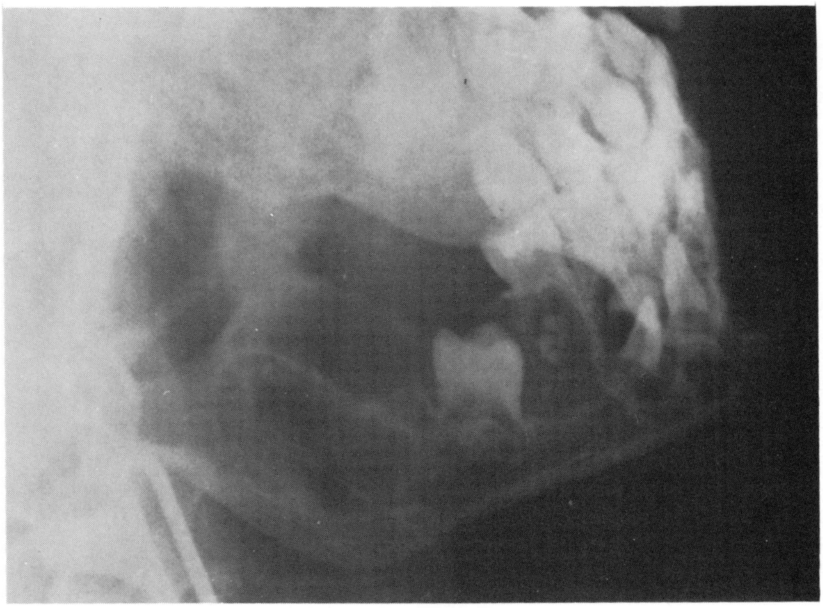

Fig. 6-54. Multiple radiolucencies in the mandible of a child with cherubism. Note enlargement of the molar area.

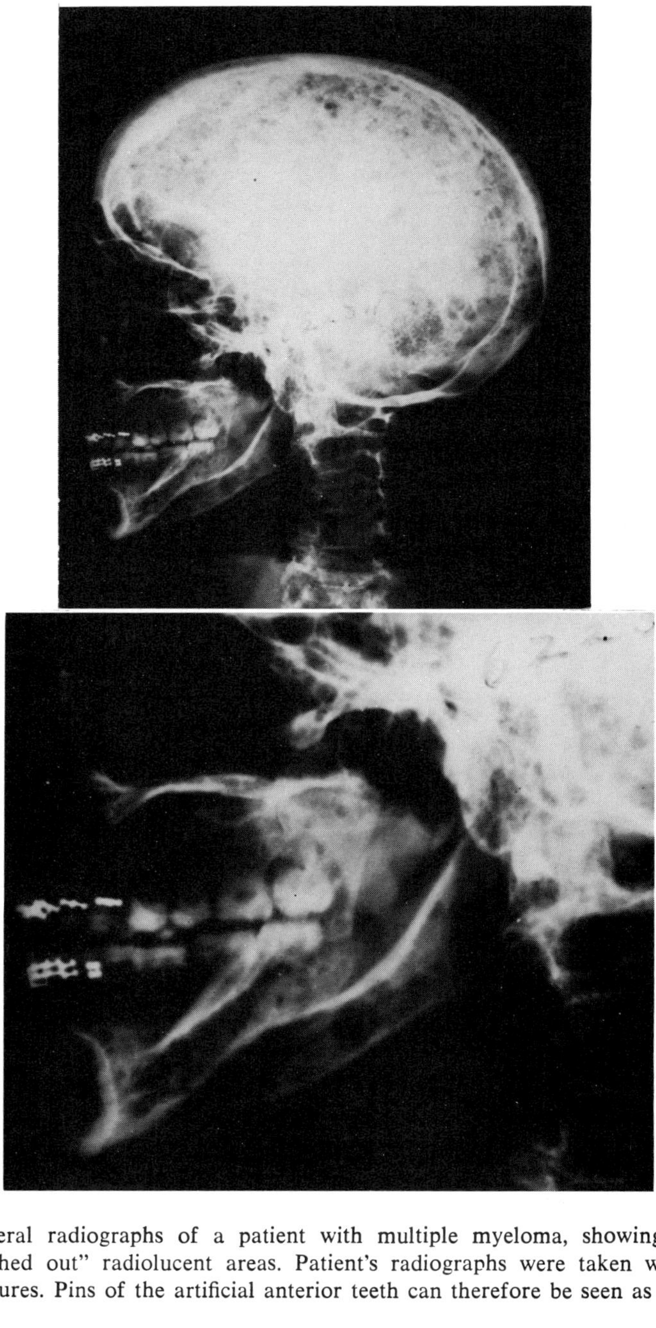

Fig. 6-55. Lateral radiographs of a patient with multiple myeloma, showing multiple but separate "punched out" radiolucent areas. Patient's radiographs were taken with full upper and lower dentures. Pins of the artificial anterior teeth can therefore be seen as radiopacities.

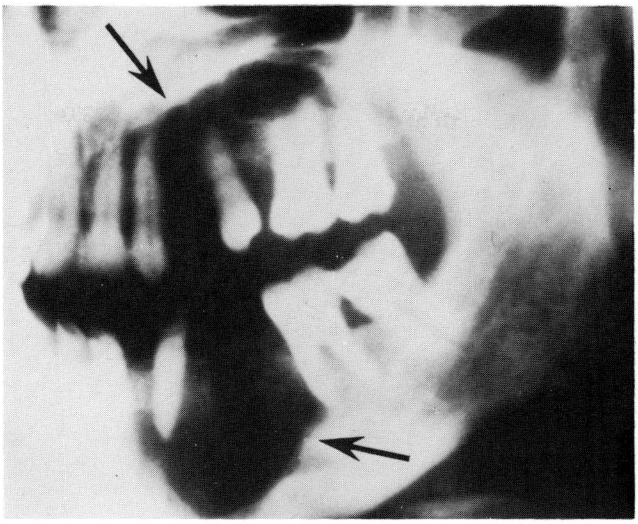

Fig. 6-56. Lateral radiograph showing two radiolucent metastatic foci of adenocarcinoma from the large intestines (colon). One focus is in the maxilla and the other in the mandible (arrows).

symptoms. The disease is hereditary and involves many members of a family. Patients are well, the jaws are the only bones affected, and the lesions begin and grow only in the first few years of life. Extraoral radiographs aided by the clinical history are often diagnostic, and in most cases surgical intervention, even for tissue biopsy, is unnecessary.

Multiple myeloma. Multiple myeloma is a malignant tumor of the bone marrow that may produce its earliest manifestation in the jaws. Patients are usually male, past 40 years of age, complain of pain in various parts of the skeleton, have weight loss, anemia, and loosening of teeth, and may show fractures. The jaws show multiple punched-out areas of radiolucency that are best demonstrated in lateral extraoral radiographs (Fig. 6-55). Such radiographs may also show similar punched-out areas in the skull. The age of the patient and the presence of neurologic symptoms distinguish this disease from other lesions in this group. Furthermore, in contrast to histiocytosis X, in which the peripheral border of the radiolucencies is often irregular, in multiple myeloma it is smooth and of regular contour.

Metastatic tumors. Malignant tumors may metastasize from different areas of the body and produce single or multiple radiolucencies in the jaws. This diagnosis, however, can be made only on biopsy. If the patient has a history of a previously treated malignant tumor, however, the presence of multiple radiolucencies in the jaws is highly suggestive of the disease (Fig. 6-56).

The important diagnostic features of lesions that appear as multiple but separate radiolucent lesions are summarized in Table 4.

Table 4. Diagnostic features of multiple but separate radiolucent lesions of the jaws

IMPORTANT CLINICAL AND RADIOLOGIC FEATURES	DIAGNOSIS
Lesions at apices of vital teeth, usually lower anteriors	Cementoma, stage I
Radiolucencies involve interradicular and interdental bone; patients include infants, children, and adults; destruction of bone around roots gives teeth "hanging in air" appearance; necrosis and ulceration of gingival tissue; loose teeth; radiolucencies, often with irregular borders	Histiocytosis X
Middle-aged patients; systemic symptoms involving weight loss, kidney disease, fatigue, fractures, increased blood calcium, and alkaline phosphatase	Hyperparathyroidism
Hereditary disease; presence of lesions in other family members; disease begins in childhood; swelling of jaws; long duration; patients in good health; migration of teeth	Cherubism
Patients older than 45 years; usually male; weight loss, anemia, leukopenia; loosening of teeth; pains in back; fractures; radiolucencies with smooth borders	Multiple myeloma
Patients usually past 30 years of age; radiolucencies with or without history of malignant disease elsewhere in the body; neurologic symptoms	Metastatic tumor

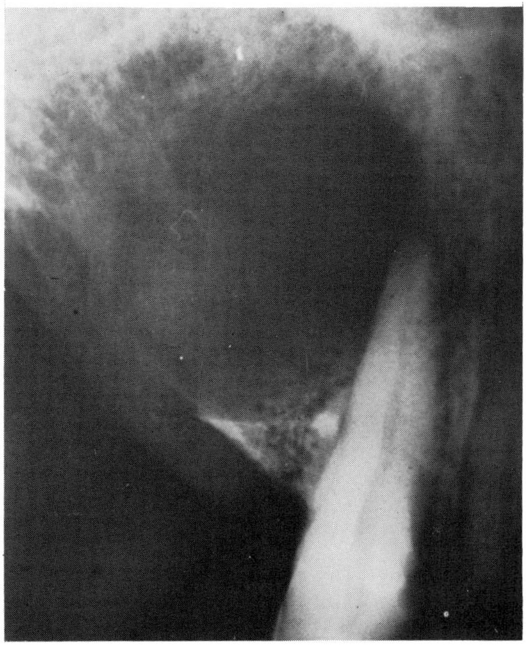

Fig. 6-57. Radiograph showing a radiolucency caused by hyperparathyroidism, which has destroyed the cortex of the maxilla.

surgically, not only to confirm the diagnosis, but also to fill this empty cavity with blood and to assure healing (Fig. 6-62).

Idiopathic bone cavity. This radiolucency occurs most frequently below the inferior dental canal of the mandible and is located just anterior to the mandibular angle (Fig. 6-63). It is asymptomatic, does not increase in size, and represents an embryonic defect. Surgical exploration is not necessary, but if attempted, it reveals a defect in the lingual cortical plate and the extension of salivary gland tissue or, less often, fat and connective tissue, from the floor of the mouth into the defect. The classic cases of this condition can be diagnosed from their radiographic appearance alone, and require no treatment. Idiopathic bone cavities, or bony defects containing salivary gland or connective tissue, can be seen in areas other than the angle of the mandible. Cases have been observed in the bicuspid area of the mandible and the maxilla (Fig. 6-64). In both these instances the defects contained salivary gland tissue and involved the lingual and the palatal plates of bone, respectively.

A

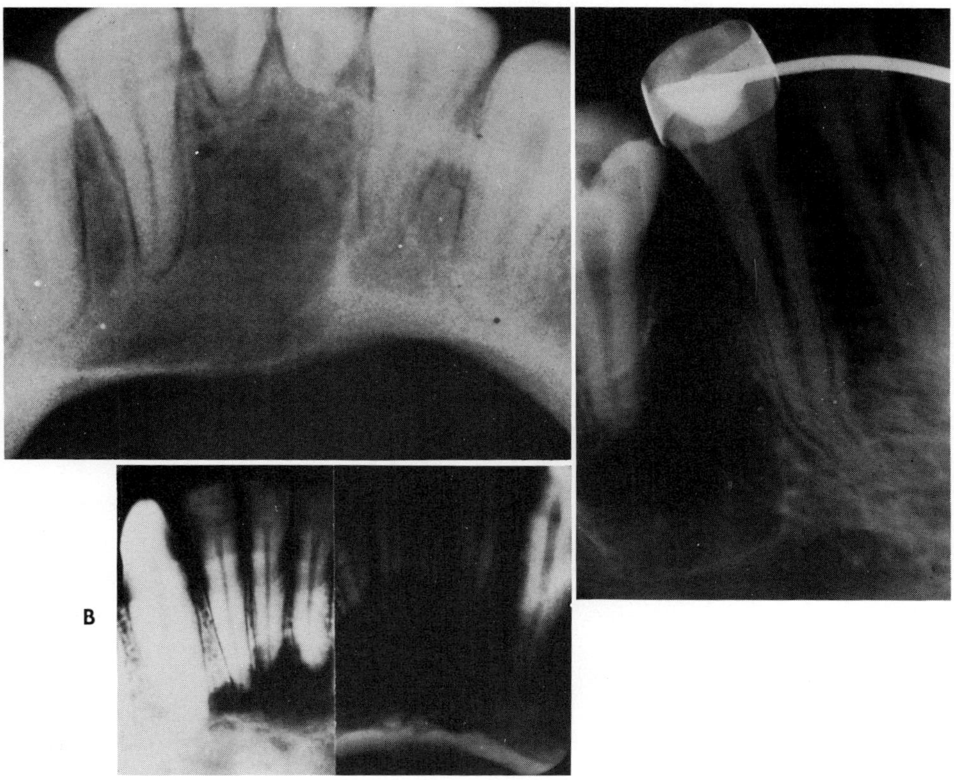

B

C

Fig. 6-61. Three cases of traumatic cyst. **A,** Occlusal view in which, because of missing permanent central incisors, the radiolucency was misdiagnosed clinically as a primordial cyst. **B,** Scalloped border of a traumatic cyst. **C,** Scalloped upper border is distinct, but diagnosis was made only on exploration.

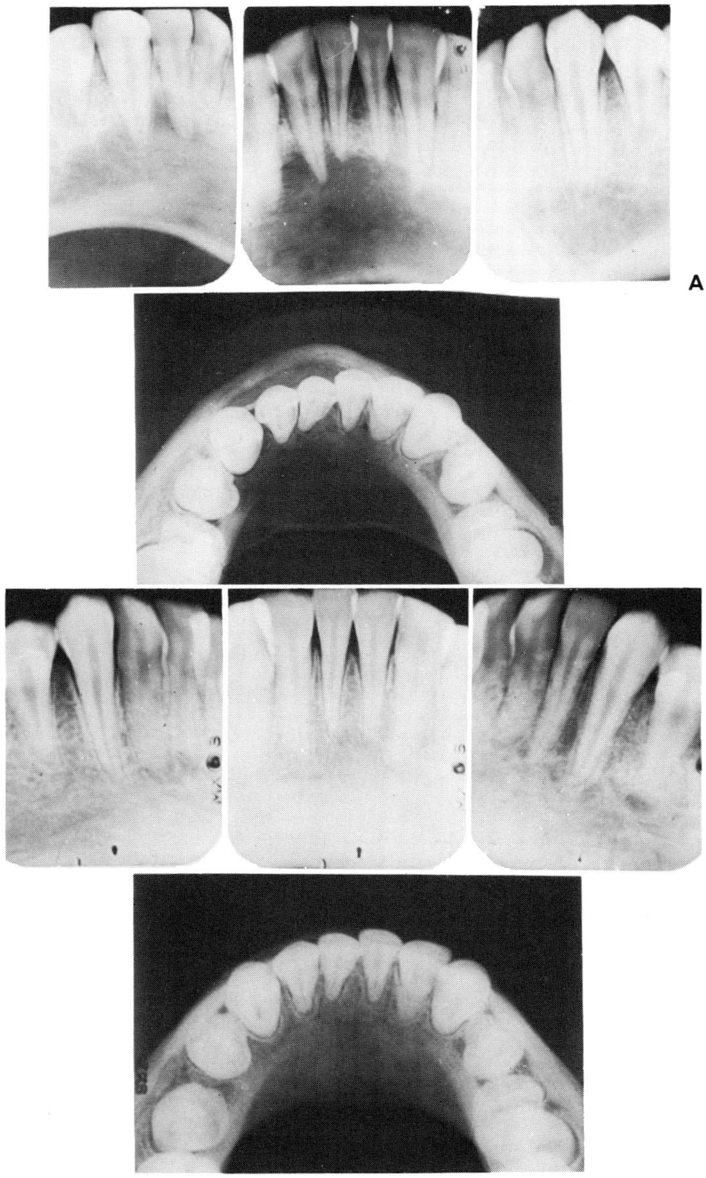

Fig. 6-62. Traumatic cyst. Intraoral and occlusal views before treatment, **A,** and after treatment, **B.** Intraoral radiographs in **A** show the scalloped border.

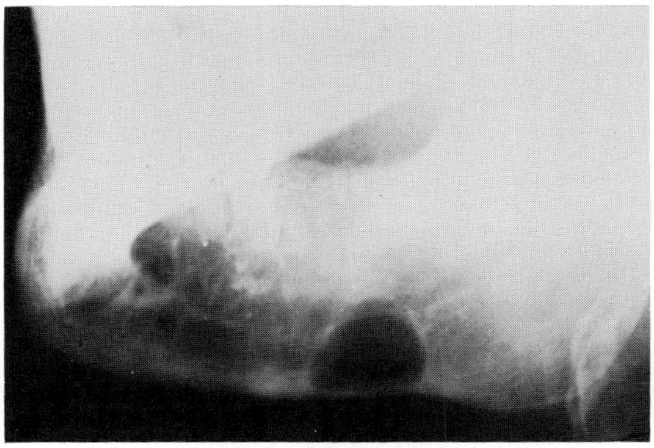

Fig. 6-63. Radiograph showing the usual location of idiopathic bone cavity.

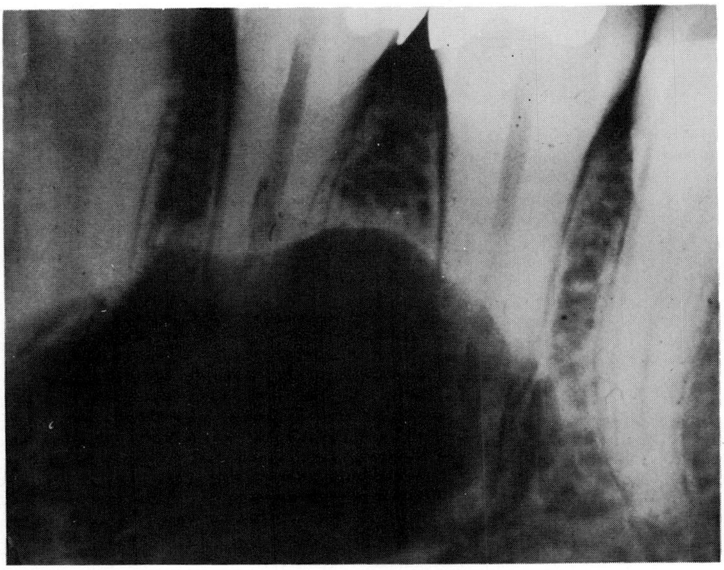

Fig. 6-64. In this rare instance a large idiopathic bone cavity was seen in a much higher location than usual. It contained salivary gland tissue and was connected to the floor of the mouth through a perforation in the lingual cortical plate of the mandible.

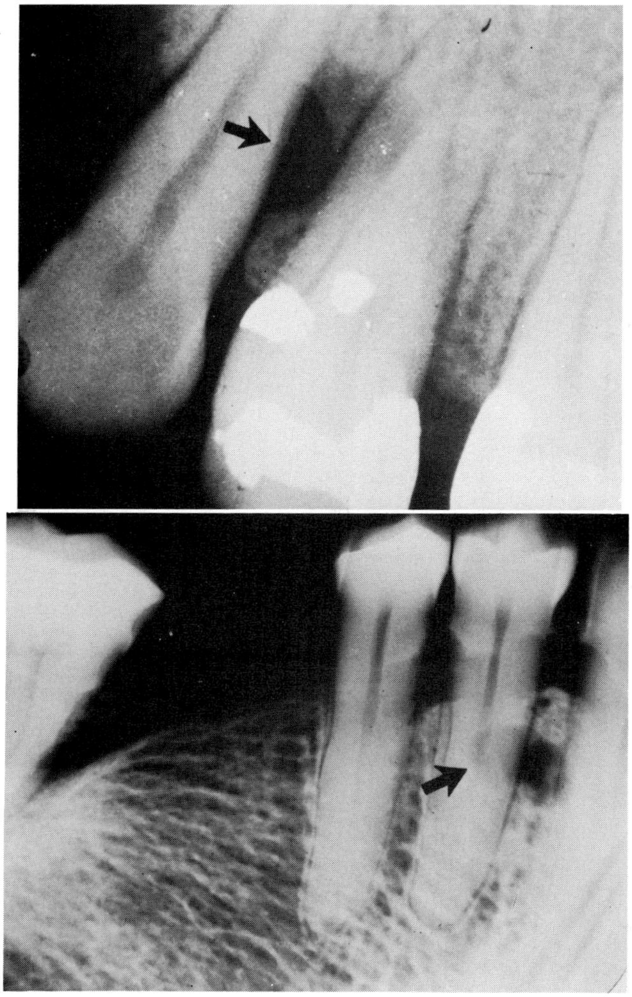

Fig. 6-65. Two cases of gingival cyst. The radiolucencies are clearly outlined (arrows).

Gingival cyst. This lesion usually presents as a pea-sized radiolucency in the cuspid and the bicuspid area and is located between the alveolar crest and apical third of the roots (Figs. 6-65 and 6-66). It is seen twice as frequently in the mandible as in the maxilla, and the greatest incidence is in the sixth decade of life. It can be felt clinically as a circumscribed elevation, and 90% of the cases involve the buccal gingiva. The cyst arises in the attached gingiva and by growth produces a cupping of the cortical plate, which produces the characteristic radiolucent shadow. The location of the radiolucency depends on the angulation employed, and the lesion is usually mistaken for the mental foramen, a lateral periodontal cyst, or a radicular cyst. Teeth in the area, however, are all vital, and this feature is important

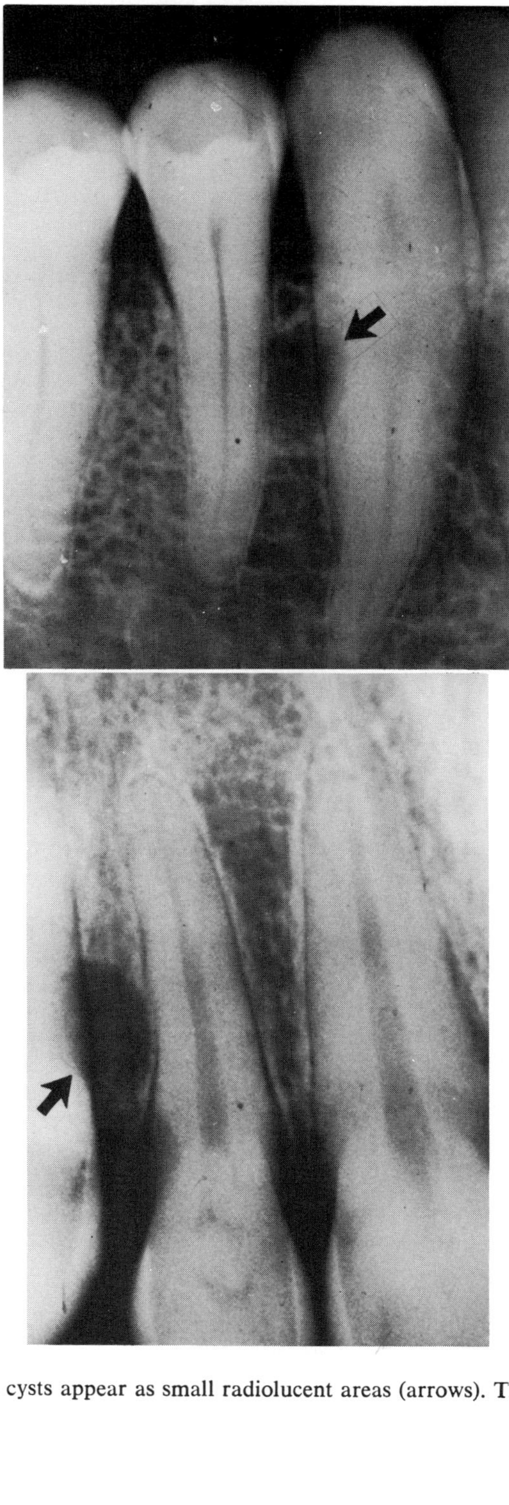

Fig. 6-66. Gingival cysts appear as small radiolucent areas (arrows). The teeth were vital.

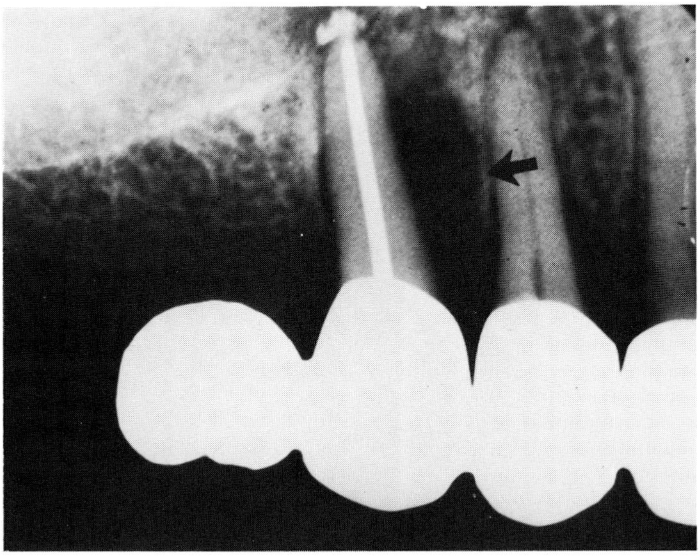

Fig. 6-67. Lateral periodontal cyst (arrow).

diagnostically. By elevating a buccal mucoperiosteal flap, a definitive diagnosis can easily be made.

Lateral periodontal cyst. The lateral periodontal cyst occurs on the lateral side of a *nonvital* tooth (Fig. 6-67). This lesion may be a radicular cyst that is associated with a lateral root canal. On the other hand, a deep periodontal pocket may produce pulpal necrosis and the development of a cystic lesion on the lateral side of the tooth (again in association with a lateral root canal). This latter condition, in which a periodontal lesion and a pulpal lesion occur together, is called the *combined* lesion and has been described on p. 102. The presence of the nonvital tooth distinguishes the lateral periodontal cyst from a gingival cyst and from uncomplicated periodontal disease.

Physiologic osteoporosis. Whenever teeth are lost in an area of the jaw, the functional stresses in bone are diminished and the bone trabeculae undergo physiologic resorption. Sometimes resorption of bone trabeculae occurs due to aging. As a result of this *physiologic bone loss,* the bone marrow spaces become larger and in intraoral radiographs appear as radiolucent "cells" (Fig. 6-68). When this phenomenon is pronounced, it may mimic an area of pathology. Osteoporosis due to physiologic factors occurs frequently in the bicuspid and molar area of the mandible and must be distinguished from disease processes.

Hematopoietic marrow. This condition is seen most frequently in the bicuspid and molar area of the mandible and usually appears as an asymptomatic, ill-defined area of radiolucency (Fig. 6-69). The teeth in the area are usually missing, but on occasion they may be present. In the latter case the pulp is vital. The radio-

A

B

C

D

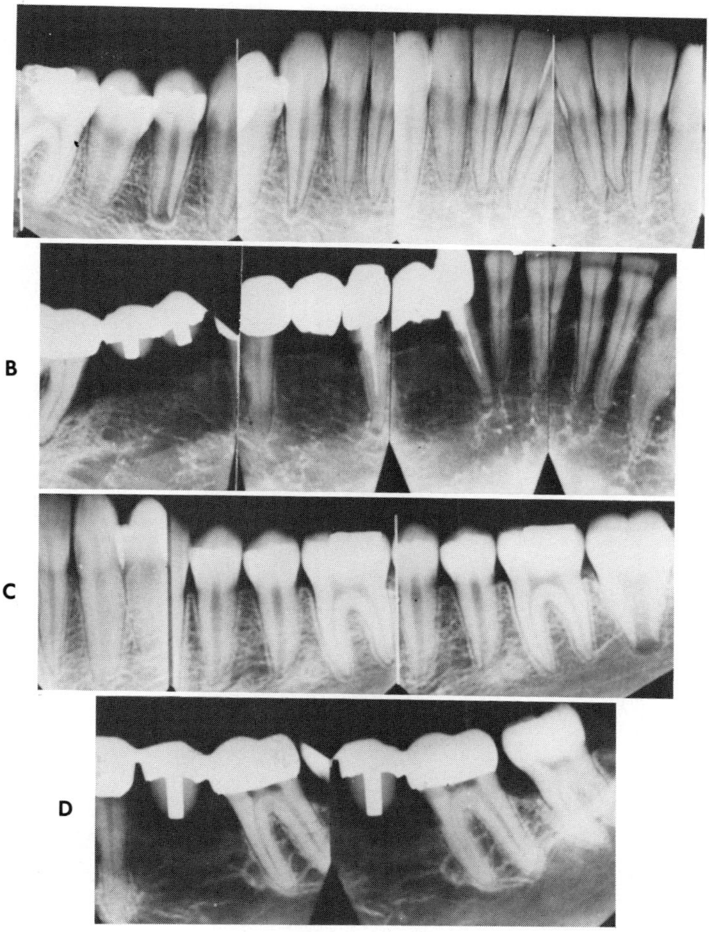

Fig. 6-68. **A** and **C,** Normal architecture of the mandible in a 12-year-old boy. **B** and **D,** Osteoporosis in a 60-year-old male patient.

lucency *does not increase in size.* It occurs more frequently in the female, and the patients are usually in the fourth decade of life or older. If the area does not increase in size, is asymptomatic, and corresponds to the description presented, it requires no therapy.

Periodontal disease. Bone loss, as evidenced by radiolucencies in the interradicular and interdental areas, is characteristic of periodontal disease, and its features are known to every dentist (Fig. 6-70). This subject was discussed in Chapter 4.

Median mandibular cyst. On extremely rare occasions a radiolucency may be seen in the midline of the mandible (Fig. 6-71). The teeth in the area are vital. Such a lesion has been called the median mandibular cyst and is believed to arise from the remnants of the fissural epithelium left in this area. It is, however, more likely that it is a primordial cyst that arises from a supernumerary tooth germ.

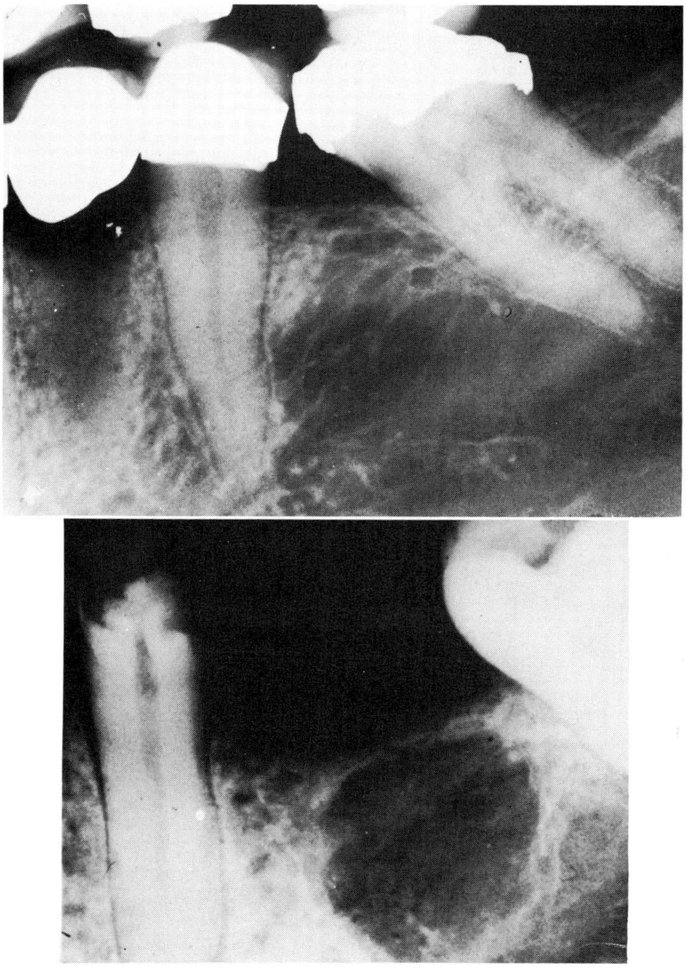

Fig. 6-69. Hematopoietic marrow appears as ill-defined radiolucencies in the bicuspid and molar area of the mandible.

From the radiographs, however, a distinction between the two is neither possible nor of any clinical importance. The lesion is treated by excision.

Central hemangioma. This extremely rare lesion appears as a moth-eaten, or ill-defined, radiolucency that involves the mandible twice as often as the maxilla (Fig. 6-72). It may be nonexpansile or it may expand the jaw. Loosening of teeth may occur, and blood may ooze from the surrounding gingiva. Radiographs may show linear trabeculations. Because of its extremely serious nature, whenever such a lesion is suspected, aspiration should be attempted and surgical intervention carried out with the most extreme caution.

Mandibular cleft. In the fetus and during the first year of life, the midline suture of the mandible can normally be seen as a zone of radiolucency (Fig. 1-6).

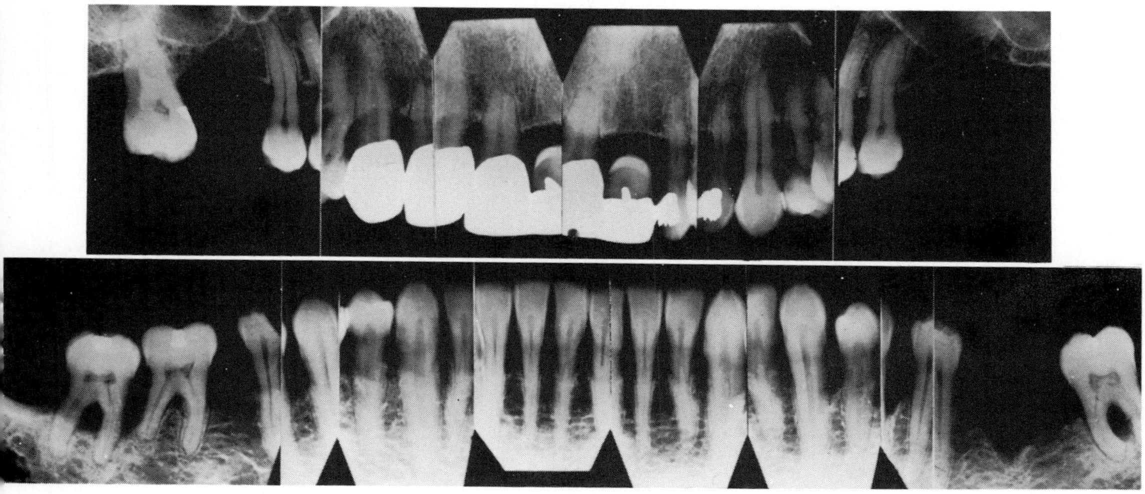

Fig. 6-70. Full-mouth intraoral radiographs showing generalized periodontal disease. In the mandibular molars, bifurcation involvement can be seen.

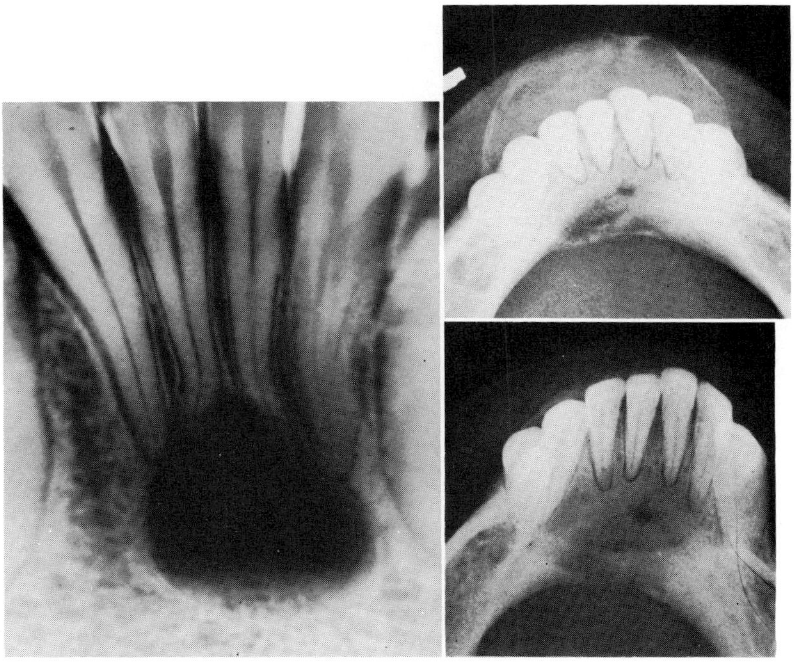

A B C

Fig. 6-71. Intraoral radiograph, **A,** and occlusal radiographs, **B** and **C,** of two cases of so-called median mandibular cyst. **B** and **C** are radiographs of the same case.

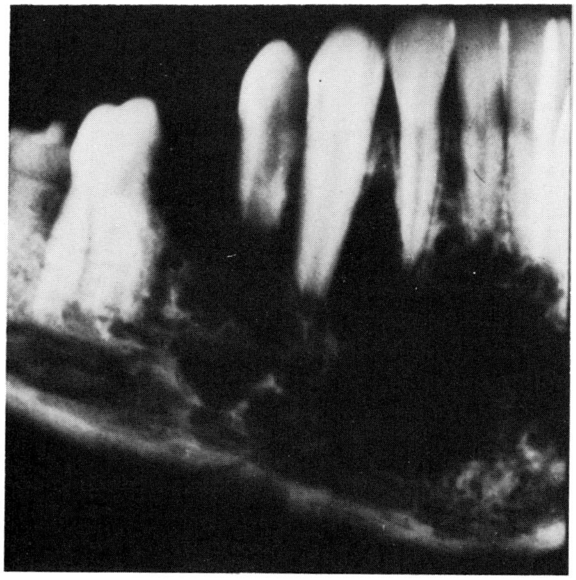

Fig. 6-72. Lateral radiographs of the mandible, showing a rare honeycombed radiolucency of a central hemangioma.

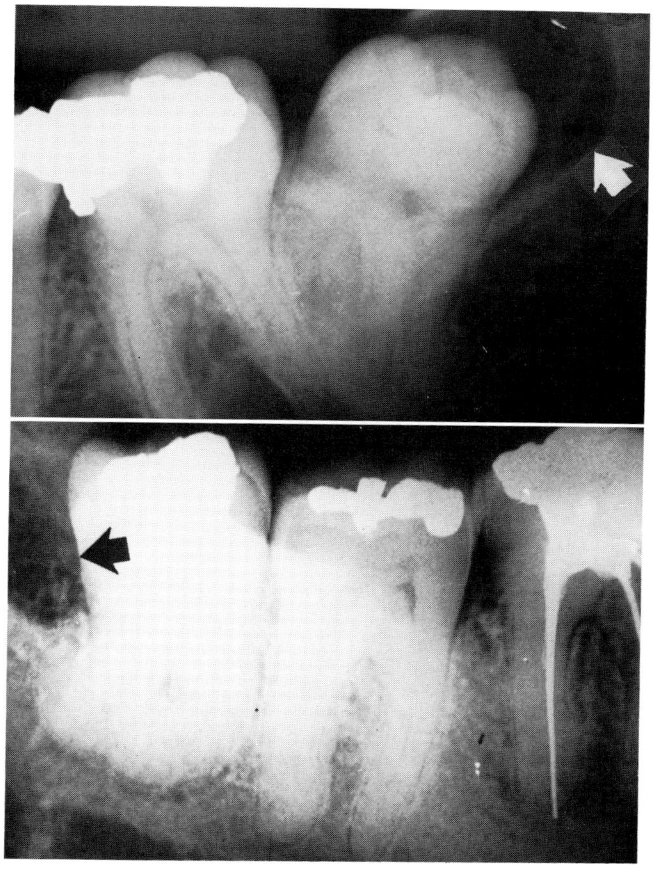

Fig. 6-73. Intraoral radiographs of the third molar area of the mandible, showing circumscribed radiolucencies (arrows) that were produced by salivary gland inclusions.

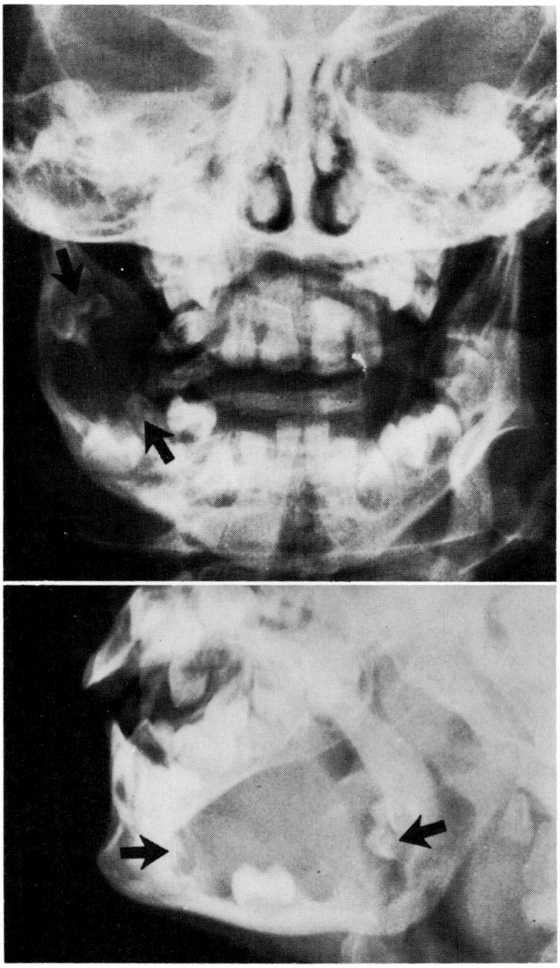

Fig. 6-74. Anteroposterior and lateral views of the jaws of a child, showing large radiolucencies caused by a mucoepidermoid tumor of salivary glands (arrows).

In a rare developmental disorder, however, it may fail to disappear and lead to the so-called midline cleft of the mandible.

Salivary gland tissue and tumors. With the exception of the gingiva and the anterior part of the hard palate, salivary gland tissue is seen everywhere in the oral mucosa. Normally, salivary glands are not included within the jaws. The salivary glands of the retromolar pad, however, develop in close proximity to the developing mandible, and some of them become enclosed within the bone. In radiographs they appear as radiolucencies in the retromolar area, and their true nature is revealed only on histologic examination (Fig. 6-73). The salivary gland tissue of the retromolar mandibular area can also produce benign and malignant salivary gland tumors that cause radiolucent shadows and that are correctly diagnosed only microscopically (Fig. 6-74). Radiolucencies in the posterior part of the mandible, which represented adenocarcinoma, mucoepidermoid tumor, adenoma, and malignant mixed tumor, have been observed (Fig. 6-74). In the maxilla, as in the mandible, salivary gland tissue may become entrapped during embryogenesis. This is consistently seen in the incisive canal and has been occasionally observed in the molar area. In addition to the presence of the salivary glands *within* the maxilla, abundant glandular tissue is seen, both on the oral and the nasal side of this bone. Salivary gland tumors of the palate or the antrum, therefore, can and do destroy the maxilla and produce radiolucent areas. Salivary gland tumors of the incisive canal have also been observed. Such cases produce radiolucent shadows.

Fractures. Fractures of the maxilla or mandible appear as radiolucent lines, and their correct diagnosis is aided by clinical history and examination. It is usually advisable to take more than one radiograph in such cases, and extraoral views are usually far more valuable than the intraoral radiographs.

REFERENCES

Abrams, A. M., Howell, F. V., and Bullock, W. K.: Nasopalatine cysts, Oral Surg. **16:** 306, 1963.

Anderson, D. E., and McClendon, J. L.: Cherubism—hereditary fibrous dysplasia of the jaws. I. Genetic considerations, Oral Surg. **15** (supp. 2):5, 1962.

Banerjee, S. C.: Metastasis to the mandible, Oral Surg. **23:**71, 1967.

Barros, R. E., Dominguez, F. V., and Cabrini, R. L.: Myxoma of the jaws, Oral Surg. **27:**225, 1969.

Bergenholtz, A., and Persson, G.: Idiopathic bone cavities, Oral Surg. **16:**703, 1963.

Bernier, J. L., and Bhaskar, S. N.: Aneurysmal bone cysts of the mandible, Oral Surg. **9:**1018, 1958.

Bhaskar, S. N.: Adenoameloblastoma: its histogenesis and report of 15 new cases, J. Oral Surg. **22:**218, 1964.

Bhaskar, S. N.: Gingival cyst and the keratinizing ameloblastoma, Oral Surg. **19:**796, 1965.

Bhaskar, S. N.: Periapical lesions—types, incidence, and clinical features, Oral Surg. **21:**657, 1966.

Bhaskar, S. N.: Bone lesions of endodontic origin, Dent. Clin. North Am., p. 521, Nov., 1967.

Bhaskar, S. N.: Oral pathology in the dental office: survey of 20,575 biopsy specimens, J. Am. Dent. Assoc. **76:**761, 1968.

Bhaskar, S. N.: Oral manifestations of metastatic tumors, Postgrad. Med. **49:**155, 1971.

Bhaskar, S. N.: Synopsis of oral pathology, ed. 4, St. Louis, 1973, The C. V. Mosby Co.

Bhaskar, S. N.: Hematopoietic marrow (unpublished data).

Bhaskar, S. N., Bernier, J. L., and Godby, F.: Aneurysmal bone cyst and other giant cell lesions of the jaws: report of 104 cases, J. Oral Surg. **17:**30, 1959.

Biesecker, J. L., and others: Aneurysmal bone cysts: a clinicopathologic study of 66 cases, Cancer **26:**615, 1970.

Burland, J. G.: Cherubism: familial bilateral osseous dysplasia of the jaws, Oral Surg. **15** (supp. 2):43, 1962.

Cash, C. D., Roger, R. Q., and Dahlin, D. C.: Metastic tumors of the jaws, Oral Surg. **14:**897, 1961.

Castigliano, S. G., and Romingen, C. J.: Metastatic malignancy of the jaws, Am. J. Surg. **87:**496, 1954.

Cataldo, E., and Meyer, I.: Solitary and multiple plasma cell tumors of the jaws and oral cavity, Oral Surg. **22:**628, 1966.

Christ, T. F.: The globulomaxillary cyst: an embryologic misconception, Oral Surg. **30:** 515, 1970.

Ciola, B., and Catena, D. L.: Midline maxillary cyst complicated by unerupted mesiodens, Oral Surg. **34:**978, 1972.

Colombo, C. S., and Boivin, Y.: Myxoma of the jaws, Oral Surg. **21:**431, 1966.

Degering, C. I.: Radiography of a lateral periodontal cyst, Oral Surg. **32:**498, 1971.

Ebling, H., and Goldenberg, N.: Central angioma, Oral Surg. **21:**9, 1966.

Ebling, H., and Wagner, J. E.: Recurrent myxoma, Oral Surg. **21:**94, 1966.

Epker, B., Merrill, R. G., and Henny, F. A.:

Breast adenocarcinoma metastatic to the mandible, Oral Surg. **28:**471, 1969.

Farquhar, R. L., and Greskovich, F. J.: Ameloblastoma, Oral Surg. **19:**145, 1965.

Fuchihata, H., Wada, T., and Inoue, T.: Radiotherapy of adenoid cystic carcinoma of the head and neck, Oral Surg. **36:**753, 1973.

Hamner, J. E., Gamble, J. W., and Gallegos, G. J.: Odontogenic fibroma, Oral Surg. **21:** 113, 1966.

Hayduk, J. W.: Hand-Schüller-Christian disease, Oral Surg. **23:**29, 1967.

Hoppe, W.: An aneurysmal bone cyst of the mandible, Oral Surg. **25:**1, 1968.

Huebner, G. R., and Turlington, E. G.: So-called traumatic (hemorrhagic) bone cysts of the jaws, Oral Surg. **31:**354, 1971.

Lalonde, E. R., and Leubke, R. G.: Radiographic analysis of periapical granulomas and radicular cysts, I.A.D.R. printed abstracts 162, 1968.

Lalonde, E. R., and Luebke, R. G.: The frequency and distribution of periapical cysts and granulomas, Oral Surg. **25:**861, 1968.

Large, N. D., Niebel, H. H., and Fredricks, W. H.: Myxoma of the jaws, Oral Surg. **13:**1462, 1960.

Lautenbach, E., and Dockhorn, R.: Osteodystrophia fibrosa generalisata (Recklinghausen's disease; hyperparathyroidism) and its effects on the jaws, Oral Surg. **25:**479, 1968.

Lichtenstein, L.: Histiocytosis X: integration of eosinophilic granuloma of bone, "Letterer-Siwe disease," and "Schüller-Christian disease" as related manifestations of a single nosologic entity, Arch. Pathol. (Chicago) **56:**84, 1953.

Meyer, I., and Shklar, G.: Malignant tumors metastatic to mouth and jaws, Oral Surg. **20:**350, 1965.

Miller, A. S., and Winnick, M.: Salivary gland inclusion in the anterior mandible, Oral Surg. **31:**790, 1971.

Papp, P., and Toth, K.: Odontogenic myxoma of the mandible, Oral Surg. **20:**82, 1965.

Parks, C. R., and Bottomley, W. K.: Lymphoblastic lymphosarcoma, Oral Surg. **33:** 297, 1972.

Pickle, D. E., Gordon, R., Scopp, I. W., and Mittelman, G. J.: Multiple myeloma: its oral manifestations, Oral Surg. **21:**347, 1966.

Rappaport, J., Shiffman, M. A., and Greaney, E. M.: Parathyroid disease, Oral Surg. **17:** 802, 1964.

Rosenberg, E. H., and Guralnick, W. C.: Hyperparathyroidism: a review of 220 previous cases, with special emphasis on findings in the jaws, Oral Surg. **15** (supp. 2):84, 1962.

Shklar, G., Taylor, R., and Schwartz, S.: Oral lesions of eosinophilic granuloma, Oral Surg. **19:**613, 1965.

Sleeper, E. L.: Eosinophilic granuloma of bone: its relationship to Hand-Schüller-Christian and Letterer-Siwe diseases, with emphasis upon oral symptoms and findings, Oral Surg. **4:**896, 1951.

Steg, R. F.: Solitary bone cyst of the mandible, Oral Surg. **20:**294, 1965.

Straith, F. E.: Metastatic adenocarcinoma of mandible, Oral Surg. **24:**1, 1967.

Straith, F. E.: Multiple myeloma, Oral Surg. **23:**294, 1967.

Symposium: Solitary bone cysts of the mandible, Oral Surg. **8:**903, 1955.

Topazian, R. G.: Central hemangioma of the mandible, Oral Surg. **18:**1, 1964.

Zegarelli, E. V., Kutschner, A. H., Napoli, N., Iurono, F., and Hoffman, P.: The cementoma, Oral Surg. **17:**219, 1964.

CHAPTER SEVEN

RADIOPAQUE LESIONS OF THE JAWS

Seven percent of all jaw lesions appear as radiopacities. In the presence of an exclusively radiopaque area, one of the following conditions should be considered:

Broken roots
Foreign bodies
Condensing osteitis
Multiple enostosis (chronic sclerosing osteomyelitis, sclerosing osteomyelitis)
Polyostotic fibrous dysplasia
Ossifying fibroma
Exostosis, torus, and osteoma
Paget's disease
Cementoma (stage III)
Unerupted teeth
Compound odontoma
Complex odontoma
Osteopetrosis
Leontiasis ossea
Caffey's disease
Garré's osteomyelitis
Thalassemia (Cooley's anemia)
Osteogenic sarcoma
Chondrosarcoma
Metastatic tumors

The important diagnostic features of these lesions are discussed.

Broken roots. A history of extraction, a resemblance to a portion of root, and a lack of growth distinguish the broken root from other lesions (Fig. 7-1). Usually the presence of the periodontal ligament can be identified. The bone surrounding these root fragments may show osteosclerosis, and in such cases they need not be removed. A broken root associated with a radiolucency implies secondary inflammation, and its removal is necessary.

Foreign bodies. Amalgam particles seen in extraction sites or areas of apical

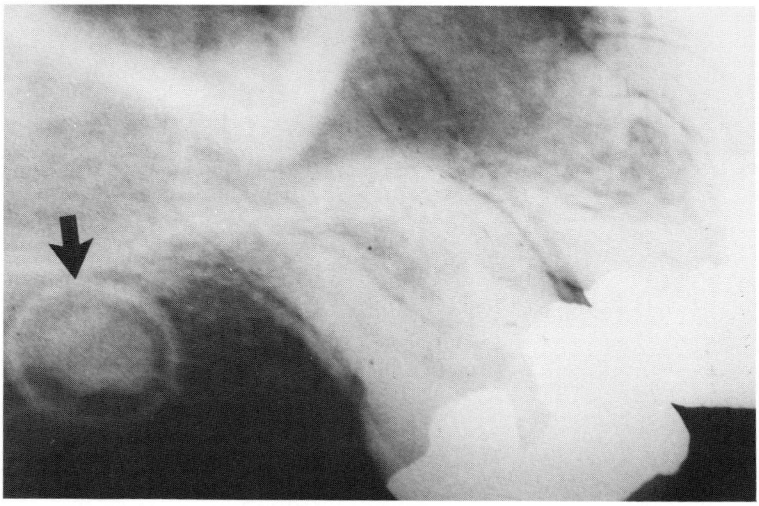

Fig. 7-1. Radiograph of a broken root fragment. Because of the horizontal position of the root, the radiopacity is surrounded on all sides by the periodontal ligament (arrow).

surgery constitute the most common radiopaque foreign bodies in the jaws (Fig. 7-2). Pieces of gutta-percha may be left in apical areas, or gutta-percha fillings may remain in the jaw after exfoliation of transplanted or reimplanted teeth (Fig. 7-3). Other foreign bodies seen in radiographs are wires, screws, pins of artificial teeth, endosseous metallic implants, broken endodontic instruments, periodontal pocket markers, endodontic implants, or portions of missiles (Figs. 7-4 to 7-6). Foreign bodies of various types may be seen in the antrum and may present as radiopaque areas (Fig. 7-7). A history of the material entering the area or surgical intervention assists in the correct diagnosis. The diagnosis of these radiopaque shadows is not difficult, and their management depends on their type. If they are associated with infection, removal is necessary.

Condensing osteitis. Condensing osteitis is perhaps the most common radiopaque lesion of the jaws. It is an ill-defined or clearly demarcated radiopacity that varies in density from that of trabecular bone to that of the dentin (Figs. 7-8 to 7-10). It is usually not as radiopaque as enamel, *and this is an important feature distinguishing it from the odontomas.*

Condensing osteitis represents a response of bone to some form of injury (e.g., low-grade infection or excessive physical stress). Although it can occur anywhere in the jaws, it is usually seen in the tooth-bearing areas, where the apical region is the preferred site. Lesions are seen most frequently in the bicuspid and molar areas of the mandible. Necrotic pulps may be associated with condensing osteitis of the periapical tissues, and this *periapical condensing osteitis* can disappear after proper endodontic therapy (Fig. 7-11).

Condensing osteitis is often discovered on routine radiographic examination and is asymptomatic. If these lesions occur near the alveolar crest of an edentulous

Text continued on p. 172.

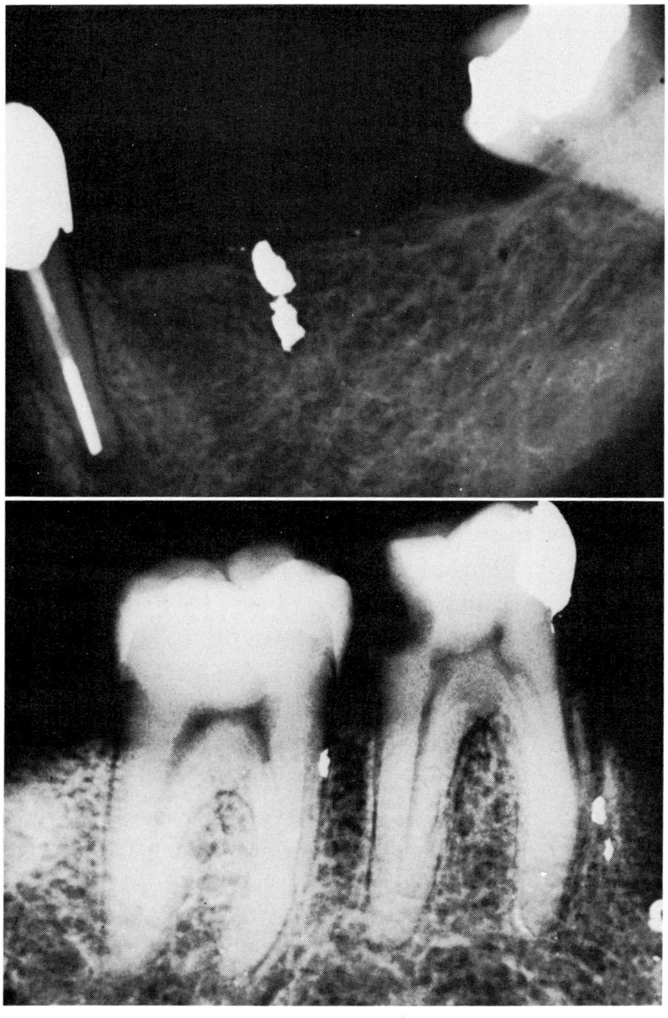

Fig. 7-2. Intraoral radiographs showing fragments of amalgam in the jaw.

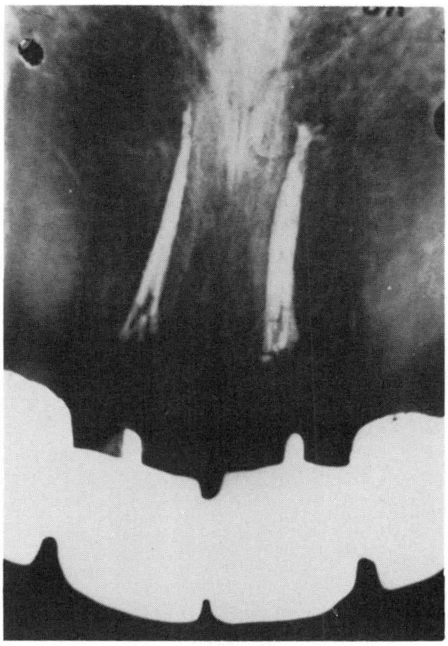

Fig. 7-3. Radiograph of the upper anterior region reveals two radiopaque structures representing gutta-percha root canal fillings. They were contained in the reimplanted teeth, which underwent external resorption and exfoliation. The root canal fillings, however, were left in bone. They have not elicited foreign body reaction.

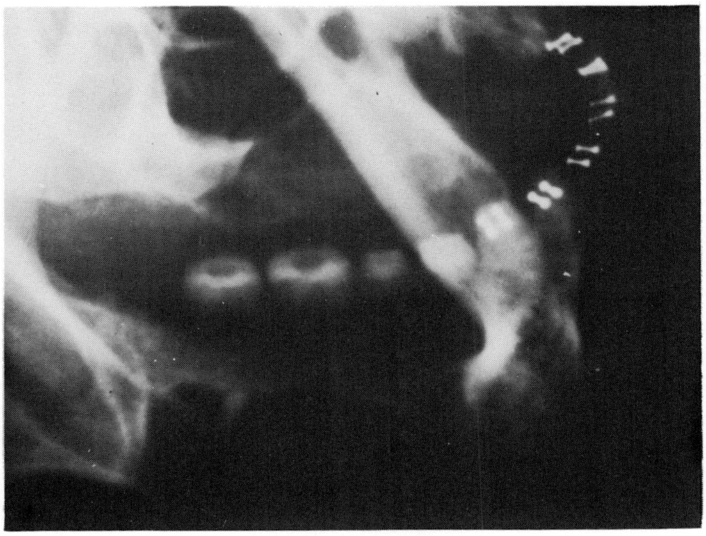

Fig. 7-4. Lateral radiograph of the jaws taken with the maxillary denture in place. Radiopaque structures are pins of the maxillary anterior teeth.

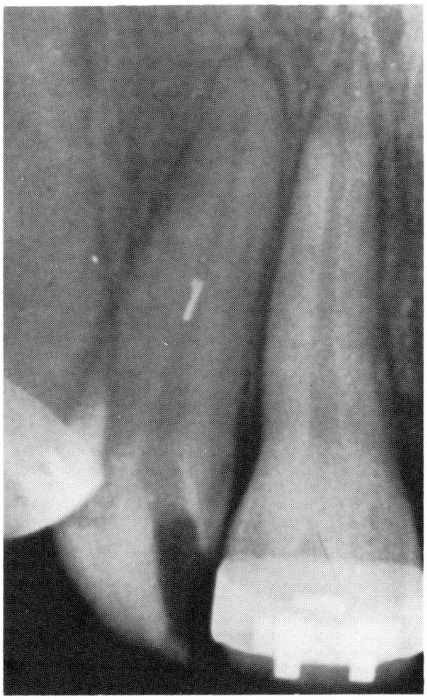

Fig. 7-5. Broken file appears as a radiopaque structure in the root canal of the lateral incisor.

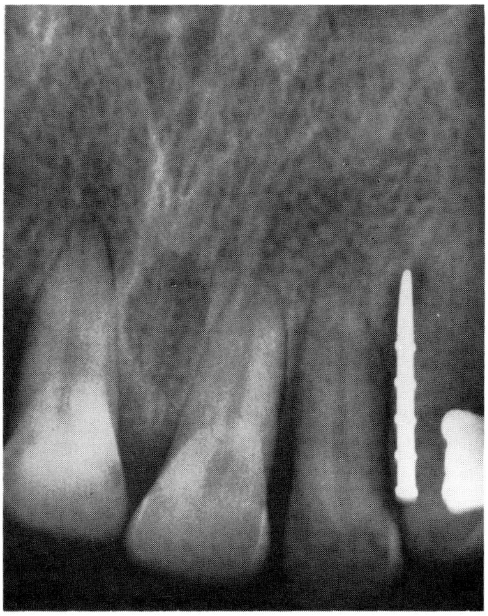

Fig. 7-6. Radiograph showing calibrated radiopaque "point" in a periodontal pocket. Such objects are often used in measuring depth of periodontal pockets.

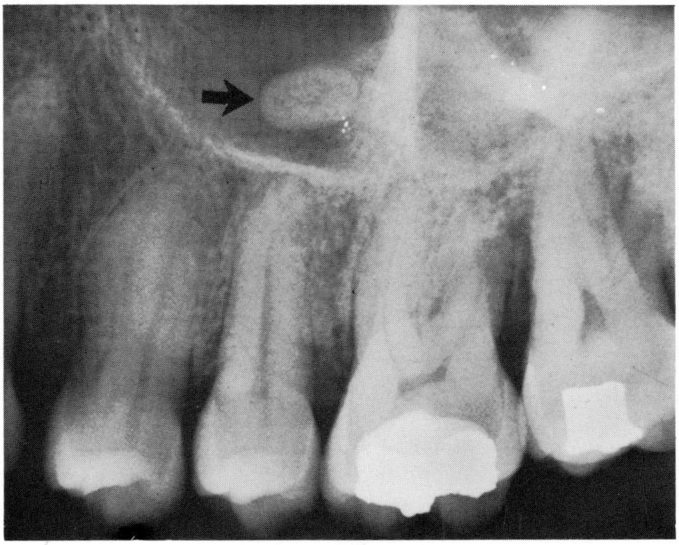

Fig. 7-7. Radiopaque foreign body in the antrum. It was asymptomatic and therefore was not removed.

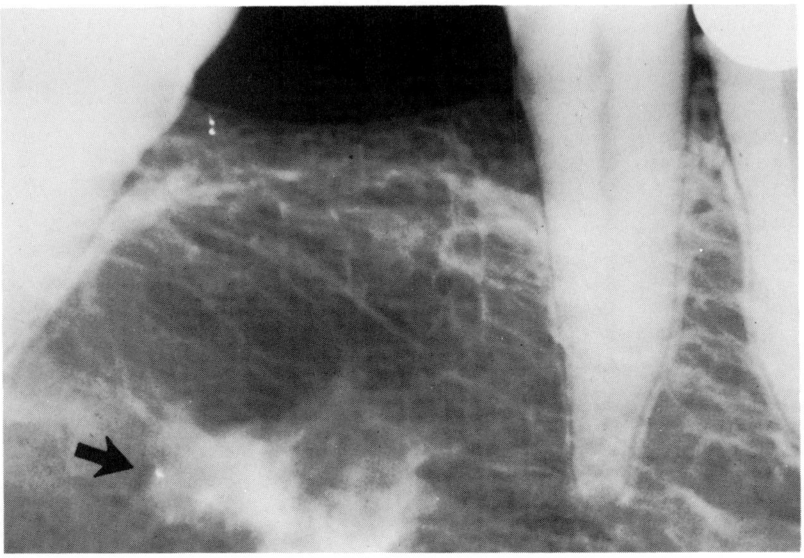

Fig. 7-8. Condensing osteitis (arrow). Radiopacity is without symptoms and does not enlarge.

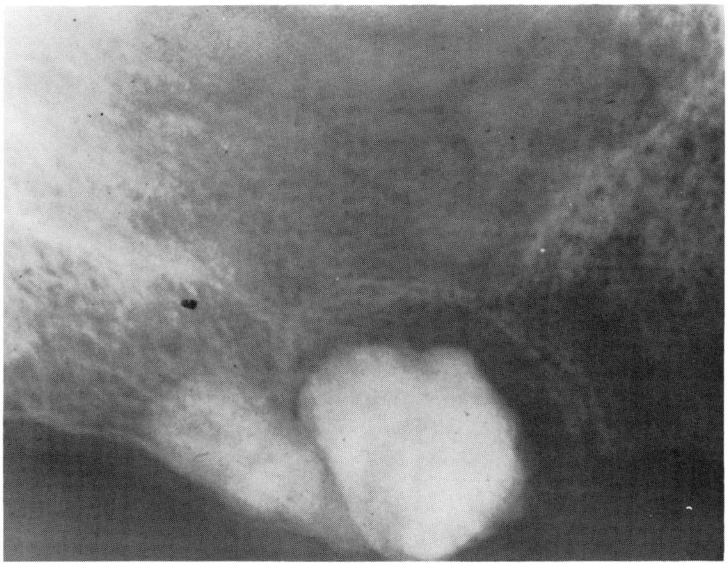

Fig. 7-9. Condensing osteitis in an area of edentulous maxillary ridge. Because of its proximity to the alveolar mucosa and the denture base, it was excised.

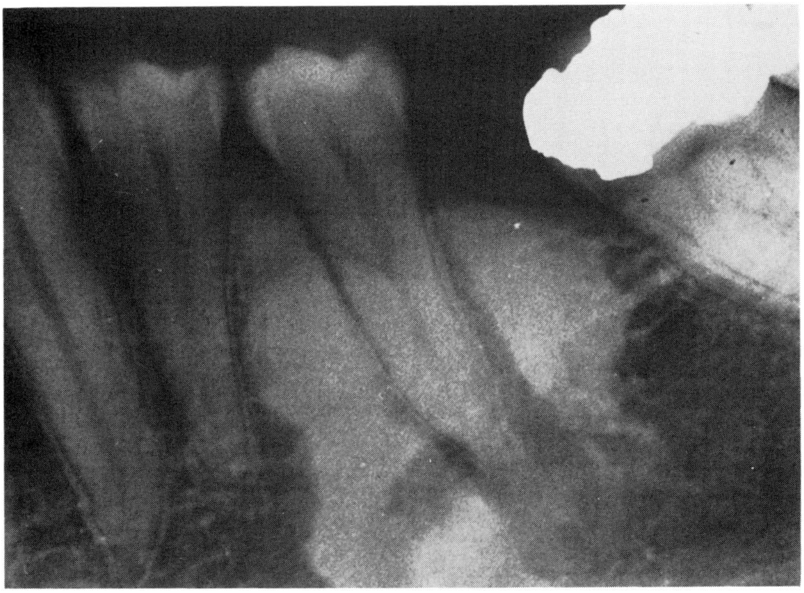

Fig. 7-10. A single asymptomatic, static radiopacity of long duration, representing condensing osteitis.

A

B

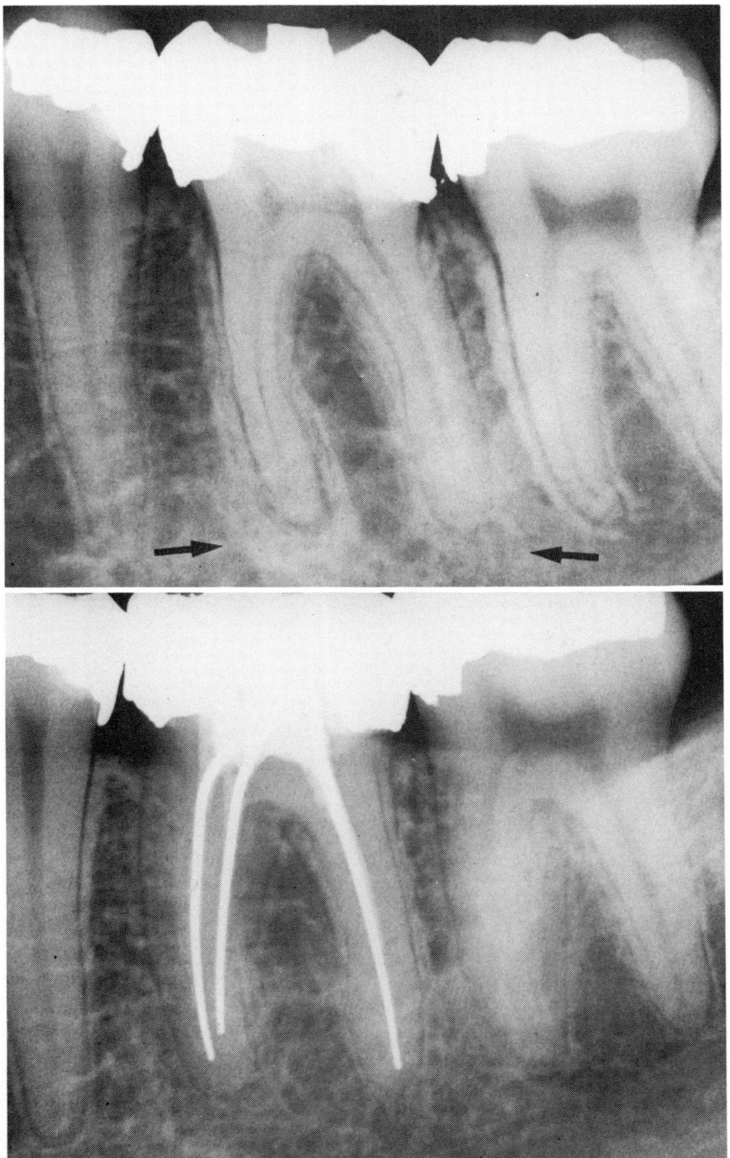

Fig. 7-11. Periapical condensing osteitis, **A,** that disappeared after root canal treatment, **B.**

A

B

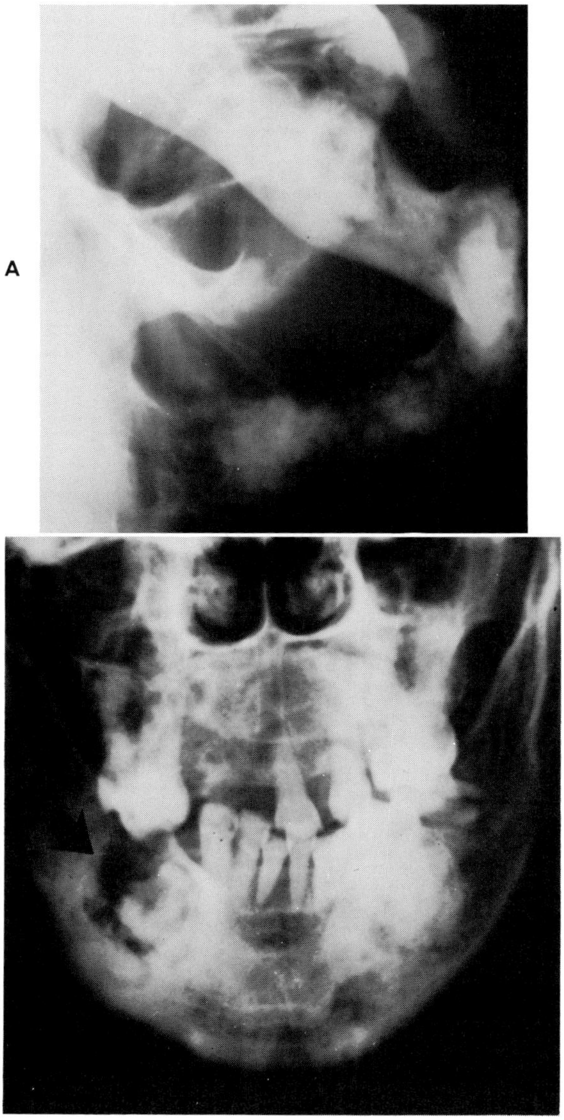

Fig. 7-12. Multiple enostosis of mandible and maxilla (two cases). **A,** Lateral radiograph of an edentulous mandible. **B,** Anteroposterior view of lesions in both jaws. Appearance of radiolucency (arrow) indicates secondary infection; such lesions should be removed.

ridge, they may undergo secondary infection. In such cases radiolucencies appear around them, and surgical removal becomes necessary.

Multiple enostosis. Also called *chronic sclerosing osteomyelitis* and *sclerosing osteomyelitis,* this condition shows multiple radiopaque masses in the jaws. Both edentulous and tooth-bearing areas of the jaws are affected (Fig. 7-12). Patients are older than 30 years of age, and the disease is more common in females. Radio-

A

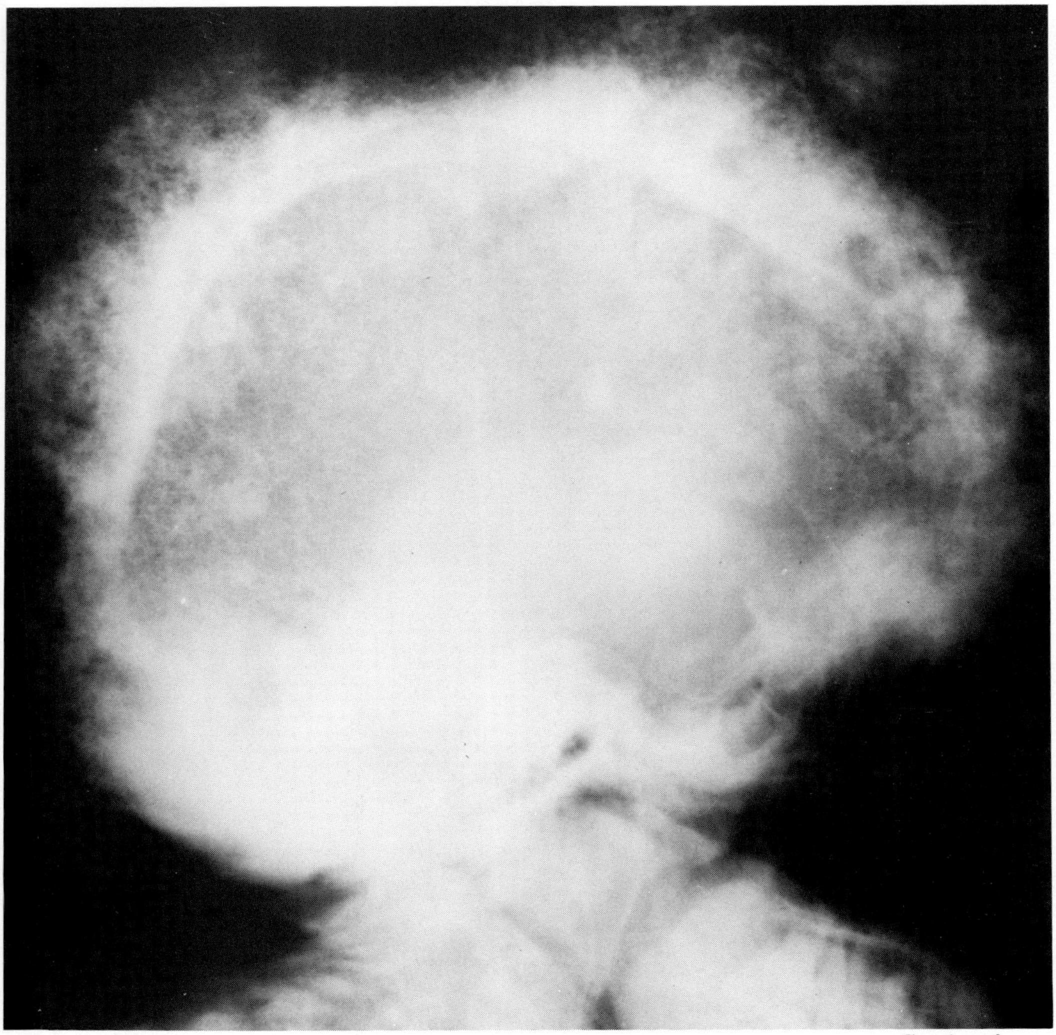

Continued.

Fig. 7-13. A, Skull of a patient with polyostotic fibrous dysplasia, revealing advanced osteosclerotic lesions. **B** and **C,** Forearms of the same patient. Note the expansion deformity and osteosclerotic lesion in the left radius, **C.**

pacities are of long duration, may expand the jaws, and unless secondarily infected are painless. A radiograph may show a cotton-wool appearance (Fig. 7-12, *A*). Normal laboratory tests and the absence of lesions in other bone, however, distinguish it from *Paget's disease* and from *polyostotic fibrous dysplasia.* Appearance of a radiolucency around one or more radiopacities indicates secondary infection, and such a change necessitates surgical intervention (Fig. 7-12, *B*). When multiple enostosis is seen in edentulous areas, the fabrication of a prosthesis should be avoided.

B 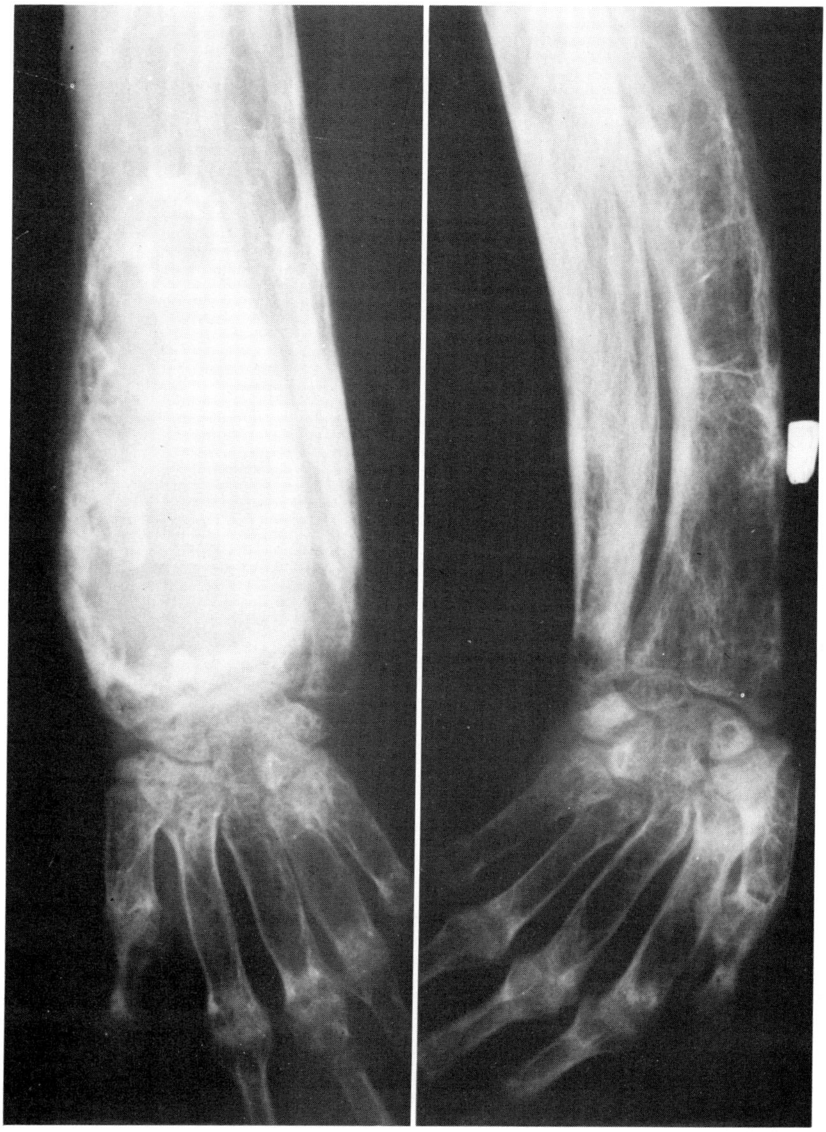 C

Fig. 7-13, cont'd. For legend see p. 173.

Polyostotic fibrous dysplasia. Polyostotic fibrous dysplasia involves multiple bones of the skeleton (Fig. 7-13). In the jaws, as elsewhere, it is characterized by expansile radiopaque lesions of varying density (Fig. 7-14). Some lesions, however, may appear radiolucent at times. Patients are children or young adults, migration of teeth is common, and lesions have slow growth. When the radiopacities involve the alveolar process, the lamina dura may disappear (Fig. 7-14). There are many other conditions, however, in which lamina dura may be lost, including hyperparathyroidism, Paget's disease, osteopetrosis, ossifying fibroma, multiple mye-

A

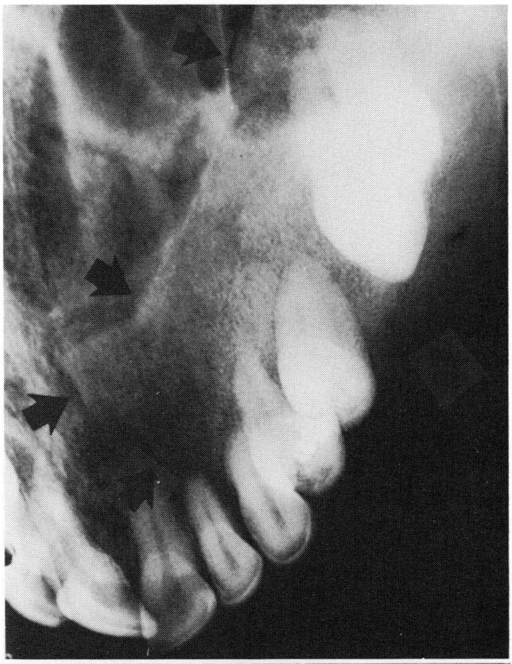

B

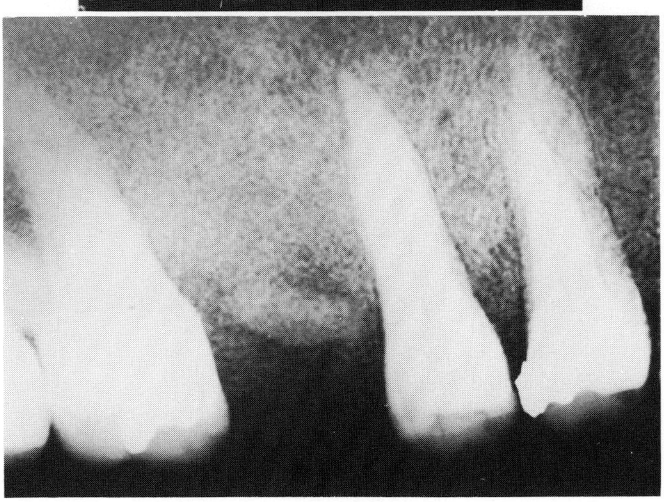

Fig. 7-14. Modified occlusal radiograph, **A,** and an intraoral radiograph, **B,** of a single lesion of fibrous dysplasia. **A,** Lesion is outlined by arrows. In **B,** note the radiopacity and the absence of lamina dura.

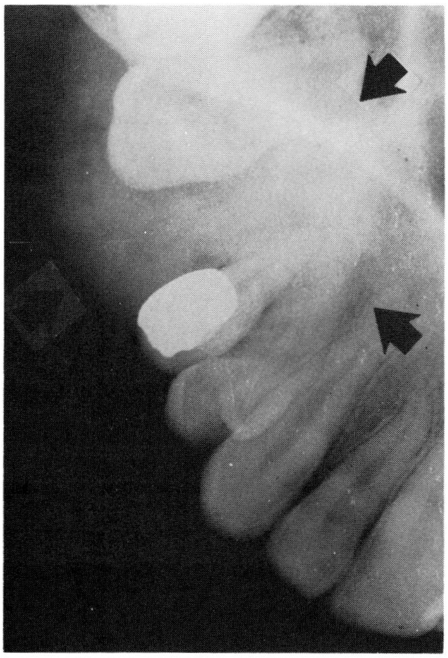

Fig. 7-15. Ossifying fibroma of the maxilla (arrows) that has produced migration of the second bicuspid and first molar teeth. Tumor is expansile but was of long duration.

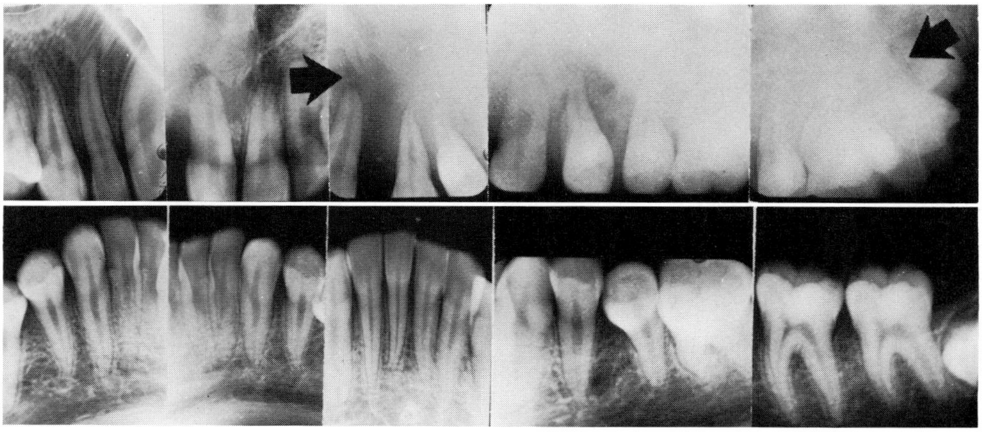

Fig. 7-16. Maxillary and mandibular intraoral radiographs showing an ossifying fibroma of the maxilla that extends from the left cuspid to the left tuberosity (arrows). Compare the tumor radiopacity with normal bony architecture seen elsewhere in the radiographs.

loma, rickets, and osteomalacia. This feature, therefore, is not of great diagnostic significance. Polyostotic fibrous dysplasia may be associated with endocrine dysfunction as well as pigmented patches on the skin, and such a symptom complex is called *Albright's syndrome*. In a differential diagnosis of this radiopacity, the in-

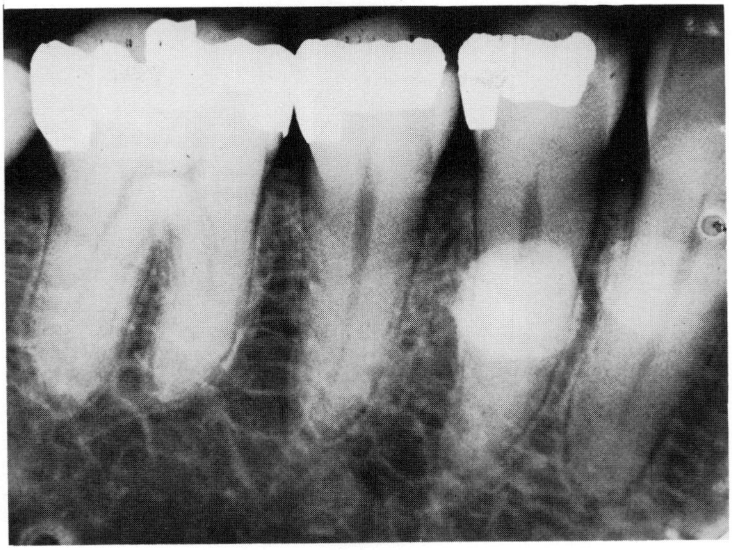

Fig. 7-17. Two tori on the lingual aspect of mandibular bicuspid teeth appear as circumscribed radiopacities. Intraoral apical radiograph.

volvement of multiple bones, in addition to the possible occurrence of endocrine disturbance and skin pigmentation, is the diagnostic feature.

Ossifying fibroma. Although ossifying fibroma is sometimes called *monostotic fibrous dysplasia,* this term should not be used for this lesion. It is always a single radiopaque lesion of dense or ground-glass opacity (Figs. 7-15 and 7-16). Patients may be of any age. The radiopacity is usually expansile (Fig. 7-15), but there are no systemic symptoms, and other bones of the skeleton are not involved. Tooth migration occurs frequently, but loosening and exfoliation of teeth are not seen (Fig. 7-15). The growth of the lesion varies from very slow to so rapid that clinically it mimics a malignant tumor. Teeth in the area may show loss of the lamina dura (Figs. 7-15 and 7-16). The solitary lesion, expansile nature, and normal blood values of calcium, phosphorus, and alkaline phosphatase distinguish ossifying fibroma from the true fibrous dysplasia and from the other radiopaque lesions.

Exostosis, torus, and osteoma. Exostoses, tori, and osteomas are related lesions, and in fact, these terms may be used interchangeably. These single or multiple radiopaque lesions occur on the *periosteal surface* of the jaws. The midline of the palate and the lingual aspect of mandibular bicuspids are the most common sites, and in these locations they are called *torus palatinus* and *torus mandibularis,* respectively (Figs. 7-17 and 7-18). They can, however, occur on the surface of any area of the mandible and maxilla. These radiopaque masses can be seen clinically and are of very slow and limited growth. In intraoral radiographs they appear as clearly outlined radiopacities and offer no diagnostic problem.

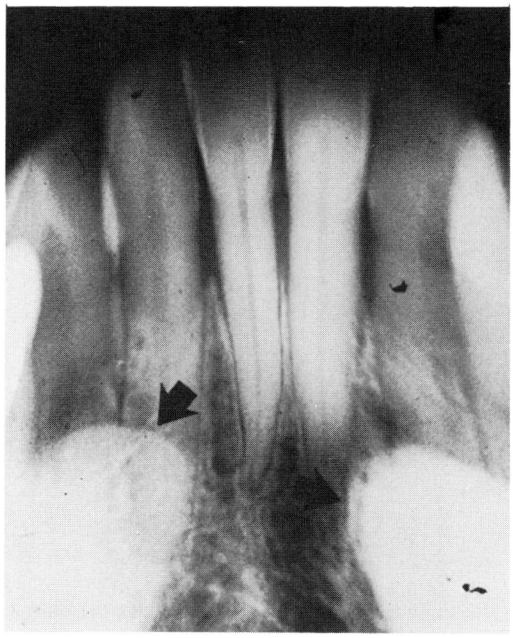

Fig. 7-18. Tori on the lingual aspect of mandibular cuspids appear as radiopaque bodies in intraoral radiographs (arrows).

Paget's disease. Paget's disease occurs in patients older than 40 years, and it involves many bones of the skeleton. Enlargement of the skull, thickening of the cranial vault (Fig. 7-19), deformity of the spine and bones of the leg, headaches, and loss of vision are only some of the many features of this disease. The jaws also show enlargement, and there is migration of teeth, which produces diastemas and gross malocclusion (Fig. 7-20). The maxilla is affected more often than the mandible. Radiographs of the skull show thickening of the cortex of the cranial vault and numerous radiopaque lesions that have a cotton-wool appearance (Figs. 7-21 and 7-22). Similar multiple lesions are seen in the jaws, and tooth migration, loss of lamina dura, and hypercementosis are frequently observed (Fig. 7-20). The jaw lesions may be diffuse and have a ground-glass appearance.

The radiographic appearance of the jaws is very similar to that seen in multiple enostosis and polyostotic fibrous dysplasia. However, it is distinguished from multiple enostosis by the presence of lesions elsewhere in the skeleton and also by elevated serum alkaline phosphatase. Paget's disease is distinguished from polyostotic fibrous dysplasia by the much older age of the patients, presence of neurologic symptoms, and absence of endocrine disturbances.

In radiographic analysis of Paget's disease the dentist must be concerned by the rapid growth of one of the radiopaque areas. Such an acceleration of growth may signify the development of an osteogenic sarcoma, which originates in about one fourth of all cases of this disease.

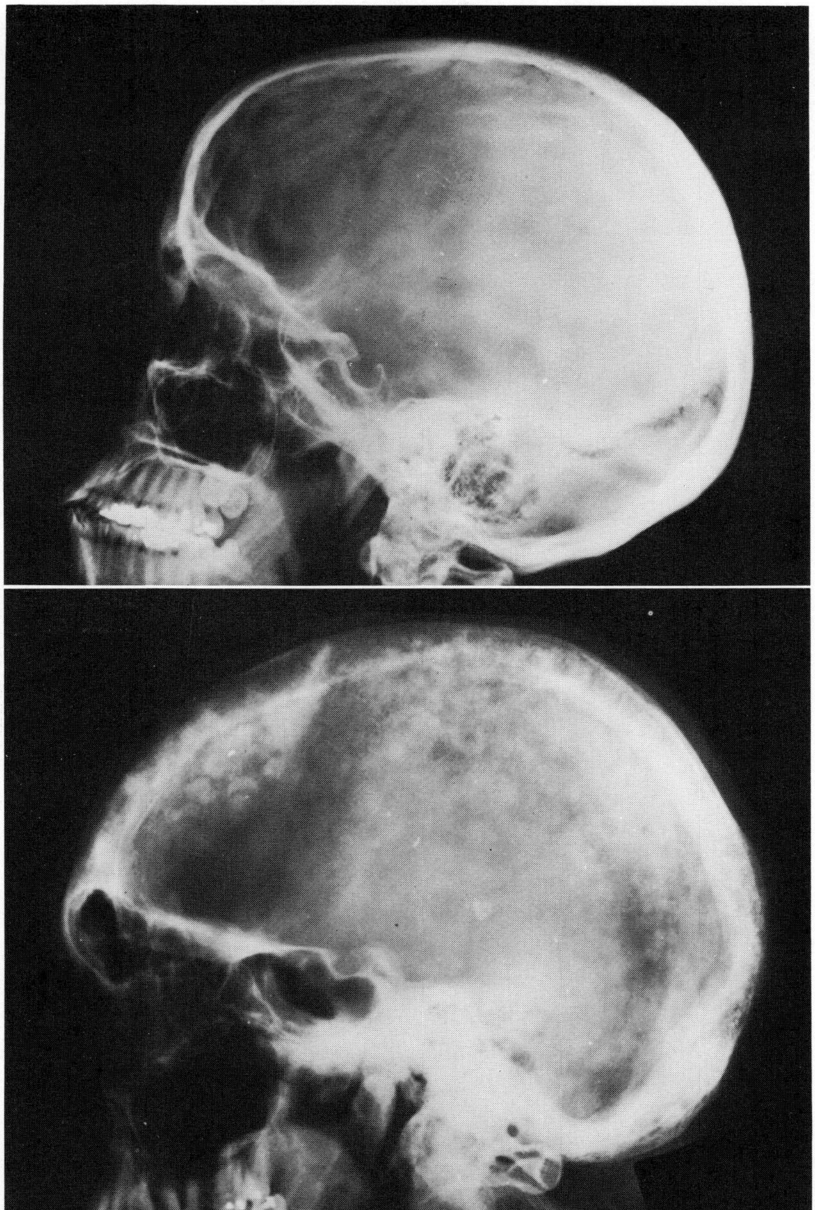

A

B

Fig. 7-19. Lateral radiographs of the normal skull, **A,** and skull in Paget's disease, **B.** Compare the thickness of the cranial vaults and cranial bases and the degree of radiopacity.

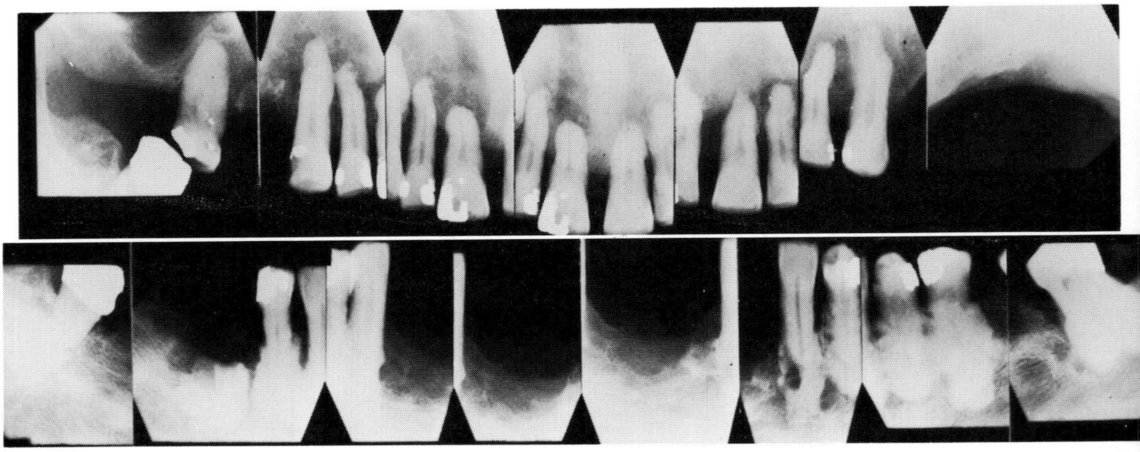

Fig. 7-20. Intraoral radiographs of the maxilla and mandible in a patient with Paget's disease. Note the dense radiopacity of the jaws, loss of lamina dura, diastemas, and hypercementosis.

Cementoma (stage III). Cementoma in the third, or last, stage appears as single or multiple circumscribed radiopaque areas at the apices of teeth (Fig. 7-23). The anterior mandibular region is the most frequently involved. Lesions are of limited growth and long duration, and occur more often in the female. Teeth are always vital. In any given case cementomas in each of the three stages may be seen (Fig. 7-23).

Unerupted teeth. Supernumerary, accessory, or normal unerupted teeth appear as radiopacities (Fig. 7-24). These structures may be in their usual location in the jaws or found far away from it. In radiographs with poor contrast it may be difficult to identify the dense radiopaque quality of enamel, and these teeth may be mistaken for lesions of other types. Usually, however, their shape is of diagnostic value.

Compound and complex odontoma. The odontogenic tumors known as compound and complex odontomas are radiopaque masses that contain enamel, dentin, and pulp. They can be distinguished from other radiopaque lesions partly by the dense radiopacity of the enamel and partly by their outline. Some of these tumors are composed of two or more small toothlike structures and are referred to as *compound odontomas* (Figs. 7-25 to 7-27). In other cases the tumor appears as an irregular, very dense (because of enamel), radiopaque, conglomerate mass of calcified tissues called a *complex odontoma* (Figs. 7-27 to 7-30). Odontomas grow slowly and are easily recognized.

Osteopetrosis. Also called Albers-Schönberg disease or marble bone disease, osteopetrosis is a hereditary disturbance that is present at birth and that involves the entire skeleton. It is characterized by normal bone formation but absence of bone resorption. As a result, bone tissue accumulates, and the bones become heavy and in radiographs appear as solid radiopaque structures with little or no

Text continued on p. 187.

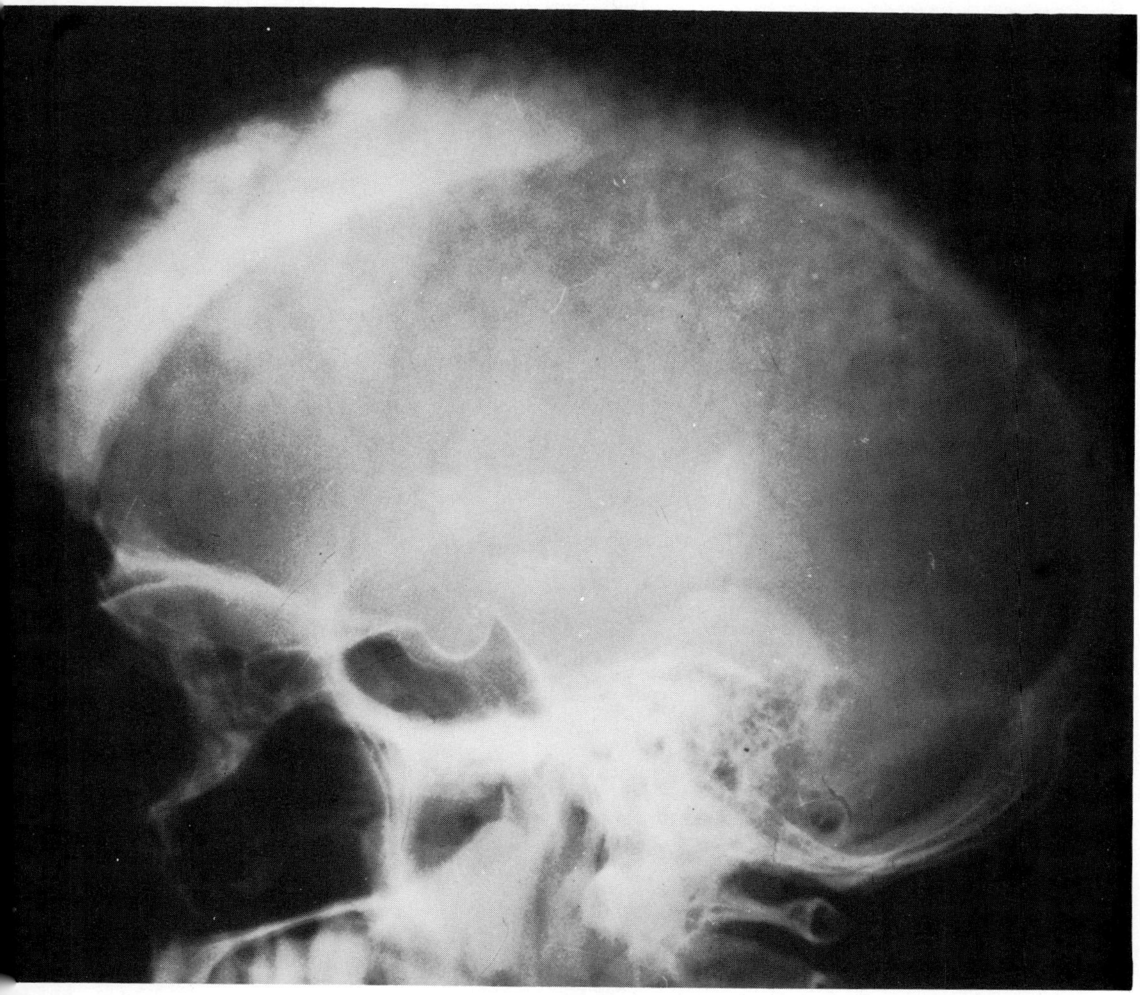

Fig. 7-21. Radiopaque cotton-wool appearance of anterior part of the cranial vault in a patient with Paget's disease.

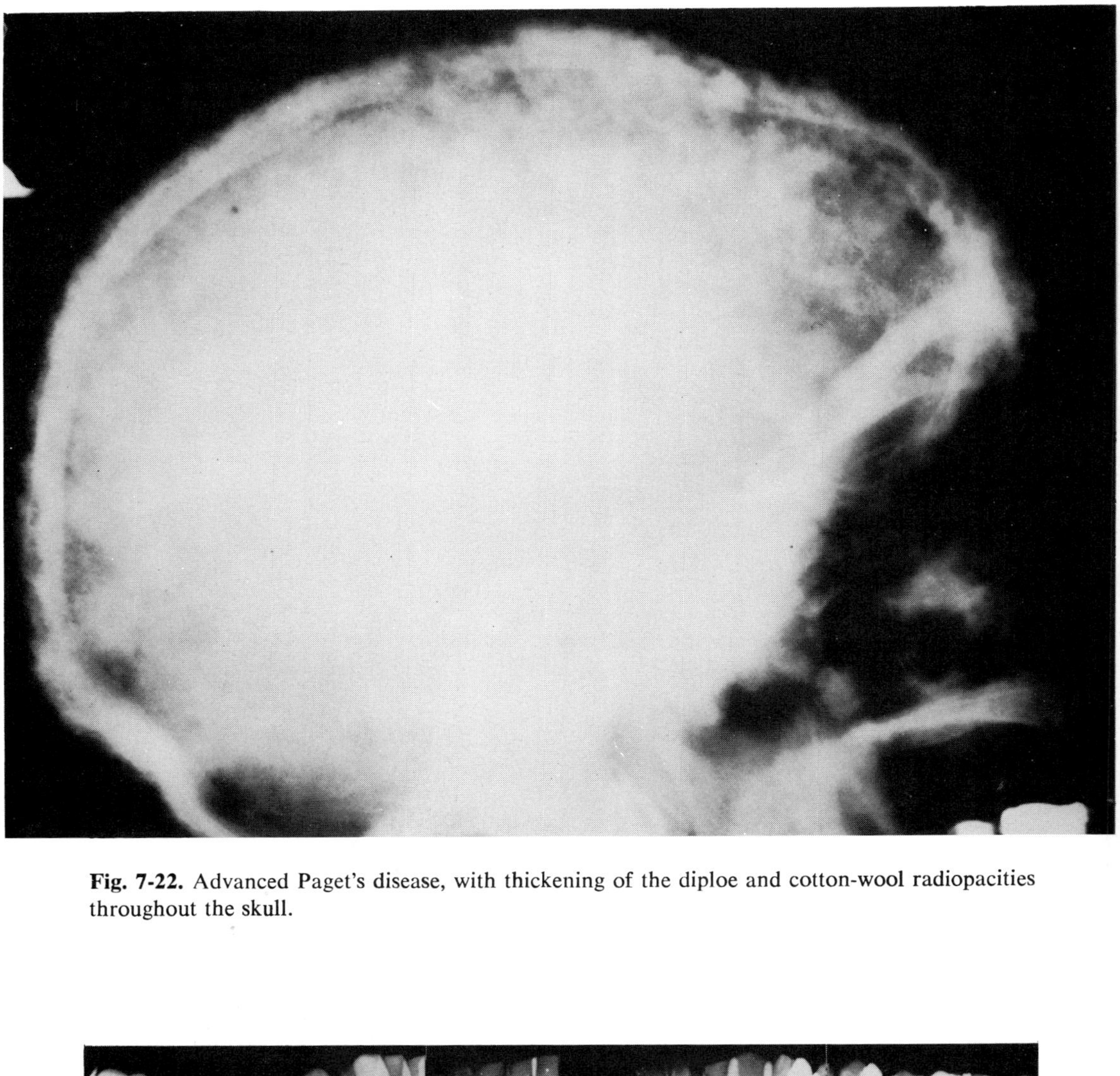

Fig. 7-22. Advanced Paget's disease, with thickening of the diploe and cotton-wool radiopacities throughout the skull.

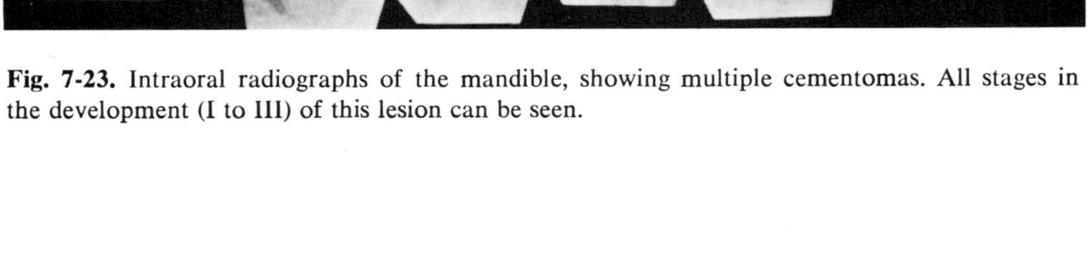

Fig. 7-23. Intraoral radiographs of the mandible, showing multiple cementomas. All stages in the development (I to III) of this lesion can be seen.

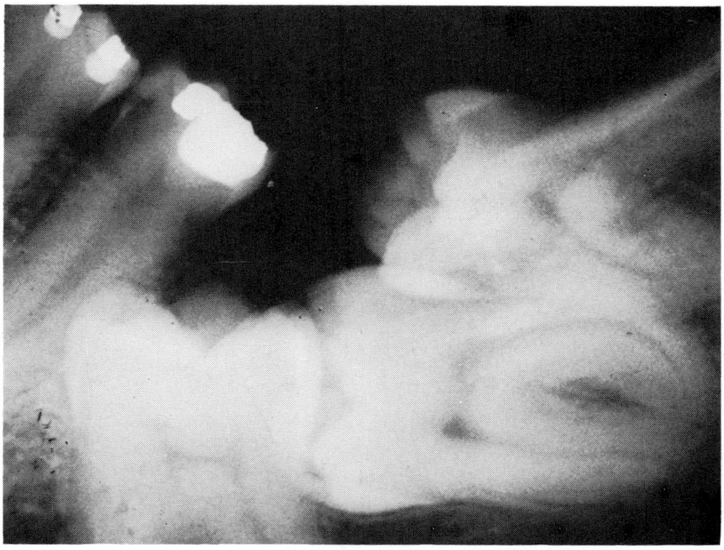

Fig. 7-24. Radiopacities produced by unerupted impacted teeth.

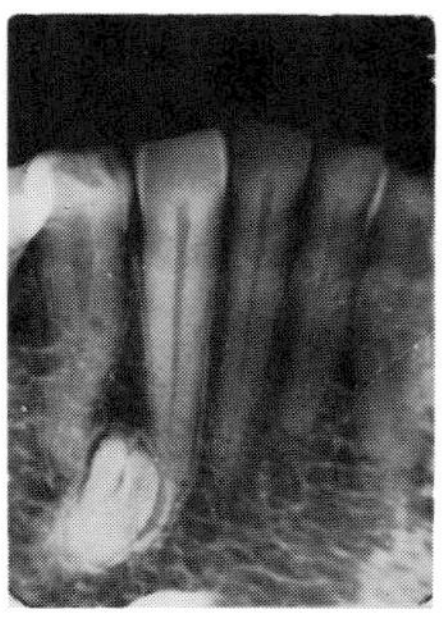

Fig. 7-25. Compound odontoma composed of two small, toothlike structures. Radiolucent border around the tumor is analogous to the periodontal ligament.

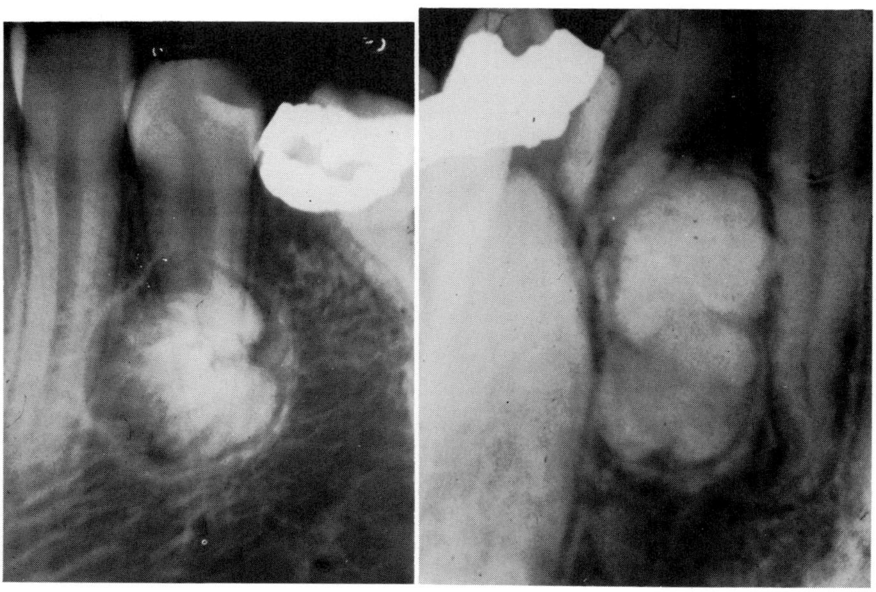

Fig. 7-26. Two cases of compound odontoma. They are both composed of many toothlike structures.

A

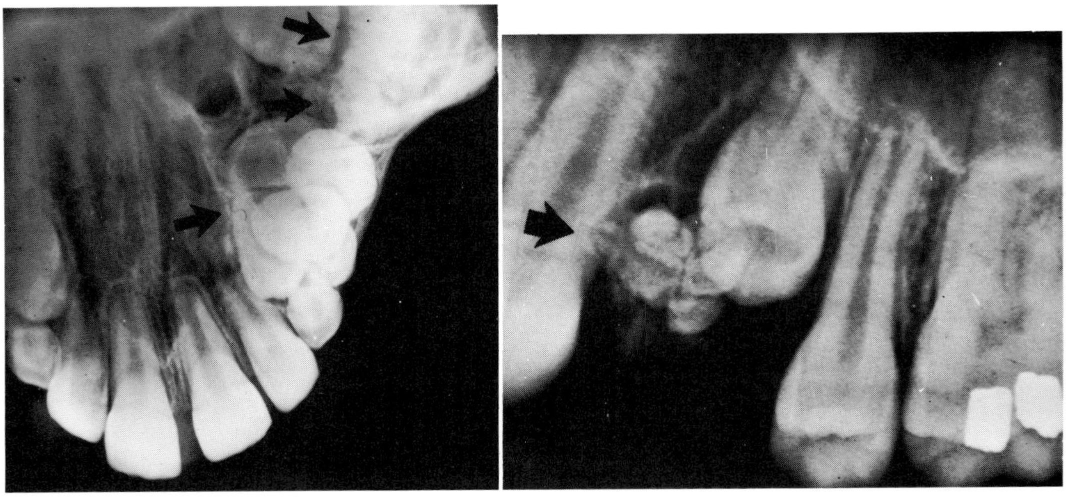

Fig. 7-27. A, Occlusal radiograph of a patient with both a compound odontoma (one arrow) and a complex odontoma (two arrows). The compound odontoma is composed of many teeth, whereas the complex odontoma is a conglomerate mass of hard and soft dental tissues. The structure above the nasolacrimal canal is an impacted tooth. **B,** Compound odontoma.

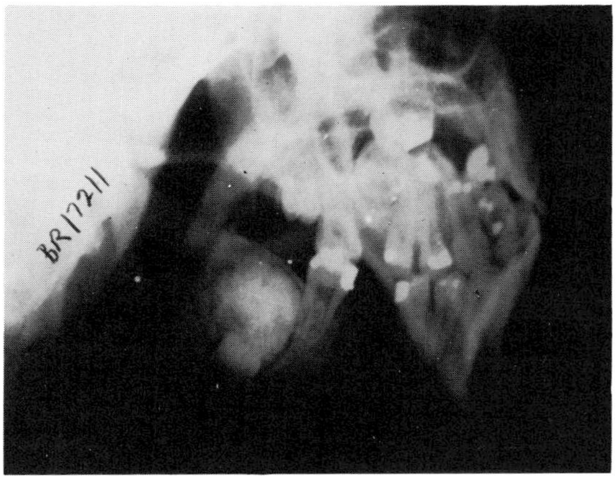

Fig. 7-28. Complex odontoma in the molar region of the mandible.

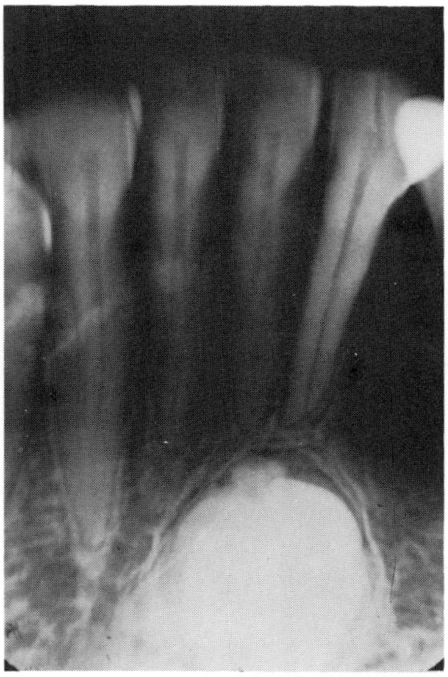

Fig. 7-29. Complex odontoma in the lower incisor area. Its dense radiopacity and size distinguish it from the cementoma.

A

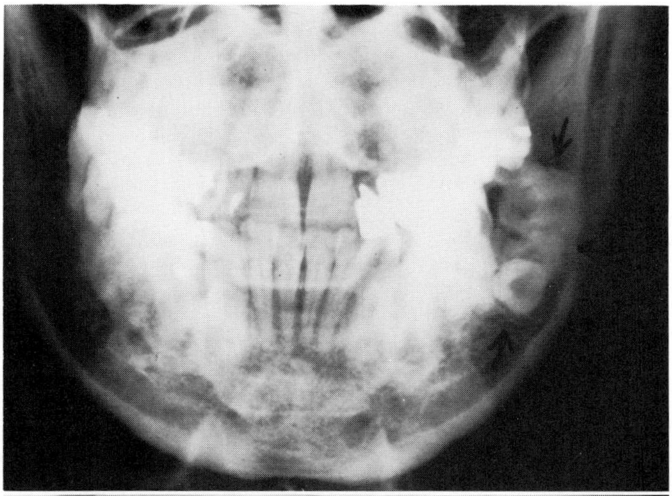

B

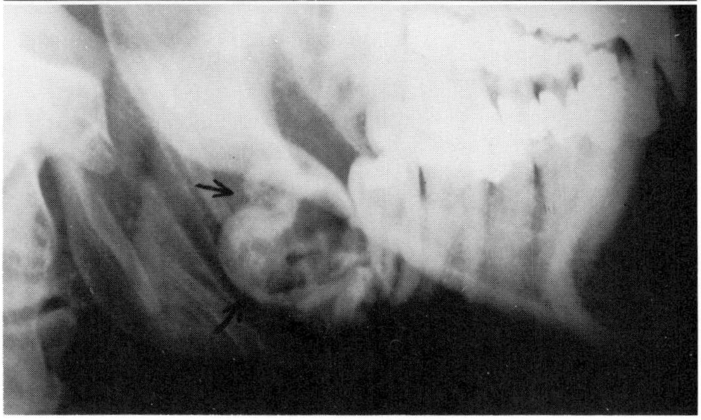

Fig. 7-30. Anteroposterior view, **A,** and lateral view, **B,** of a complex odontoma. In **B** the tumor appears to be impinging on the inferior dental canal.

A

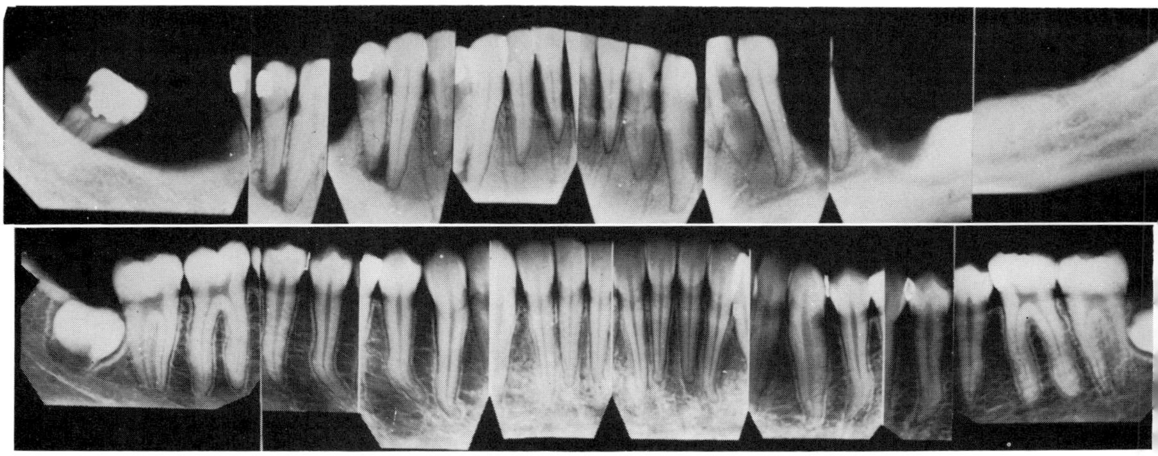

B

Fig. 7-31. Intraoral radiographs of the mandible in marble bone disease, **A,** show far greater radiopacity than the normal, **B.** In **A,** bone trabeculae cannot be identified.

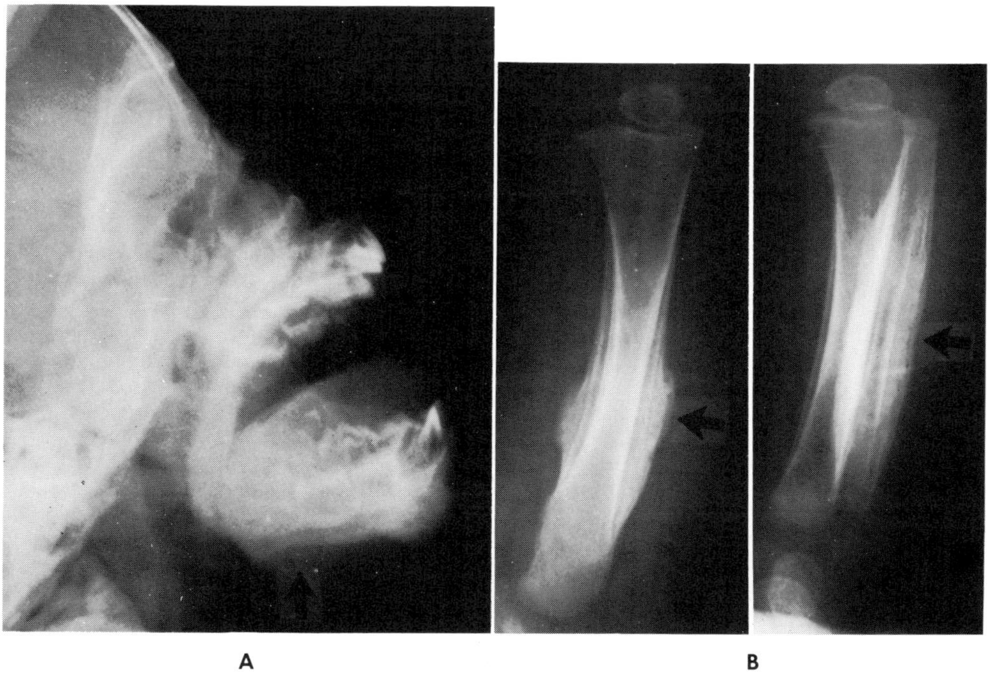

A B

Fig. 7-32. Caffey's disease reveals radiopacity along the lower border of mandible, **A. B,** Cortices of the tibia and fibula show marked thickening (arrows).

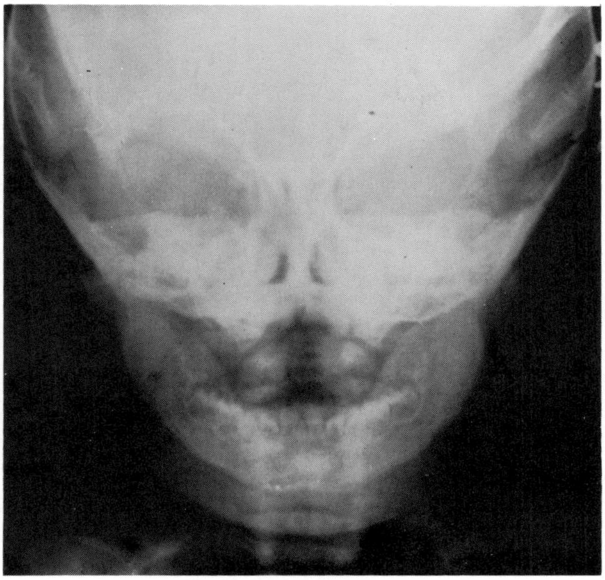

Fig. 7-33. Anteroposterior view of the skull in Caffey's disease, showing marked radiopaque thickening of the lower border of the mandible.

bone marrow. In the skull, the diploë is thick and densely radiopaque. The jaws show radiopacity, loss of lamina dura, and abnormal location of teeth (Fig. 7-31). Extraction sites heal very slowly. The dense radiopacity of most or all parts of the skeleton and the presence of the disease from birth are the diagnostic features.

Leontiasis ossea. Leontiasis ossea is a developmental disorder that starts in childhood, is progressive, and affects the upper face. It is characterized by osteopetrosis-like changes that are limited to the maxilla, nasal, frontal, and zygomatic bones. Radiographs show dense radiopacities and may be associated with disturbances of vision and hearing.

Caffey's disease. This abnormality of unknown etiology involves patients in the first year of life, usually under 6 months of age. The mandible is involved in more than 75% of the cases, and the ulna, clavicle, and other long bones are involved less often. Children have fever and leukocytosis and are irritable. Radiographs show radiopaque enlargement or thickening of the lower border of the mandible and thickening of the cortex of the other affected bones (Figs. 7-32 and 7-33). The age of the patient and the characteristic radiographic appearance of the mandible and the long bones are diagnostic. The disease requires no therapy.

Garré's osteomyelitis. Garré's osteomyelitis is essentially a *proliferative sclerosing type of periostitis.* It is more common in the mandible and usually occurs along its lower border. Patients are children and young adults, and the enlargement of the lower border of the jaw occurs in response to some centrally located inflammatory lesion, such as abscess, cyst, or osteomyelitis. Radiographs show radiopacity on

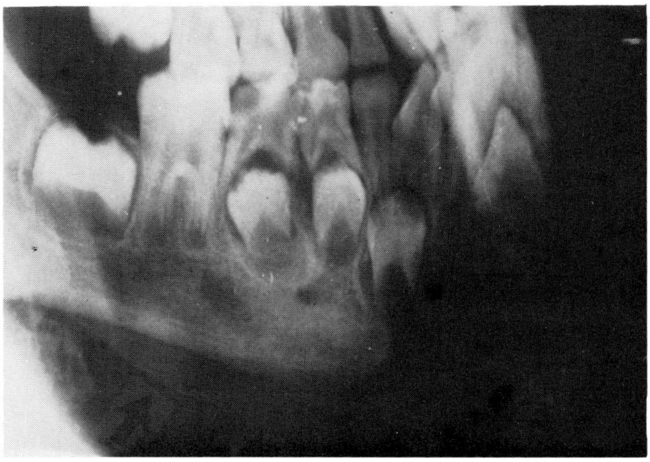

Fig. 7-34. Garré's osteomyelitis is characterized by a radiopaque thickening of the lower border of mandible (arrow).

A

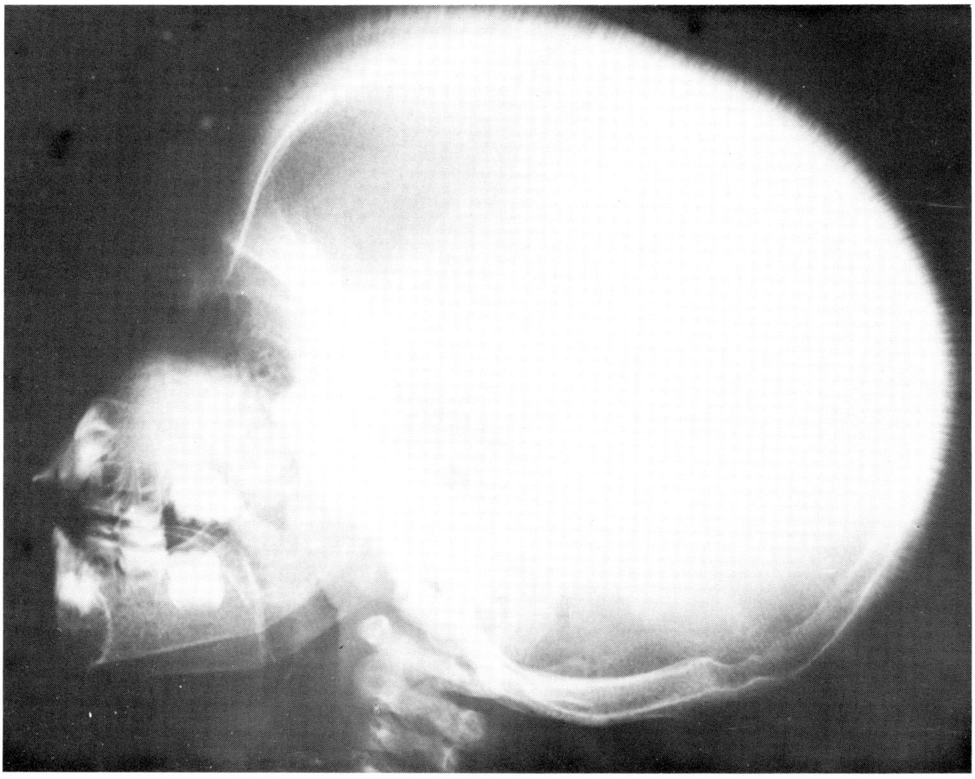

Fig. 7-35. Lateral, **A,** and anteroposterior, **B,** radiographs of the skull in a patient with Cooley's anemia. Note the "hair on end" appearance of the cranial vault.

B

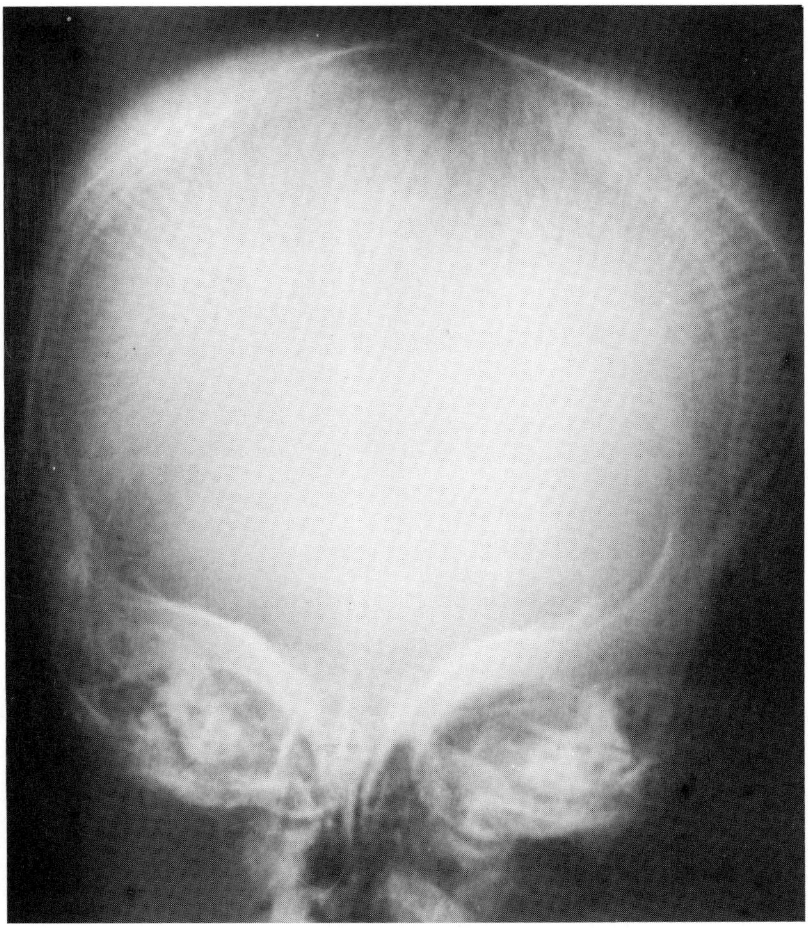

Fig. 7-35, cont'd. For legend see opposite page.

the periosteal side of the affected bone (Fig. 7-34). Except for the treatment of the apparent cause of the periosteal bone deposition, this condition does not require any therapy.

Thalassemia (Cooley's anemia). Thalassemia, a type of hemolytic hereditary anemia, occurs among the Mediterranean races and is characterized by yellow skin, weakness, and enlargement of liver and spleen. Some patients have a mongoloid appearance. Radiographs of the skull show thickening of diploë and vertical radiopaque trabeculae on the surface of the cranial vault, which give it a "hair on end" appearance (Fig. 7-35). These radiopaque trabeculae start from the inner table of the cranial vault and extend beyond the outer surface. The jaws are enlarged and show many dense, irregular, coarse trabeculations (Fig. 7-36), and the maxillary antrum may be obliterated. The bones of the hands and feet may also show a peculiar characteristic, lattice type of trabeculation (Fig. 7-37).

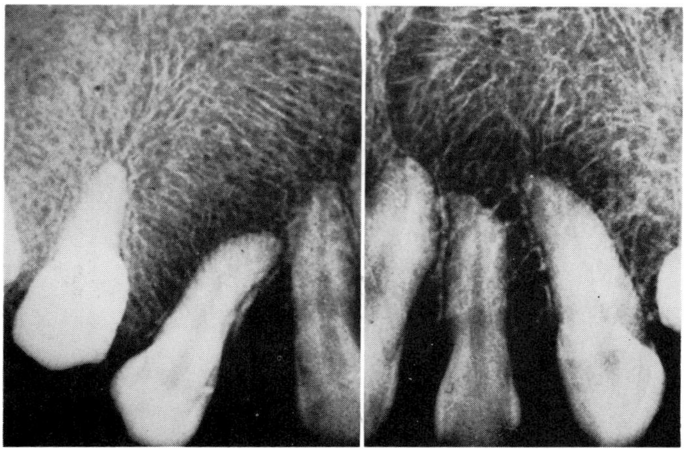

Fig. 7-36. Radiograph of the maxilla in Cooley's anemia. Note peculiar, coarse, radiopaque trabeculations of bone.

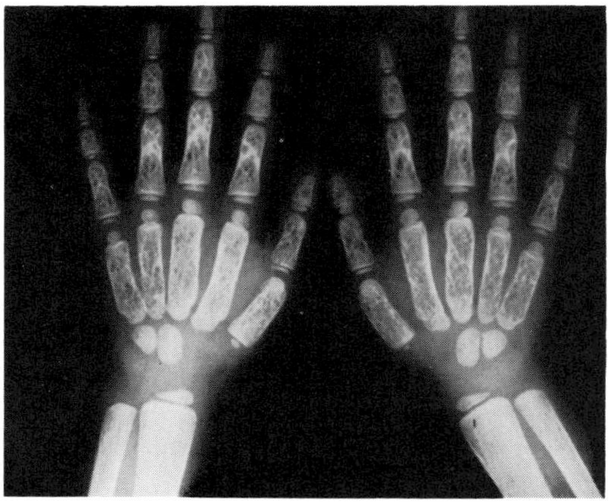

Fig. 7-37. Radiograph of the hands in a patient with Cooley's anemia, showing dense radiopaque trabeculae.

Osteogenic sarcoma. Osteogenic sarcoma, a malignant tumor of bone, is characterized by rapid growth, migration and loosening of teeth, ulceration, pain, and paresthesia. It occurs in patients who are between 10 and 30 years of age. Although some osteogenic sarcomas, like the osteolytic osteogenic sarcoma, may be radiolucent, the majority show radiopacities of varying density (Figs. 7-38 to 7-40). Widening of the periodontal space of teeth in the area of the tumor is believed to be the earliest radiographic sign (Figs. 7-41 and 7-42). The radiopacity destroys the cortex of the affected bone and extends into soft tissues (Figs. 7-38 to 7-40). Radiating radiopaque striae from the cortex of the affected bone give the radiograph the so-called "sunray" appearance (Figs. 7-38 and 7-39). However, it is not seen in all tumors (Fig. 7-40). The rapid growth, neurologic symptoms, and

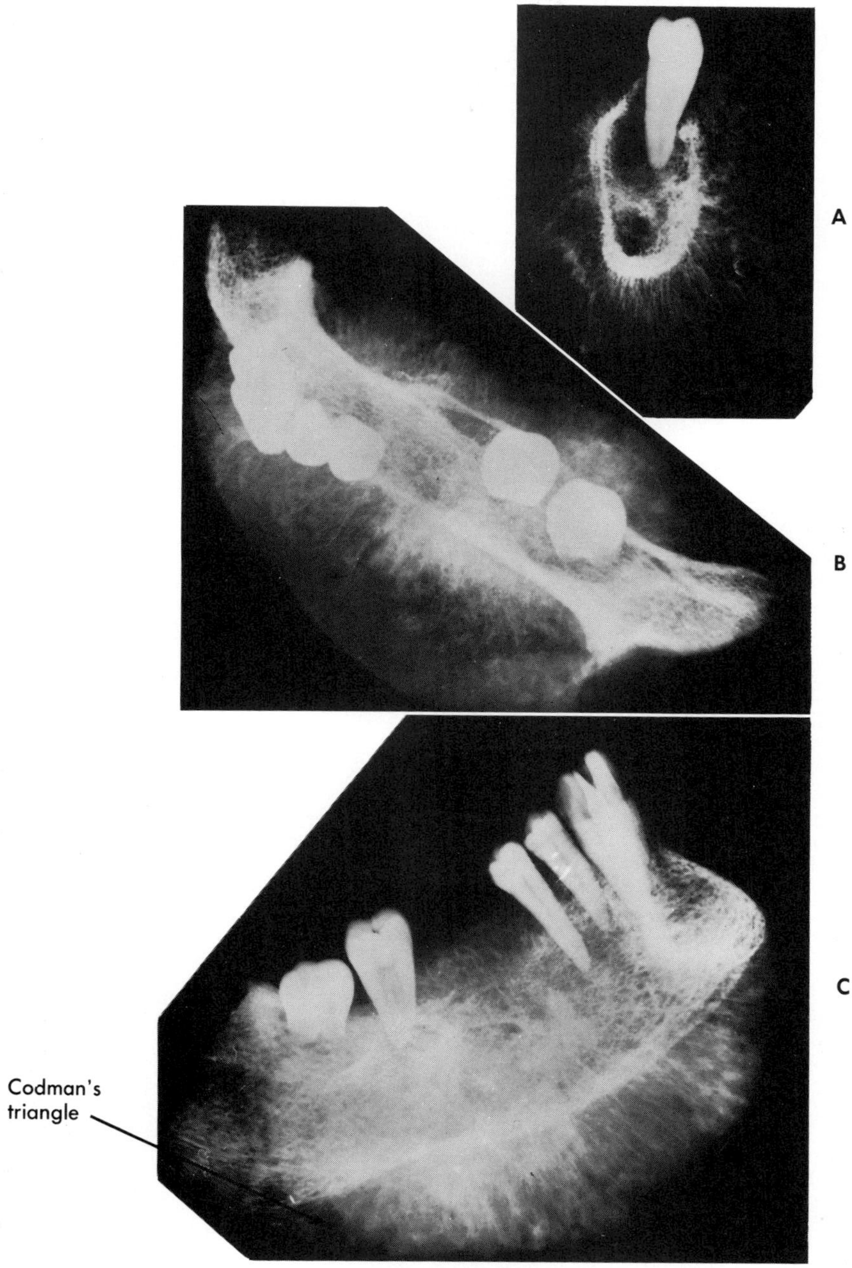

Fig. 7-38. Anteroposterior view, **A,** occlusal view, **B,** and lateral view, **C,** of a part of the mandible resected because of osteogenic sarcoma. In all three views the "sunray" effect can be seen. This type of radiopacity grows rapidly and violates the cortical plates of the jaws. In **C** note so-called Codman's triangle.

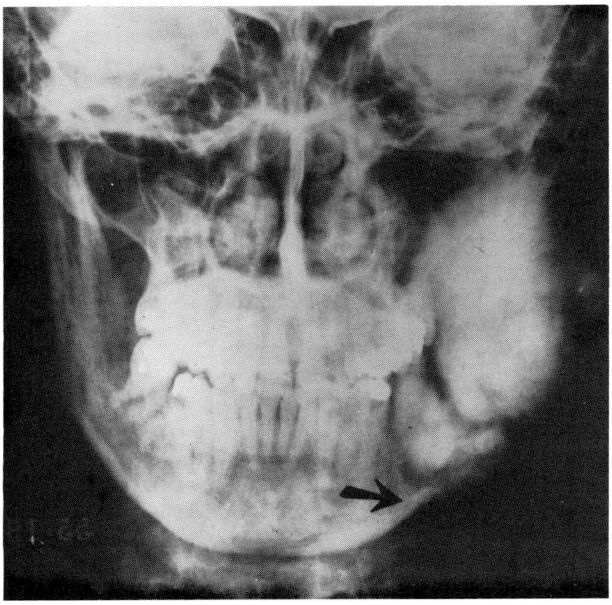

Fig. 7-39. Anteroposterior view of the skull, showing the radiopacity of an osteogenic sarcoma. Note the sunray effect and the destruction of the cortical plate beyond the arrow.

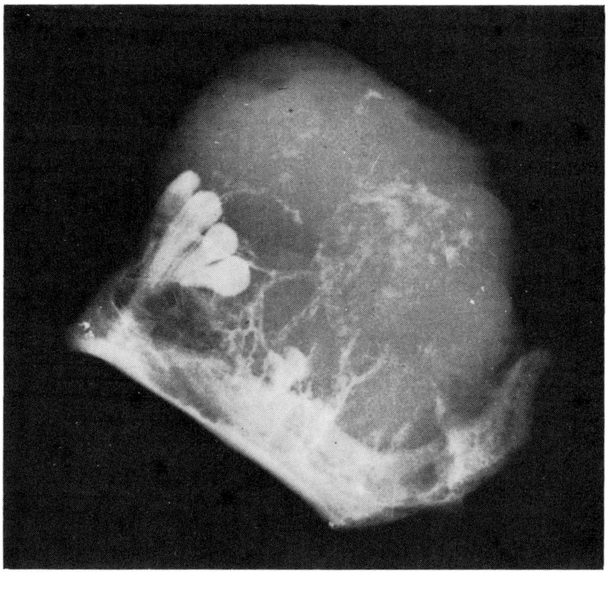

Fig. 7-40. Radiograph of a mandible resected for an osteogenic sarcoma. Note that the radiopacity of this tumor is less dense than that of tumors seen in Figs. 7-38 and 7-39.

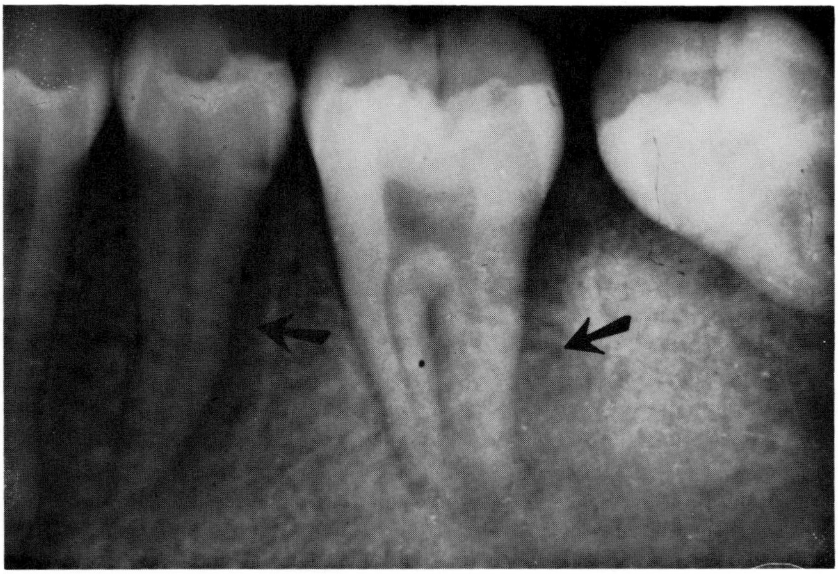

Fig. 7-41. Intraoral radiograph of an osteogenic sarcoma. Note the widening of the periodontal ligament (arrow) in two areas. This feature is believed to be an early diagnostic sign of the osteosarcoma and the chondrosarcoma.

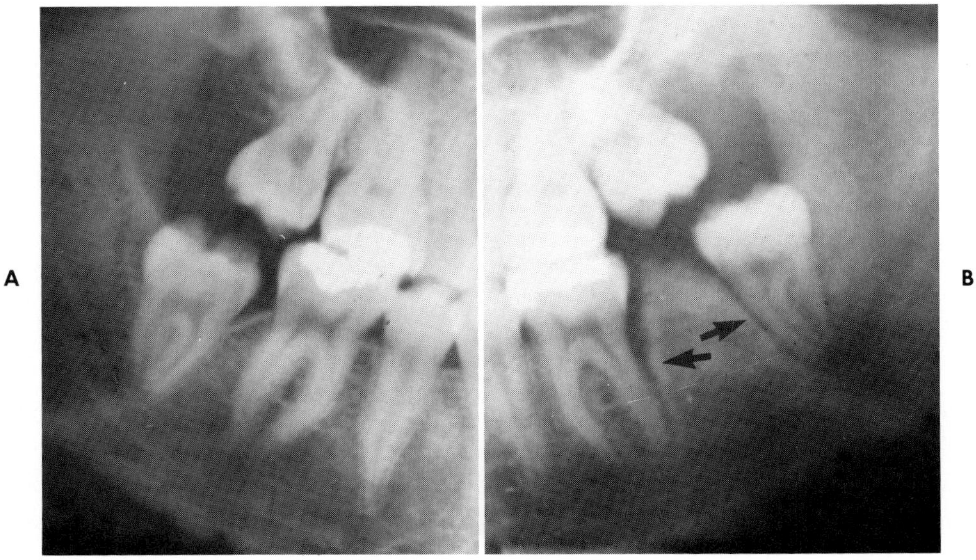

Fig. 7-42. Normal, **A,** and tumor side, **B,** in a patient with osteogenic sarcoma. In **B** note the widening of the periodontal spaces (arrows).

A

B

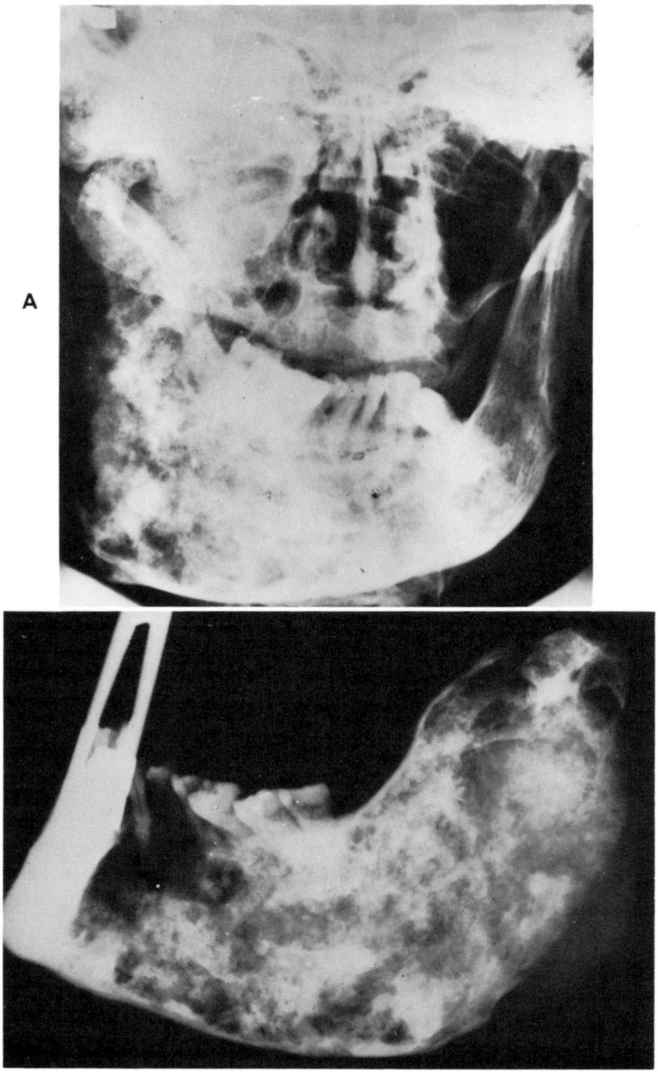

Fig. 7-43. Anteroposterior view, **A,** and lateral view, **B,** of a chondrosarcoma. In **B** the tumor has been excised. The rapid growth of the tumor and the destruction of the cortex distinguish a chondrosarcoma from an ossifying fibroma.

sunray effect, when present, are diagnostic features. In some cases of osteogenic sarcoma, in which the tumor extends beyond the cortex of the bone, it raises the surrounding periosteum, and in the triangular area between the periosteum and the underlying bone, new bone formation occurs and a triangular radiopaque area, called Codman's triangle, appears (Fig. 7-38).

Chondrosarcoma. A chondrosarcoma resembles an osteogenic sarcoma and cannot be distinguished from it radiographically (Fig. 7-43). As in the osteosar-

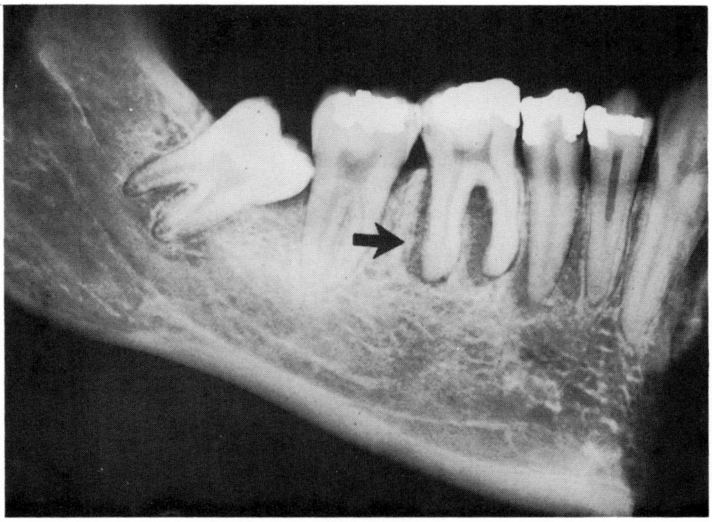

Fig. 7-44. In this lateral radiograph of an excised mandible with chondrosarcoma, the widening of the periodontal ligament (arrow) of the first molar is clearly seen. This feature is believed to be highly suggestive of chondrosarcomas and osteosarcomas.

Table 5. Diagnostic features of radiopaque lesions of the jaws

LESION	IMPORTANT CLINICAL AND RADIOGRAPHIC FEATURES
Broken roots	Shape and clinical history
Foreign bodies	Shape and clinical history
Condensing osteitis	Location, absence of symptoms, absence of growth, usually nonexpansile radiopacity
Multiple enostosis	Multiple lesions, long duration, patient older than 30 years, absence of lesions elsewhere in skeleton
Polyostotic fibrous dysplasia	Multiple bones involved, patient young; endocrine disturbances
Ossifying fibroma	Single lesion, migration of teeth, expansive growth
Exostosis, torus, and osteoma	Slow or limited growth, and periosteal location
Paget's disease	Patient older than 40 years; male; multiple cotton-wool radiopacities; involvement of skull and other bones of skeleton
Cementoma (stage III)	Small size of lesion, apical location; vital teeth, absence of symptoms, mandibular incisor location
Unerupted teeth	Anatomic shape
Compound odontoma	Multiple toothlike structures in one location
Complex odontoma	Single lesion, clear border, radiopacity of enamel, absence of or slow growth
Osteopetrosis	Presence since birth, dense radiopacity of entire skeleton
Leontiasis ossea	Presence since birth, dense radiopacity in upper facial bones only, optic and auditory disturbances
Caffey's disease	Patients under 1 year of age; enlargement and radiopacity of lower border of mandible
Garré's osteomyelitis	Single radiopacity on periosteal side of an inflammatory lesion within jaw; patients children and young adults
Thalassemia (Cooley's anemia)	History, hair-on-end appearance of skull; coarse trabeculation of jaws and bones of hand and feet
Osteogenic sarcoma and chondrosarcoma	Rapid growth; radiopacity destroys cortex; sunray effect, widening of periodontal ligament, pain, ulceration
Metastatic tumors	History of prostatic or breast cancer

coma, one of the earliest signs of this tumor is said to be the widening of the periodontal ligament (Fig. 7-44).

Metastatic tumors. Metastatic foci of adenocarcinoma of the prostate and rarely of the breast may cause local radiopacities. However, they are a rare occurrence, and clinical history is of diagnostic significance.

• • •

The most important diagnostic features of various radiopaque lesions of the jaws are shown in Table 5.

REFERENCES

Bethart, H., and Fitch, H. B.: Caffey's disease, Oral Surg. **16:**622, 1963.

Bhaskar, S. N.: Synopsis of oral pathology, ed. 3, St. Louis, 1969, The C. V. Mosby Co.

Bhaskar, S. N., and Cutright, D. E.: Multiple enostosis, J. Oral Surg. **26:**321, 1968.

Boyne, P. J.: Incidence of osteosclerotic areas in the mandible and maxilla, J. Oral Surg. **18:**486, 1960.

Caffey, J.: Infantile cortical hyperostoses, J. Pediatr. **29:**541, 1946.

Catena, D. L., and Glick, G. L.: Monostotic fibrous dysplasia with dental anomalies, Oral Surg. **32:**136, 1971.

Chaudhry, A. P., Robinovitch, M. R., Mitchell, D. F., and Vickers, R. A.: Chondrogenic tumors of the jaws, Am. J. Surg. **102:**403, 1961.

Gage, S. M., Stein, M., and Radcliffe, R. B.: Paget's disease, Oral Surg. **20:**616, 1965.

Gomez, A. C., Youmans, R. D., and Chambers, R. G.: Osteogenic sarcoma of the mandible: a method of treatment, Am. J. Surg. **100:**613, 1960.

Hayes, R. L.: Ossifying fibroma, Oral Surg. **19:**633, 1965.

Keen, E. G., Sammartino, C. A., and Johnson, E. S.: Chronic sclerosing osteomyelitis of the mandible, J. Am. Dent. Assoc. **76:**597, 1968.

Kolas, S., Halperin, V., Jefferis, K., Huddleston, S. D., and Robinson, H. B. G.: The occurrence of torus palatinus and torus mandibularis in 2,478 dental patients, Oral Surg. **6:**1134, 1953.

Pell, G. J., Shafer, W. G., Gregory, G. T., Ping, R. S., and Spear, L. B.: Garré's osteomyelitis of the mandible, J. Oral Surg. **13:**248, 1955.

Potdar, G. G.: Osteogenic sarcoma of the jaws, Oral Surg. **30:**381, 1970.

Potdar, G. G., and Srikhande, S. S.: Chondrogenic tumors of the jaws, Oral Surg. **30:**649, 1970.

Poyton, H. G., and Davey, K. W.: Thalassemia, Oral Surg. **25:**564, 1968.

Prowler, J. R., and Smith, E. W.: Dental bone changes occurring in sickle cell diseases and abnormal hemoglobin traits, Radiology **65:**763, 1955.

Smith, N. H. H.: Albers-Schönberg disease (osteopetrosis), Oral Surg. **22:**69, 1966.

Smith, R. M.: Osteopetrosis (Albers-Schönberg disease, marble bones, osteosclerosis fragilis generalisata), Oral Surg. **20:**298, 1965.

Tillman, H. H.: Paget's disease of bone, Oral Surg. **15:**1225, 1962.

CHAPTER EIGHT

RADIOLUCENT AND RADIOPAQUE (MIXED) LESIONS OF THE JAWS

The third and last group of lesions of the jaws are partly radiolucent and partly radiopaque. They comprise about 1% of all jaw lesions and therefore are the rarest of the three groups. Since many radiopaque lesions may temporarily go through this phase, lesions described in this chapter have also been referred to in Chapter 7.

A partly radiolucent and partly radiopaque lesion implies that bone destruction and formation of calcified tissue are occurring concomitantly or alternately. Such lesions can arise in one of three ways: (1) a radiolucent lesion such as cementoma or Paget's disease may gradually "mature" into a radiopaque mass, and during this process may appear partly radiolucent and partly radiopaque, (2) a radiopaque lesion such as condensing osteitis may become secondarily infected, suppurate, destroy bone, and become partly radiolucent and partly radiopaque, or (3) the lesion may begin as a mixed lesion. Certain rare odontogenic tumors such as the ameloblastic odontoma are lesions of this type.

Thus there are some members of this group that begin as radiolucencies, others that begin as radiopacities, and some that begin as "mixed" lesions. In a differential diagnosis of such radiographs the clinical features are of great significance. The following belong to this group:

- Cementoma (stage II)
- Ossifying fibroma
- Condensing osteitis
- Polyostotic fibrous dysplasia
- Cystic odontoma
- Ameloblastic odontoma
- Multiple enostosis
- Paget's disease
- Broken roots
- Osteogenic sarcoma
- Chondrosarcoma
- Osteoradionecrosis
- Rare lesions
  - Calcifying epithelial odontogenic tumor
  - Keratinizing and calcifying ameloblastoma
  - Metastatic carcinomas of the prostate and the breast

Cementoma (stage II). Cementoma is described on pp. 106 and 133. The presence of vital teeth, the periapical location, and the multiplicity of lesions are all of

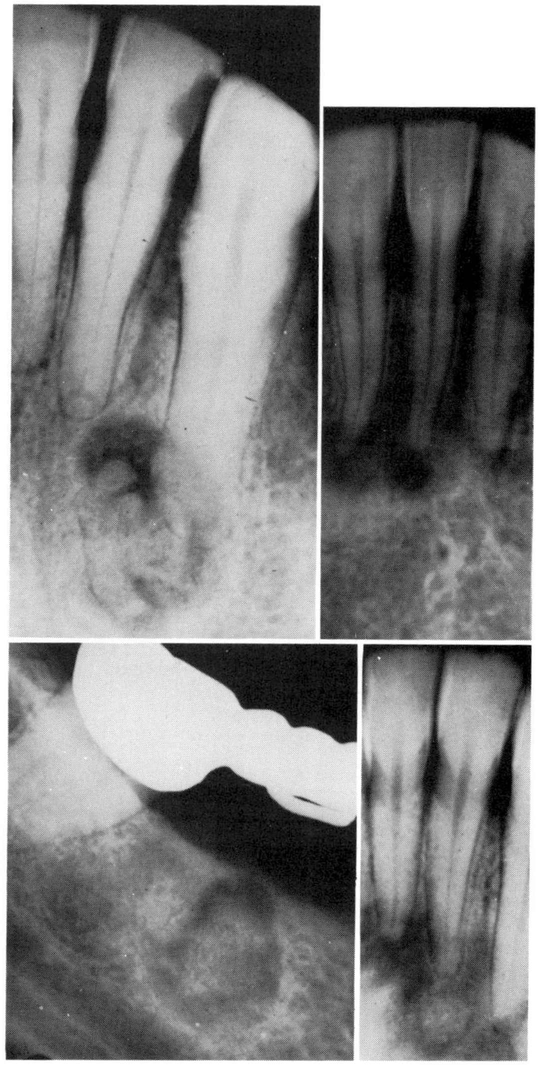

Fig. 8-1. Four cementomas in stage II. Note radiolucent/radiopaque (mixed) lesions.

diagnostic value. Stage II precedes the final radiopaque appearance of this odontogenic tumor (Fig. 8-1).

Ossifying fibroma. By far the vast majority of ossifying fibromas are radiopaque lesions. On extremely rare occasions, however, a lesion with a sparse amount of bone formation, radiographed in a very early stage, may appear either radiolucent, or partly radiolucent and partly radiopaque (Figs. 8-2 and 8-3). Clinically, the facts that these lesions are solitary, are of long duration and slow growth, occur usually in the young adult, and produce expansion of the jaw are valuable aids in diagnosis. For additional features of this tumor, see p. 177.

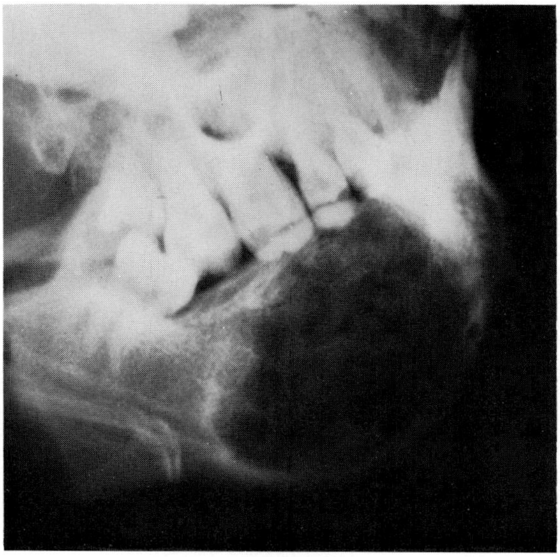

Fig. 8-2. Radiolucent/radiopaque appearance of an ossifying fibroma.

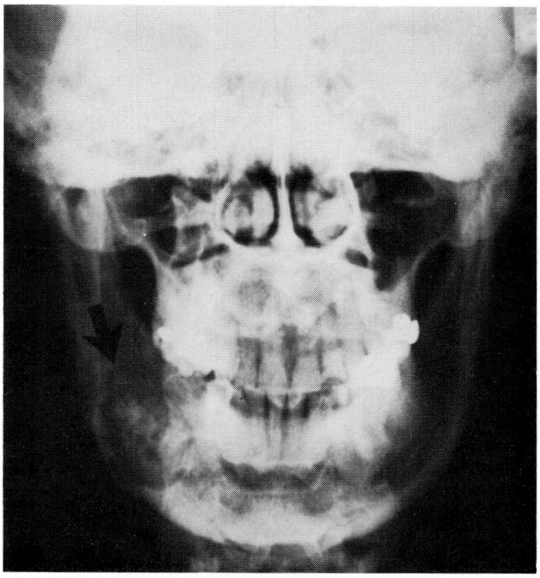

Fig. 8-3. Ossifying fibroma (arrow) seen as a radiolucent/radiopaque shadow in an antero-posterior view.

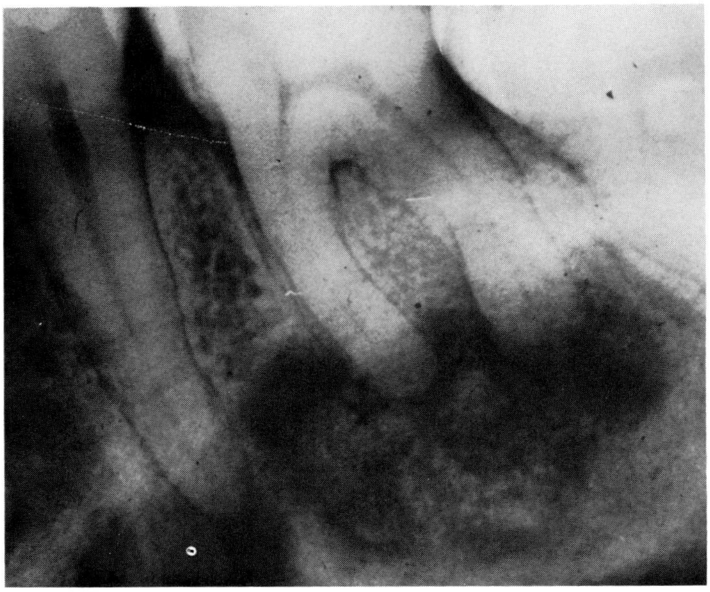

Fig. 8-4. Intraoral apical radiograph showing radiopaque/radiolucent features of condensing osteitis.

Condensing osteitis. Condensing osteitis has been described on p. 165. Usually this lesion is irregularly radiopaque. On occasion, however, it may undergo secondary infection, and the ensuing bone destruction produces a radiolucency. Such lesions appear as partly radiolucent and partly radiopaque (Fig. 8-4). Diagnostic features are the long history, the sudden appearance of pain and suppuration in an area of previous radiopacity, the presence of sequestration in advanced cases, and the location in the bicuspid and molar area. When a radiopaque lesion develops a radiolucent zone, surgical removal should be accomplished promptly.

Polyostotic fibrous dysplasia. Polyostotic fibrous dysplasia may show partly radiolucent and partly radiopaque lesions. This condition has been discussed on p. 174.

Cystic odontoma. The compound and complex odontomas are lesions of slow growth and are radiopaque (described on p. 180). On rare occasions one of them may undergo a cystic change. Under these circumstances a compound odontoma (having multiple toothlike structures) is surrounded by a radiolucency and is called a cystic compound odontoma (Fig. 8-5). On the other hand, if a complex odontoma (conglomerate mass of radiopaque tissues) becomes cystic and is associated with a radiolucency, it is called a cystic complex odontoma (Figs. 8-6 and 8-7). A differential diagnosis between these two types of cystic odontomas can easily be made from the radiographs.

When odontomas are near the alveolar crest, some of them may undergo secondary inflammation, and the resulting osteitis destroys the surrounding bone. As a result, a radiolucency develops in relation to these lesions. Such cases can be dis-

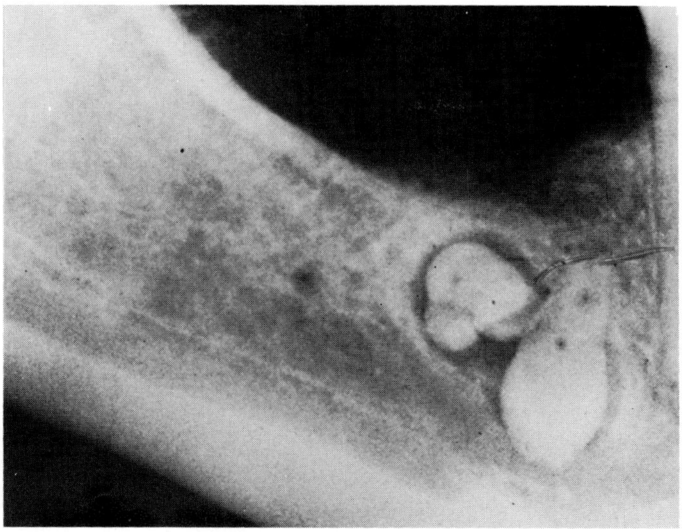

Fig. 8-5. Intraoral radiograph of the mandible, showing a cystic compound odontoma.

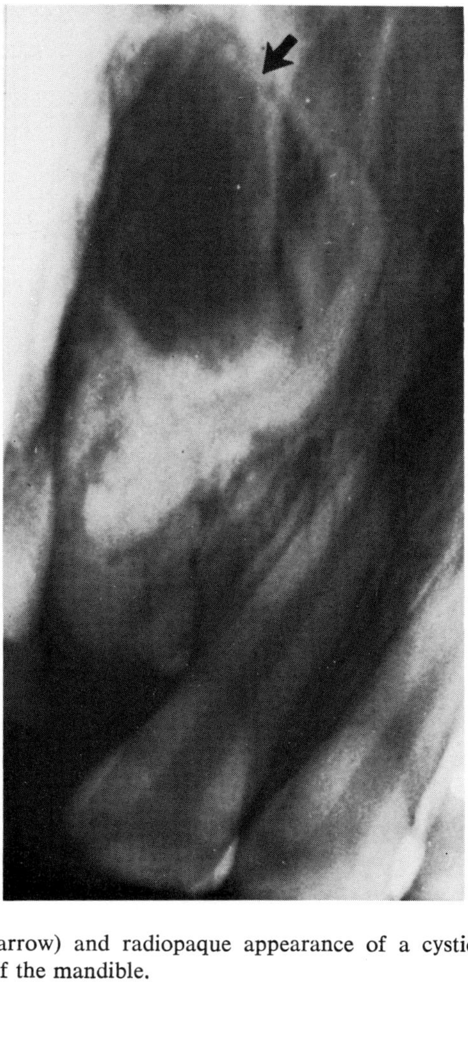

Fig. 8-6. Radiolucent (arrow) and radiopaque appearance of a cystic complex odontoma in the lateral incisor area of the mandible.

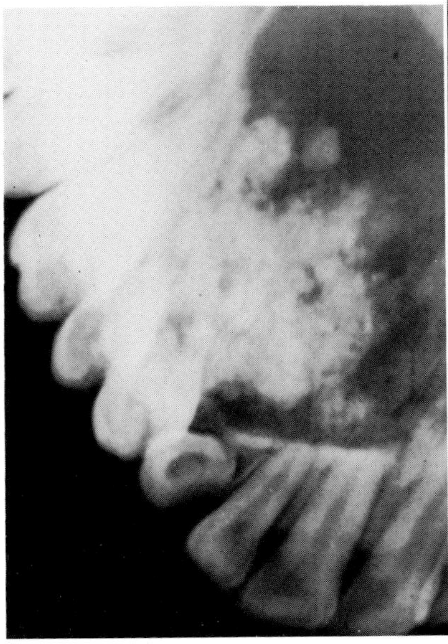

Fig. 8-7

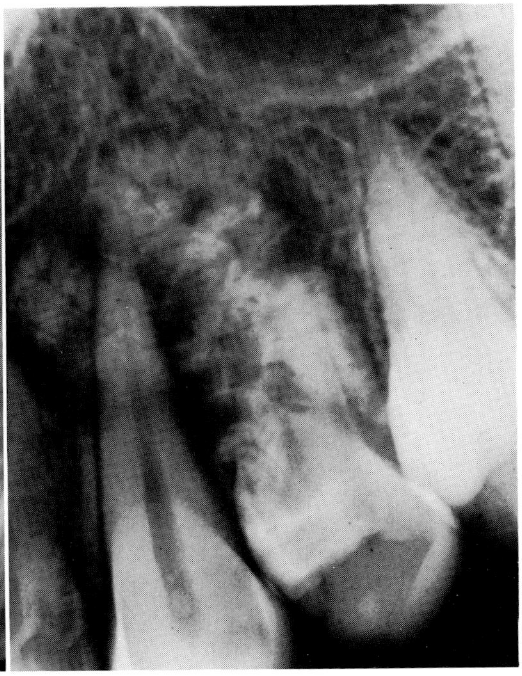

Fig. 8-8

Fig. 8-7. Occlusal radiograph of the maxilla, showing an unusually large cystic complex odontoma. Note radiopaque/radiolucent character.
Fig. 8-8. Circumscribed radiolucent/radiopaque lesion, the ameloblastic odontoma. In this case the calcified portion is greater than the noncalcified part.

tinguished from the cystic odontomas by the presence of pain or purulent exudate, and they should be promptly removed.

Ameloblastic odontoma. Ameloblastic odontoma is a rare, slowly growing odontogenic tumor that occurs in childhood or in young adulthood, and the maxilla is involved more frequently than the mandible. The radiograph shows an irregular area of radiopacity associated with a radiolucent area of varying size (Figs. 8-8 to 8-10). In some cases a large radiolucency with only a few foci of radiopacity may be seen (Fig. 8-11). In a differential diagnosis, however, a radiopacity of the density of enamel seen in a partly radiopaque and partly radiolucent lesion narrows the choice between the ameloblastic and the cystic odontoma. Radiographically, a distinction between these two lesions is sometimes impossible, but it is not essential to proper therapy.

Multiple enostosis. The usual radiographic features of multiple enostosis, or chronic sclerosing osteomyelitis, were described on p. 172. When one of these radiopaque masses becomes secondarily infected, it appears as a partly radiopaque and partly radiolucent lesion (see Fig. 7-12). Although radiographically this con-

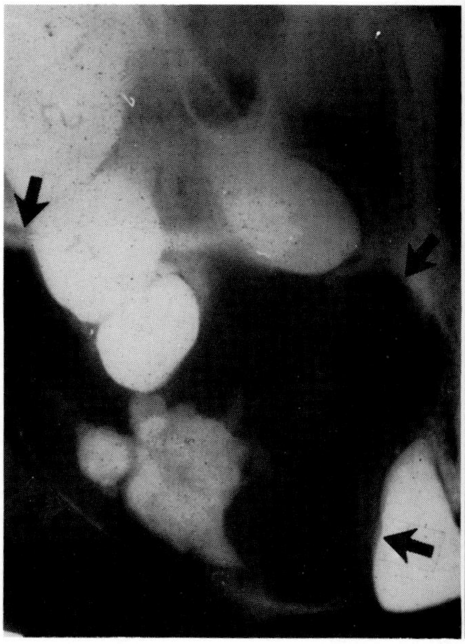

Fig. 8-9

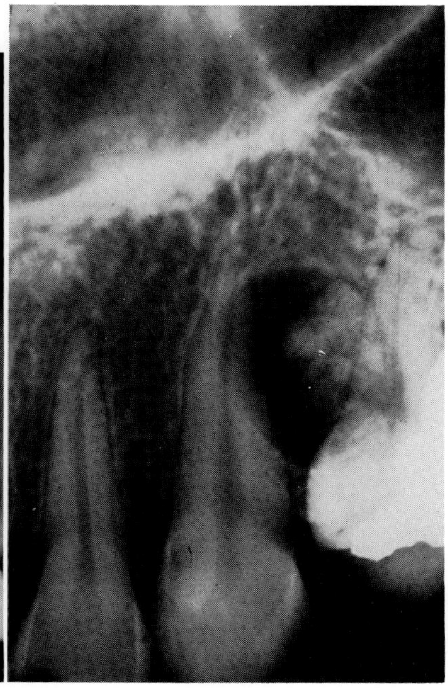

Fig. 8-10

Fig. 8-9. Occlusal view of an ameloblastic odontoma in which the uncalcified portion is far in excess of the calcified part. Arrows outline the boundary of the tumor.
Fig. 8-10. Intraoral radiograph of the cuspid area of the maxilla, showing a radiolucent/radiopaque ameloblastic odontoma.

dition mimics Paget's disease, the abscence of lesions elsewhere in the skeleton and the presence of normal serum alkaline phosphatase aid in the differential diagnosis. Since multiple enostosis usually occurs in patients with poor dental care, teeth are often lost because of caries or periodontal disease, and the radiopaque masses lie close to the alveolar crest. In such instances the use of a denture may produce pressure, ulceration of the overyling mucosa, and secondary infection. Appearance of a radiolucency in conjunction with foci of multiple enostosis is an undesirable development, and such an area should be excised.

Paget's disease. The diagnostic features of Paget's disease are described on p. 178. Although primarily characterized by multiple radiopaque masses, in early stages one or more of the foci of Paget's disease may present as radiolucent and radiopaque areas. The radiolucencies represent the areas where normal bone is destroyed and replaced by connective tissue, whereas the radiopaque areas represent regions of intense bone activity. In known cases of Paget's disease, rapidly growing radiolucencies should be suspected of malignant degeneration and should be looked on with great concern.

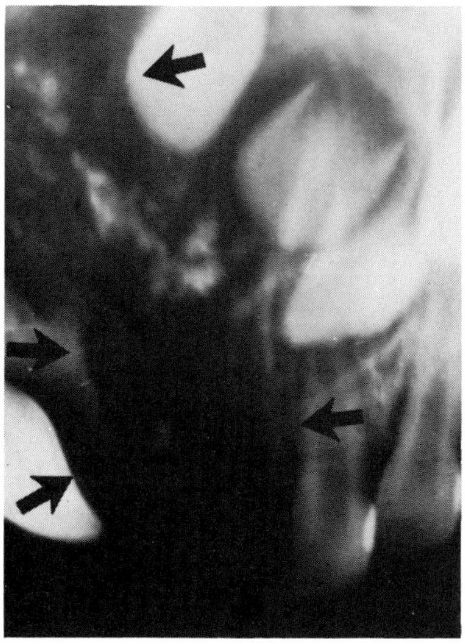

Fig. 8-11. Radiograph of an ameloblastic odontoma in the maxilla of a child, showing a large radiolucency with only a few small radiopaque foci. Arrows mark the periphery of the lesion.

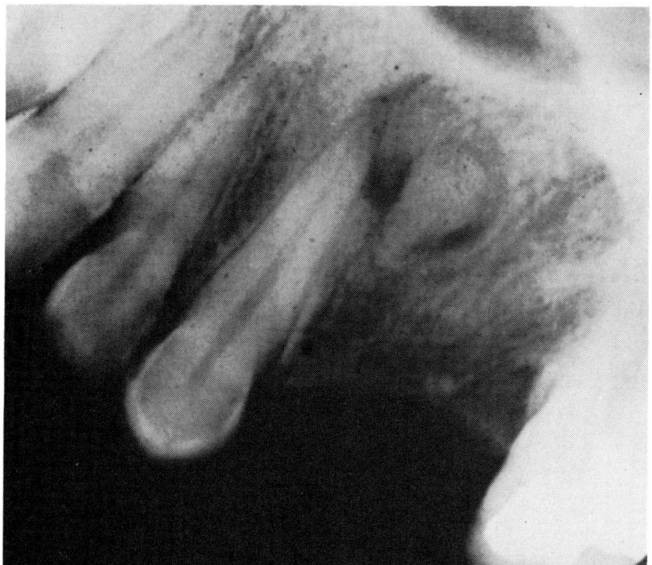

Fig. 8-12. Broken root (radiopaque), with surrounding area of secondary inflammation (radiolucent).

Broken roots. Secondary infection of broken roots produces a partly radiolucent and partly radiopaque (mixed) lesion. The clinical history, location, and appearance of the radiopaque area assist in arriving at the correct diagnosis (Fig. 8-12).

Osteogenic sarcoma. Osteogenic sarcoma was discussed under radiopacities of the jaws (p. 190). Since in this malignant lesion there are varying amounts of soft and hard tissues, the degree of radiopacity varies not only from lesion to lesion but also at different times in the same lesion. Although, as the name implies, the osteogenic sarcoma is supposed to produce bone, some members of this group produce very little calcified material and consist predominantly of soft tissue. The radiographic appearance of the osteogenic sarcoma, therefore, ranges widely and varies from a densely radiopaque lesion to one that is predominantly radiolucent (Figs. 7-38 to 7-40). Any single radiolucent/radiopaque lesion that grows rapidly and is associated with pain or other neurologic symptoms should arouse one's suspicion of an osteogenic sarcoma.

Chondrosarcoma. A chondrosarcoma (described on p. 194), although usually a radiopaque lesion, may appear partly radiolucent and partly radiopaque (Fig. 5-6). Patients are between 25 and 50 years of age, and the lesion occurs more often in the mandible than the maxilla. Tumors occur as a single focus, show rapid growth, and may be accompanied by neurologic symptoms and by migration or loosening of teeth. Like osteogenic sarcomas, chondrosarcomas vary widely in the relative amount of calcified material, and therefore the degree of radiopacity varies in different tumors and at different times in the same tumor.

Osteoradionecrosis. Radiation is often used in the primary treatment of some malignant oral tumors. It is also used as an adjunct or palliative therapy in inoperable oral malignancies. Radition therapy in doses sufficient to affect malignant lesions produces deleterious effects on the jaws. A high dosage of radia-

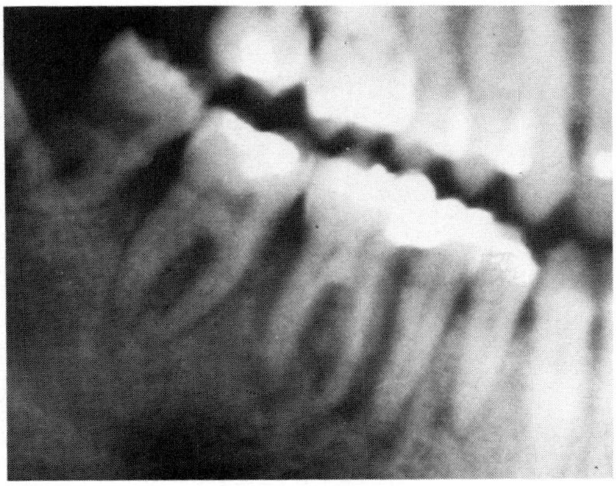

Fig. 8-13. Radiograph of a patient who was treated for a carcinoma of the tongue with high dosage of radiation (6000 r). Note radiolucency around the roots of teeth and radiopaque foci elsewhere in the bone.

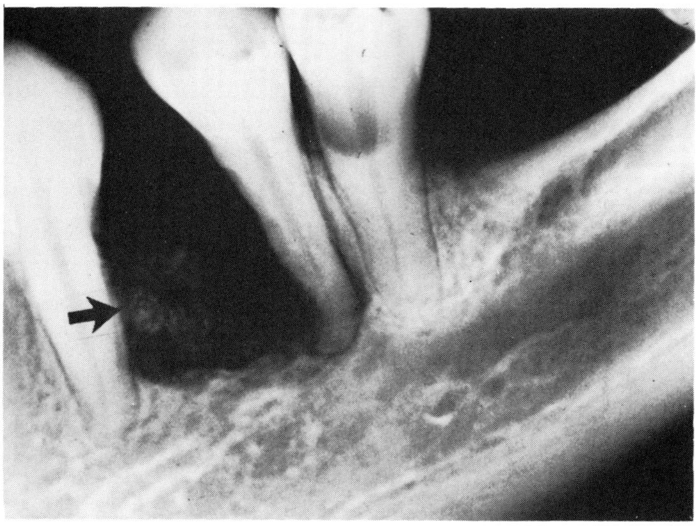

Fig. 8-14. Rare odontogenic lesion, a calcifying epithelial odontogenic tumor, in the cuspid area of the mandible. The arrow points to minute radiopaque foci.

A

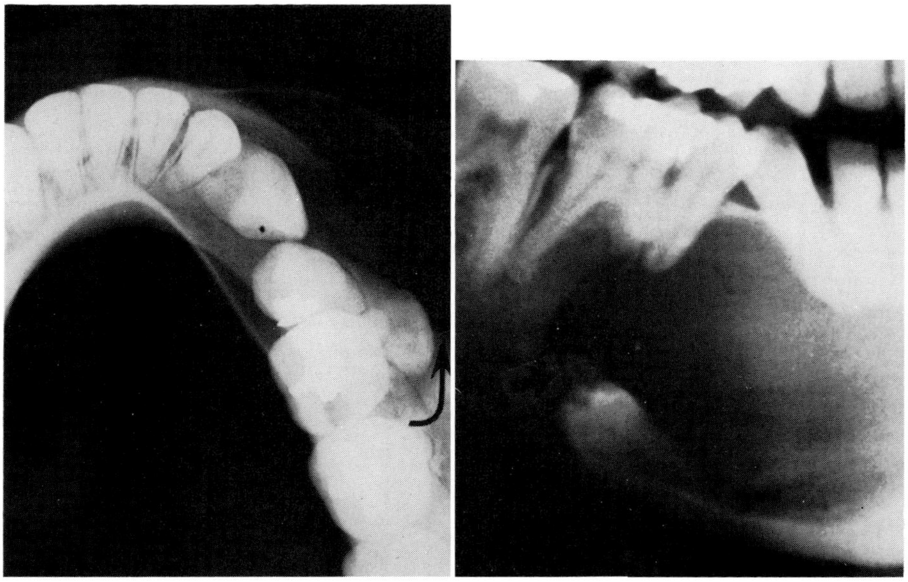

B

Fig. 8-15. Large calcifying epithelial odontogenic tumor of the mandible, seen in an occlusal view, **A,** and a lateral view, **B.** In this predominantly radiolucent lesion an impacted tooth and minute specks of radiopacity can be seen (arrows). Note that in **A,** the lesion has "expanded" but has not destroyed the cortex.

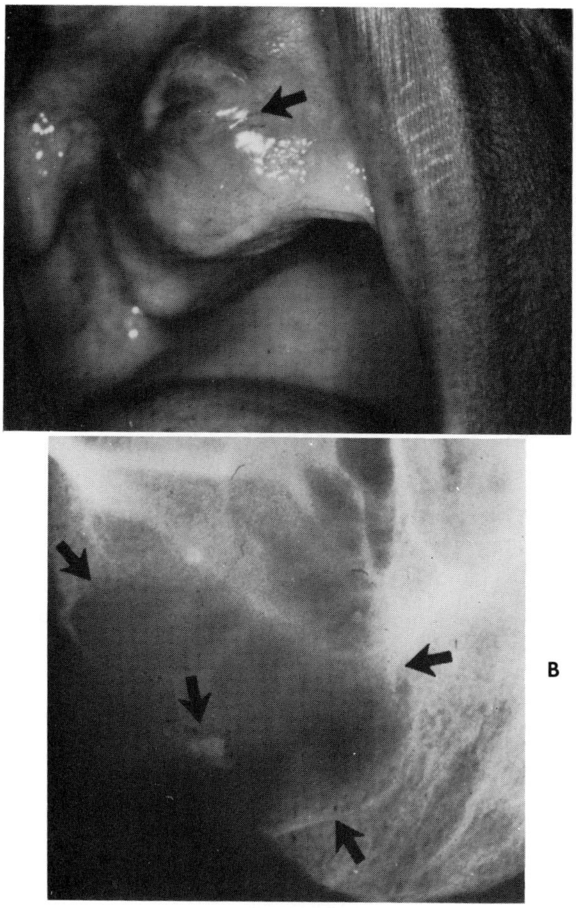

Fig. 8-16. Clinical view, **A,** and radiographic view, **B,** of a calcifying and keratinizing ameloblastoma (also called calcifying and keratinizing odontogenic cyst). Although predominantly a radiolucent lesion, it also contains radiopaque calcified foci (center arrow).

tion destroys cells of the bone and bone marrow and lowers resistance of the jaws to infection and injury for many years. Thus, extraction of teeth many years after radiation may be followed by infection and sequestration. Since teeth and periodontal pockets are sources of infection, extraction of all teeth in the subject field is usually a highly recommended procedure in patients scheduled to receive radiation therapy. Otherwise, radiation therapy may be followed by caries and periodontal disease, which in turn produce infection of apical areas and prolonged and catastrophic bone destruction. Edentulous areas are more resistant to the deleterious effects of therapeutic cancer radiation.

The radiographs of the radiated jaws show an early stage of radiopacity that soon is accompanied by radiolucent areas (Fig. 8-13). The radiopaque/radiolucent lesions are accompanied by sequestration and sometimes by pain. They may be localized or widespread. When teeth are present in the area, the destruction of alveolar bone is frequently seen (Fig. 8-13). *Osteoradionecrosis,* as the jaw lesions of radiation are called, is thus characterized by radiolucent/radiopaque lesions that offer no diagnostic problem because of the clinical history of radiation therapy. Radiation caries has been described on p. 68.

Rare lesions. There are some rare lesions that have a partly radiopaque and partly radiolucent appearance. One of them is the so-called *calcifying epithelial odontogenic tumor,* which occurs in both male and female, is seen usually in the *third or later decade* of life, may be expansile, and may be associated with an impacted tooth (Figs. 8-14 and 8-15). Lesions occur in the mandibular bicuspid and molar area and in the radiographs show a radiolucent area with varying amounts of minute or large radiopaque foci (Figs. 8-14 and 8-15).

A second lesion, called the *keratinizing and calcifying ameloblastoma* or the *keratinizing and calcifying odontogenic cyst,* is predominantly a radiolucent lesion in which, however, minute specks of radiopacity can be recognized (Fig. 8-16). The lesion grows very slowly, and its diagnosis is usually made on tissue examination.

Last, there are two malignant tumors which, in their rare metastatic foci to the jaws, may give a partly radiolucent and partly radiopaque shadow. They are the *metastatic carcinomas of the prostate and the breast.* The history of the patient, the presence of pain or other neurologic symptoms, and the rapid growth of the lesion are of diagnostic assistance.

REFERENCES

Bhaskar, S. N.: Synopsis of oral pathology, ed. 4, St. Louis, 1973, The C. V. Mosby Co.

Bhaskar, S. N., and Cutright, D. E.: Multiple enostosis, J. Oral Surg. **26:**321, 1968.

Chaudhry, A. P., Holte, N. D., and Vickers, R. A.: Calcifying epithelial odontogenic tumor, Oral Surg. **15:**843, 1962.

Forsberg, A., Lagergren, C., and Martensson, G.: Ameloblastic odontoma, Oral Surg. **14:** 726, 1961.

Frissell, C. T., and Shafer, W. G.: Ameloblastic odontoma: report of case, Oral Surg. **6:**1129, 1953.

Gage, S. M., Stein, M., and Radcliffe, R. B.: Paget's disease, Oral Surg. **20:**616, 1965.

Keen, E. G., Sammartino, C. A., and Johnson, E. S.: Chronic sclerosing osteomyelitis of the mandible, J. Am. Dent. Assoc. **76:** 507, 1968.

Olech, E., and Alvares, O.: Ameloblastic odontoma, Oral Surg. **23:**487, 1967.

Smith, J. F., and Blankenship, J.: The calcifying odontogenic cyst, Oral Surg. **20:** 624, 1965.

Zigarelli, E. V., Kutschner, A. H., Napoli, N., Iurono, F., and Hoffman, P.: The cementoma, Oral Surg. **17:**219, 1964.

PART FOUR

SOFT TISSUES

CHAPTER NINE

RADIOGRAPHY OF ORAL SOFT TISSUES

As a rule, radiographs of oral soft tissues are of no great interest to the dentist. On occasion, however, either by accident or by design, routine intraoral or extraoral radiographs of the oral regions reveal lesions in the oral soft tissues. On other occasions, the dentist may introduce radiopaque materials (solid or liquid) into soft tissues and take radiographs for diagnostic purposes. Soft tissue lesions seen in radiographs include the following:

- Lesions of salivary glands
  - Sialography
  - Sialoliths (salivary calculi, or stones)
  - Chronic obstructive adenitis
  - Salivary gland tumors
  - Ranula
  - Mikulicz's disease
  - Sjögren's syndrome
  - Congenital sialoangiectasis
- Miscellaneous soft tissue lesions
  - Periodontal pockets
  - Peripheral fibroma with calcification
  - Foreign bodies
  - Phlebolith
  - Trichinosis
  - Furuncles
  - Myositis ossificans
  - Scleroderma
  - Calcified lymph nodes
  - Dermoid cyst
  - Emphysema

LESIONS OF SALIVARY GLANDS

Sialography. By introducing about 1 ml. of a radiopaque, iodine-containing oil (such as Lipiodol or Ethiodol) in the duct of the parotid or the submaxillary

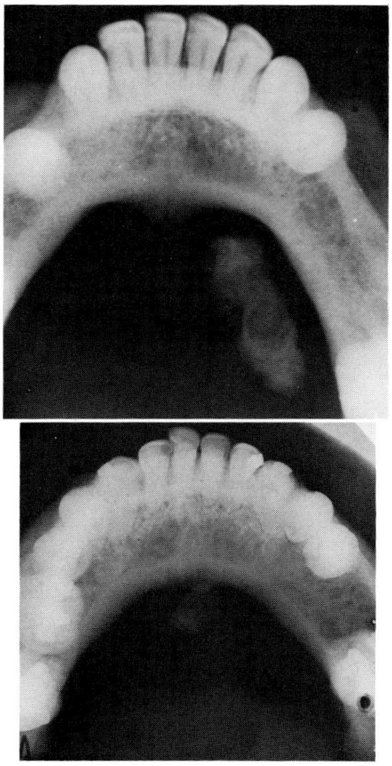

Fig. 9-1. Occlusal radiographs of two cases of sialolithiasis of the submaxillary gland.

gland, the duct system of these organs can be radiographically demonstrated. This procedure is called *sialography*. For sialography of the parotid and submaxillary glands, a lateral and a lateral oblique projection are respectively the most revealing angulations. Sialography is sometimes given a great deal of emphasis, and it is suggested that one can make meaningful diagnoses by examining these radiographs. This, however, is not the case. In establishing a correct interpretation of a salivary gland lesion, the clinical history and, if necessary, the biopsy are the reliable methods of diagnosis. Since sialography does carry some hazard (such as forceful injection of the media, leakage into the surrounding tissue, and foreign body reactions) and some patient discomfort, its use should be discouraged.

Sialoliths (salivary calculi, or stones). Sialoliths, or salivary calculi, occur far more frequently in the submaxillary duct than in the parotid or other ducts. Submaxillary calculi are best seen in occlusal radiographs, where they appear as lightly radiopaque structures of varying shape and size (Figs. 9-1 and 9-2). On rare occasions a calculus may be found within the submaxillary gland. Calculi in the gland are best seen in lateral oblique projections of the mandible. Salivary calculi in the parotid gland or its duct are rare. When they are suspected, a lateral extraoral film or an intraoral film placed between the cheek and the first maxillary molar area shows the stone. The radiopacity of the stones varies widely and depends

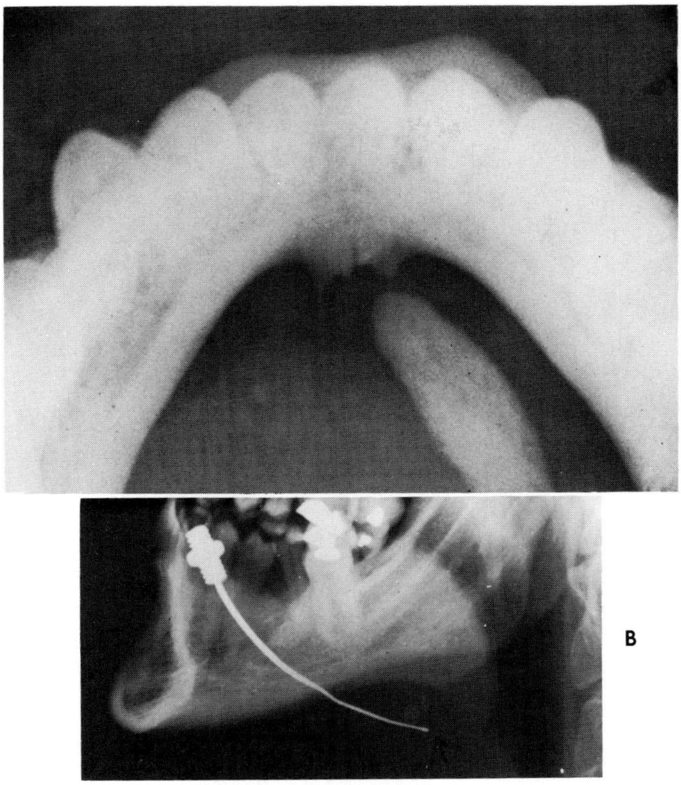

Fig. 9-2. Occlusal view, **A,** and lateral view, **B,** of sialoliths in the submaxillary gland ducts. In **B** a cannula has been inserted up to the point of duct obstruction caused by two small stones (arrow).

on their degree of calcification. It should be remembered, however, that in early stages the salivary "stones" are uncalcified, consist only of a protein matrix, and therefore are radiolucent. Clinical symptoms of an obstructed duct and obstructive adenitis do not always imply that a radiograph will reveal the sialolith.

It is when the duct obstruction is suspected but radiographs fail to reveal a radiopaque sialolith that a radiograph, after a careful injection of a contrast medium into the duct, should be considered.

Chronic obstructive adenitis. Sialograms taken of the normal parotid and submaxillary glands show a duct system that has the appearance of a symmetrical tree. The branches of the duct extend evenly in all directions to the capsule and are of uniform width (Fig. 9-3, *A*). In chronic obstructive sialadenitis, the duct system undergoes few or many constrictions and periductal fibrosis. The degree of constriction varies with the type and duration of sialadenitis. In such cases, sialograms either fail to show any duct system at all or show a varying number of constrictions or irregularities in the outline of ducts (Fig. 9-3, *B*). In some cases the radiopaque material pools proximally to the ductal constrictions, and the sialograms show a grapelike design (Fig. 9-4).

A

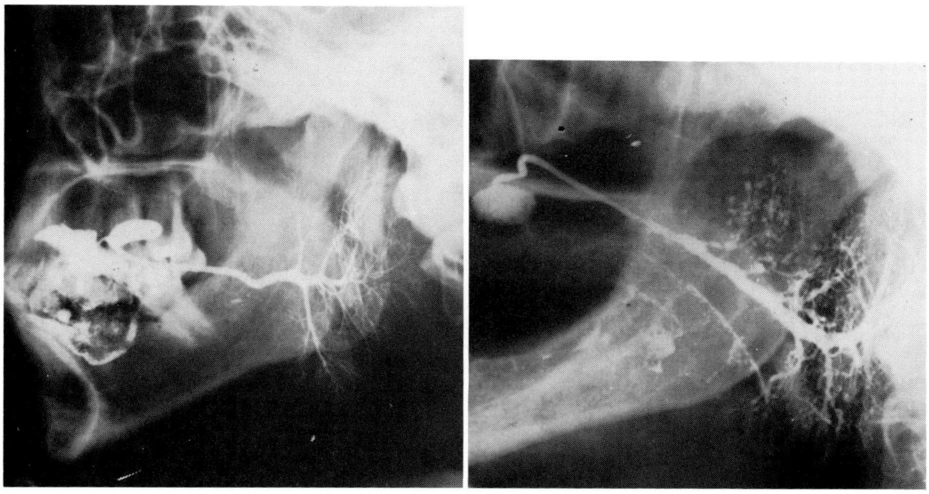

B

Fig. 9-3. A, Sialogram of the normal duct system of the parotid. Note a treelike pattern. **B,** Sialogram of a parotid with early obstructive adenitis. Note a disruption of the normal smooth outline and even distribution of ducts.

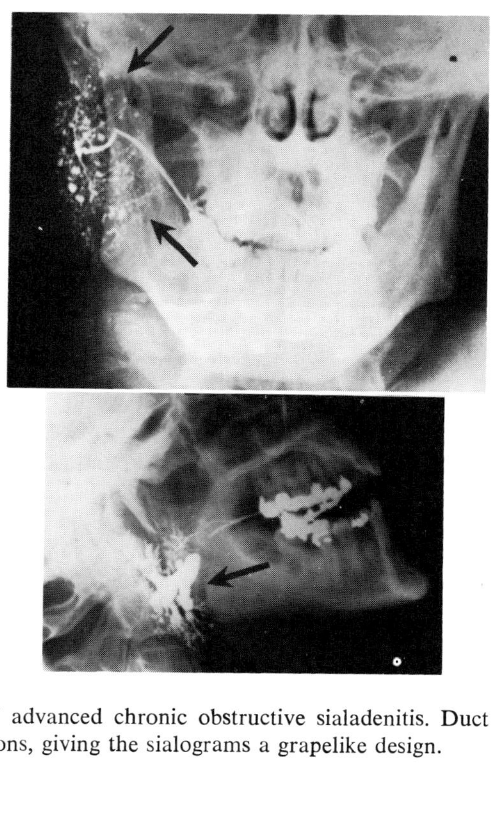

Fig. 9-4. Two cases of advanced chronic obstructive sialadenitis. Duct system is replaced by numerous saclike dilations, giving the sialograms a grapelike design.

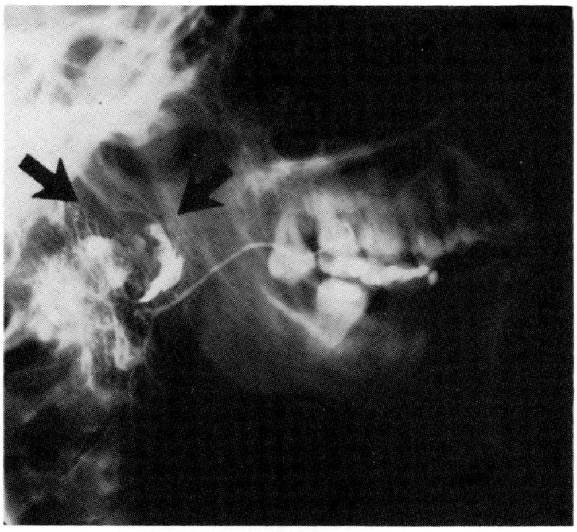

Fig. 9-5. Sialogram showing a salivary gland tumor. Note that in the area of the arrows there is a circumscribed zone devoid of ducts. This area contained a salivary gland tumor.

A

B

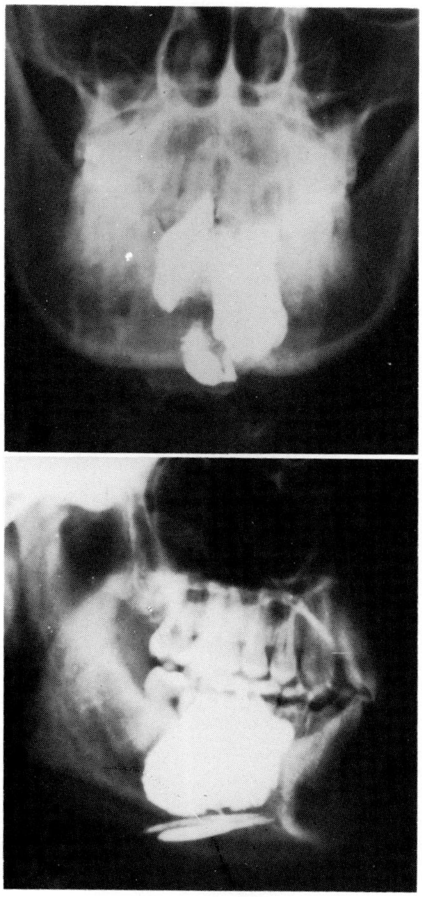

Fig. 9-6. Two cases showing an anteroposterior view, **A,** and a lateral view, **B,** of the ranula. The radiopaque material outlines the size and shape of the lesions.

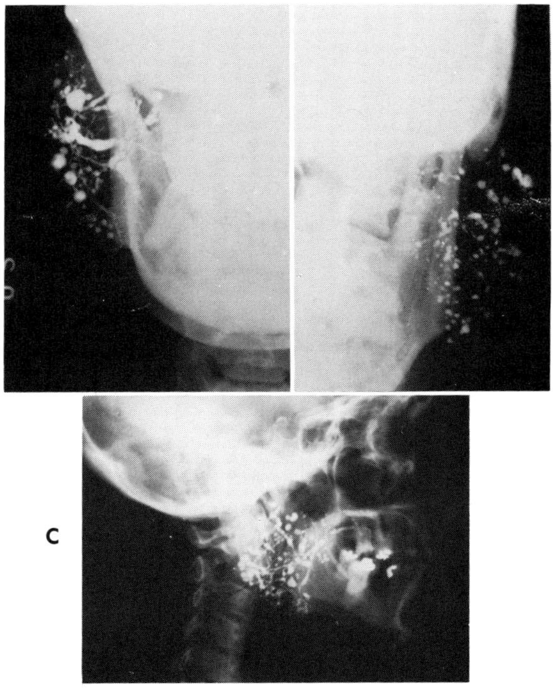

Fig. 9-7. **A** and **B,** Anteroposterior views of the parotid in Mikulicz's disease. They show how the entire duct system of the parotid has been replaced by small, grapelike clusters of radiopacities. Microscopically, these areas represent microcysts. **C,** Lateral view of a parotid in Sjögren's syndrome. The sialogram resembles that seen in sialadenitis and Mikulicz's disease.

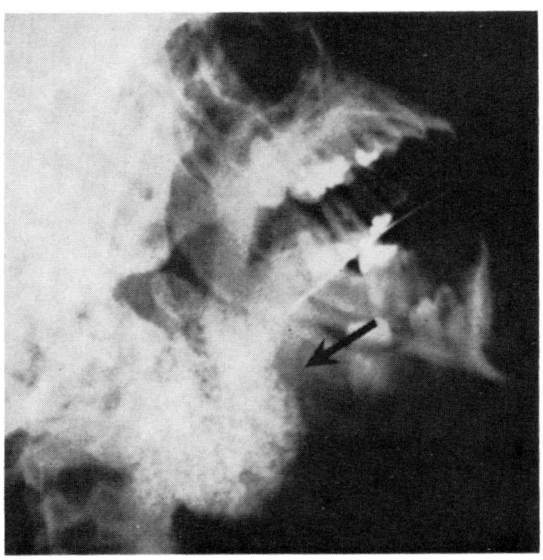

Fig. 9-8. Advanced case of Sjögren's syndrome, in which the entire gland has been replaced by microcysts that appear as radiopaque "pebbles."

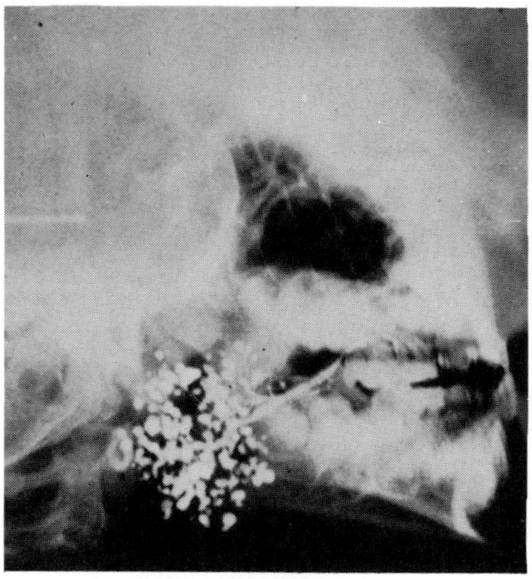

Fig. 9-9. Sialogram of the parotid of a child, showing congenital sialoangiectasis. Note grapelike radiopacities.

Salivary gland tumors. There are many different types of benign and malignant tumors that affect the salivary glands. As a rule they occur more often in the parotid gland than in other major glands.

A tumor occupies space that is normally filled with the duct system and acini. A sialogram of a gland that contains a tumor, therefore, shows the absence of the duct system in that area and a disruption in the symmetry of its normal pattern (Fig. 9-5). Such a radiograph shows an area of radiolucency in an otherwise radiopaque pattern of branching ducts and indicates that a ductless mass has replaced the normal glandular tissue. Whether this is a benign or a malignant tumor, a primary or a metastatic lesion, or an enlarged intraglandular lymph node cannot be established from a sialogram. This must be done by tissue examination. It is thus apparent that a sialogram is of limited value in the diagnosis of salivary gland tumors.

Ranula. Sialography is not necessary to diagnose a ranula. However, if an anteroposterior or a lateral radiograph is taken after these lesions have been injected with contrast media, their size and outline can be demonstrated with ease (Fig. 9-6).

Mikulicz's disease and Sjögren's syndrome. Somewhat similar sialograms are seen in the late stages of two allied diseases that occur in the adult and in aged individuals: Mikulicz's disease and Sjögren's syndrome. In these conditions the duct system of the parotid gland (and sometimes of the submaxillary gland) shows multiple cystlike dilations, and the sialograms show multiple radiopaque pools, or grapelike clusters (Fig. 9-7). In some cases the entire gland may be replaced by nodular radiopaque accumulations of the contrast medium (Fig. 9-8). In a patient who shows the alterations of the normal duct pattern, therefore, it is difficult to distinguish between chronic obstructive sialadenitis and various stages of Mikulicz's disease and Sjögren's syndrome. This distinction must be made from clinical history and symptoms.

Congenital sialoangiectasis. In a congenital malformation of the parotid gland, the duct system shows many saclike dilations that can easily be demonstrated in sialograms (Fig. 9-9). The latter show many saccular clusters of radiopacity. The age of the patient, however, is of diagnostic significance.

MISCELLANEOUS SOFT TISSUE LESIONS

Periodontal pockets. The depth and topography of a periodontal pocket can be demonstrated by inserting a radiopaque object such as a gutta-percha point or a calibrated steel point into the pocket and taking an intraoral radiograph (Chapter 4). Such radiographs are the only means by which long-term comparisons of the débridement and therapy of the periodontal disease can be made.

Peripheral fibroma with calcification. The peripheral fibroma is a soft tissue tumor of the gingiva that usually arises from the interdental papilla and contains varying amounts of calcified material. Radiographs taken of this soft tissue growth, therefore, show varying degrees of radiopacity (Fig. 9-10).

A

B

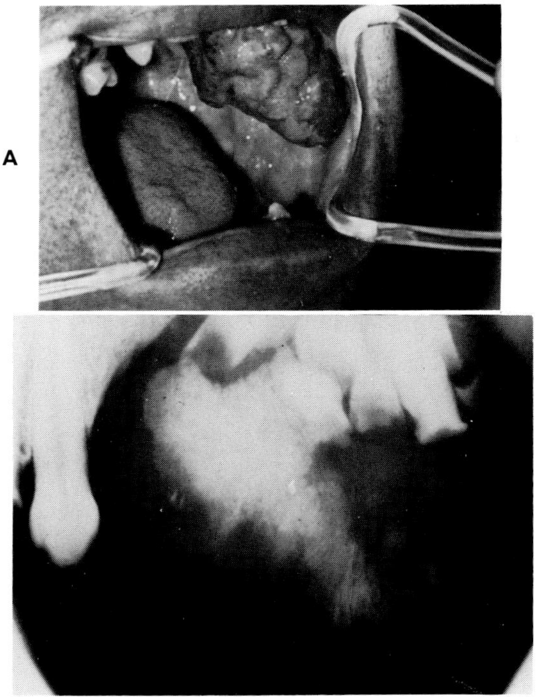

Fig. 9-10. Clinical view, **A,** and radiographic view, **B,** of a peripheral fibroma with calcification. This soft-tissue tumor of the gingiva shows varying amounts of radiopacity.

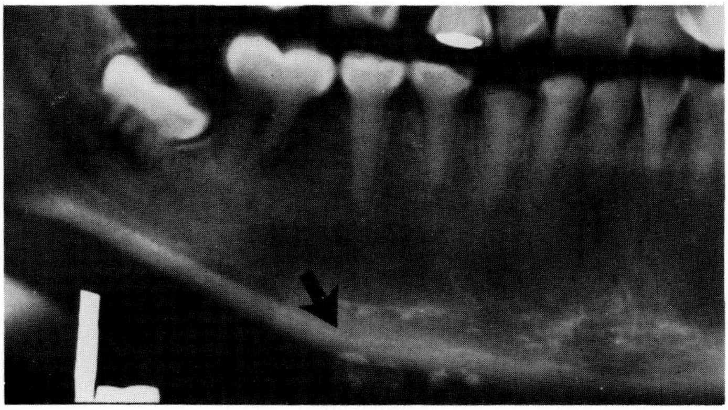

Fig. 9-11. Panorex view of a patient with dentinogenesis imperfecta. The facial skin of this patient had four furuncles, which appeared in the radiograph as small radiopaque bodies (arrow).

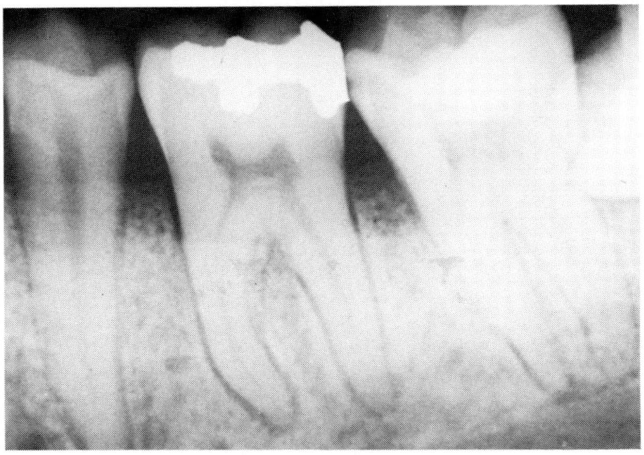

Fig. 9-12. Radiograph of the jaw in a case of scleroderma. Note widening of the periodontal space.

Foreign bodies. Foreign bodies in soft tissues are often found in routine intraoral or extraoral radiographs. Some of the foreign bodies found in soft tissues are amalgam particles, wires, and parts of missiles.

Phlebolith. Calcified thrombi in a vein or in a hemangioma of soft tissues appear as a radiopaque focus. The presence of such a radiopacity in a clinically visible hemangioma offers no diagnostic problem. Phleboliths in the very rare central hemangiomas of bone are not easily identified.

Trichinosis. Under extremely rare circumstances the *Trichinella spiralis* may infest the tongue, and in old infections the trichinae may become encapsulated and calcify. In radiographs they may appear as opaque areas.

Furuncles. Furuncles on the face may appear in radiographs as small radiopaque bodies (Fig. 9-11).

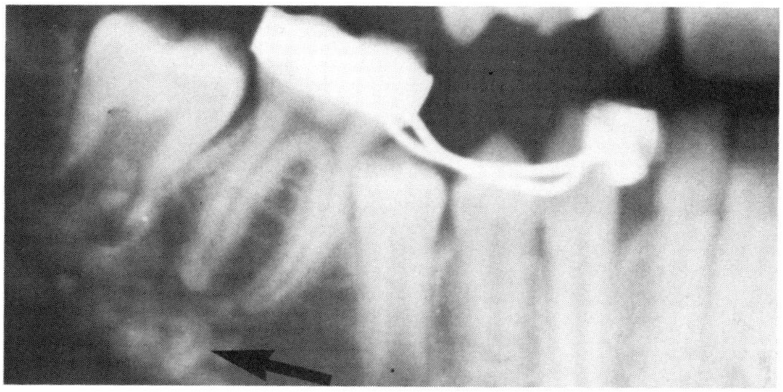

Fig. 9-13. Panographic radiograph showing calcified foci in the first and second molar area. These foci were not within the jaw but represented calcified foci in the regional lymph nodes (arrow).

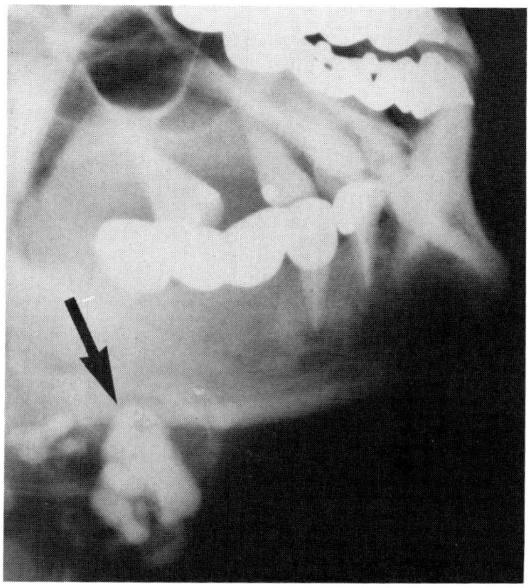

Fig. 9-14. A lateral jaw radiograph showing calcified cervical lymph nodes. This area represented calcified healed tubercular foci (arrow).

Myositis ossificans. This disease of the muscles may involve the masseter and is characterized by calcifications. Radiographs of the area may show radiopacities.

Scleroderma. This rare disease of the skin is characterized by atrophy, stiffening, and limiting of the mobility of the area. Calcifications also occur, and when the disease affects the facial areas, calcifications may be seen in the oral radiographs. Clinical history and examination assist in making the correct diagnosis.

The radiographs of the jaws sometimes show widening of the periodontal space, which is especially prominent in posterior teeth (Fig. 9-12). When these teeth are extracted, the dense periodontal ligament remains adherant to the root surface.

Calcified lymph nodes. Calcified cervical and facial lymph nodes as seen in

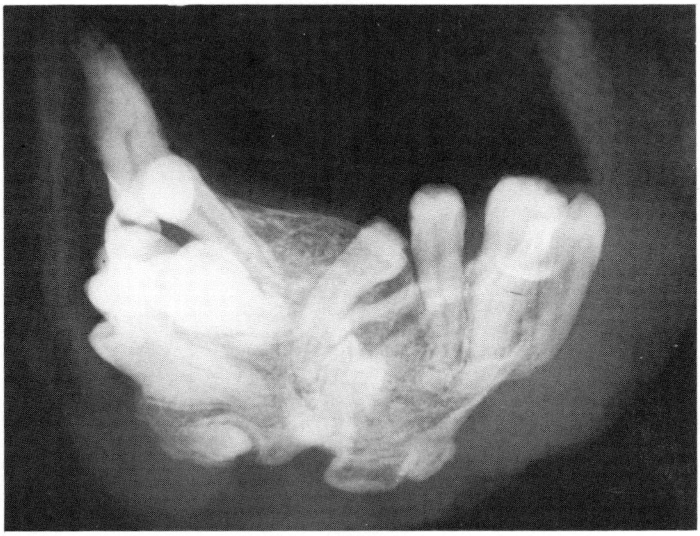

Fig. 9-15. Radiograph of a dermoid cyst of the ovary.

healed tubercular or chronic inflammatory lesions may be seen in oral radiographs (Figs. 9-13 and 9-14). Depending on the angle at which the radiographs are made, these calcified structures may be superimposed on the jaws and can be mistaken for jaw lesions (Fig. 9-13). Clinical history, examination, and radiographs taken from other directions are of diagnostic value.

Dermoid cyst. Dermoid cysts of the ovary show calcified dental structure (Fig. 9-15).

Emphysema. When air or gases are trapped in soft tissues the condition is referred to as emphysema. It is associated with swelling that begins to subside in a few days. The area may show crepitus. Emphysema may occur after tooth extraction, endodontic therapy, or restorative procedures. This condition may follow forceful use of air jet on traumatized tissues. Radiographs show single or multiple areas of radiolucency. Clinical examination and history assist in making the correct diagnosis.

REFERENCES

Bhaskar, S. N.: Synopsis of oral pathology, ed. 4, St. Louis, 1973, The C. V. Mosby Co.

Blair, G. S.: Hydrostatic sialography, Oral Surg. **36:**116, 1973.

Buchignani, J. S., and Shimkiu, P. M.: Subtraction sialography: an improved and simplified technique, Oral Surg. **31:**828, 1971.

Chomenko, A. G., and Caulfield, J. J.: Projected artifacts viewed on soft-tissue dental radiographs, Oral Surg. **34:**838, 1972.

Lee, J. L., and Bordenca, C. M.: Self-inflicted air emphysema of the face and neck, Oral Surg. **36:**603, 1973.

Nealon, F. H.: Scleroderma: oral manifestations, Oral Surg. **24:**310, 1967.

Poyton, H. G., and Arora, B. K.: Radiologic evidence of surgical emphysema, Oral Surg. **36:**129, 1973.

Scopp, I. W., and Schlagel, E.: Scleroderma: its orofacial manifestations, Oral Surg. **15:** 1510, 1962.

INDEX